"This book offers a reflective, self-critical examination of MSF as one of the world's most iconic humanitarian organisations, which can't be more timely as the aid sector faces acute crises and must radically evolve to remain fit for purpose."

Gilles Carbonnier, *Professor of Development Economics, The Geneva Graduate Institute*

"MSF's ability to engage in uncompromising introspection remains fascinating! A collective book that provides an insight into the organisation's ability to confront its own practices. These are relevant questions for the entire humanitarian sector as it navigates the challenges ahead."

Jean-Baptiste Richardier, *President of the Board of Directors, Humanitarian Alternatives and Co-Founder of Handicap International / Humanity & Inclusion*

"*Humanitarian Myths and Hubris* is a critical guide for the entire MSF movement at a moment when our principles, positioning, and practices are under growing strain. It is both a mirror and a map – inviting us to renew our mission with clarity, humility, and solidarity."

Wacuka Maina, *The LEAF Charity*

"This volume offers an insightful perspective on humanitarian action through a medical NGO's lens, critically exploring contemporary challenges. Reflecting a sustained commitment to the continued reappraisal of humanitarian aid, it is an essential read for anyone working, studying, teaching, or simply interested in the field."

Alexandre Hermet, *Faculty Member, Sciences Po Toulouse*

Humanitarian Myths and Hubris

This collective work offers a critical analysis of contemporary humanitarian action, through the prism of Médecins Sans Frontières/Doctors Without Borders (MSF).

Initially created to provide healthcare to the most vulnerable populations in crisis-stricken countries, MSF has grown from just a few dozen members in 1971 to a movement of over 67,000 people with an annual budget of over 2 billion euros. But in today's rapidly evolving global landscape, many of the founding principles and myths surrounding its creation are questioned or undermined. The post-COVID era has been marked by a reinforcement or acceleration of pre-existing trends that continue to challenge the work of humanitarian organisations: restrictive, or indeed hostile, state policies; the presence of non-state actors in counter-terrorism contexts; questionable adherence to international humanitarian law. MSF must also address several key issues, such as combating discrimination, defining its position with regard to protest movements in countries of intervention, confronting challenges related to climate change and global health security, and safeguarding patients' personal data.

Drawing on the viewpoints of practitioners, analysts, and academics, this book will be an essential read for anyone engaged in or curious about humanitarian action.

Duncan McLean is currently a Senior Researcher with MSF's Research Unit on Humanitarian Stakes and Practices (UREPH), based in Geneva. Holding a PhD in history, he has published widely on the humanitarian sector, regularly lectures at universities throughout Europe, and is on the editorial board of the *Journal of Humanitarian Affairs*.

Françoise Duroch began working in the humanitarian field in the early 1990s with Handicap International, then with MSF. She has spent 15 years researching gender-based violence and holds a PhD in social sciences. She is a lecturer at several universities and currently coordinates the MSF Switzerland research unit in Geneva.

Amy Mavor holds master's degrees in languages from the University of Edinburgh and translation from Université Rennes 2, and has worked since 2018 as Publishing and Editing Officer at MSF Switzerland's research unit.

Routledge Humanitarian Studies

The Routledge Humanitarian Studies series in collaboration with the International Humanitarian Studies Association (IHSA) takes a comprehensive approach to the growing field of expertise that is humanitarian studies. This field is concerned with humanitarian crises caused by natural disaster, conflict or political instability and deals with the study of how humanitarian crises evolve, how they affect people and their institutions and societies, and the responses they trigger.

We invite book proposals that address, amongst other topics, questions of aid delivery, institutional aspects of service provision, the dynamics of rebel wars, state building after war, the international architecture of peacekeeping, the ways in which ordinary people continue to make a living throughout crises, and the effect of crises on gender relations.

This interdisciplinary series draws on and is relevant to a range of disciplines, including development studies, international relations, international law, anthropology, peace and conflict studies, public health and migration studies.

Forced Migration and Humanitarian Action
Operational Challenges and Solutions for Supporting People on the Move
Edited by Lorenzo Guadagno and Lisette R. Robles

Understanding Humanitarian Diplomacy
Principles and Practice
Edited by Hafize Zehra Kavak

An Introduction to Humanitarian Action
Edited by Katrin Radtke and Kristina Roepstorff

Humanitarian Myths and Hubris
A Critical Self-Portrait from Médecins Sans Frontières
Edited by Duncan McLean, Françoise Duroch, and Amy Mavor

For more information about this series, please visit: www.routledge.com/Routledge-Humanitarian-Studies/book-series/RHS

Humanitarian Myths and Hubris

A Critical Self-Portrait from Médecins Sans Frontières

Edited by
Duncan McLean, Françoise Duroch, and Amy Mavor

Routledge
Taylor & Francis Group
LONDON AND NEW YORK

Designed cover image: © Rash BRAX

First published 2026
by Routledge
4 Park Square, Milton Park, Abingdon, Oxon OX14 4RN

and by Routledge
605 Third Avenue, New York, NY 10158

Routledge is an imprint of the Taylor & Francis Group, an informa business

For Product Safety Concerns and Information please contact our EU representative: GPSR@taylorandfrancis.com
Taylor & Francis Verlag GmbH, Kaufingerstraße 24, 80331 München, Germany.

British Library Cataloguing-in-Publication Data
A catalogue record for this book is available from the British Library

ISBN: 978-1-032-89329-7 (hbk)
ISBN: 978-1-032-89324-2 (pbk)
ISBN: 978-1-003-54224-7 (ebk)

DOI: 10.4324/9781003542247

Typeset in Sabon
by Taylor & Francis Books

The views expressed in this book are those of the individual contributors and do not necessarily reflect the positioning of Médecins Sans Frontières.

Contents

List of Figures x
Notes on Contributors xi
Foreword xiv
Acknowledgements xvi
Abbreviations xvii

Introduction: Humanitarianism in Retreat? 1
DUNCAN MCLEAN

PART I
Elements of Change and Continuity 7

1 Good and Bad Victims? A Matter of Choice 9
THIERRY ALLAFORT-DUVERGER, MARIE-HORTENSE KOUDIKA, AND FRANÇOISE DUROCH

Zoom-in: Healthcare without Borders: Navigating Securitisation and Exclusion of Migrants 24
REEM MUSSA

2 The Evolution of How MSF Treats People 31
KARSTEN EMMANUEL NOKO AND MARC DUBOIS

3 Hostility to Aid Actors: Normalising Transgression? 51
STEPHEN CORNISH, ALEJANDRO POZO, AND DUNCAN MCLEAN

Zoom-in: Security Management with Locally Hired Staff: A Collaboration with Gaps? 68
MAHAMAT SEID ARABI

PART II
Navigating Expectations 75

4 From Technique to Technicity: Evolving Aims in MSF's Medical Practice 77
JACOB BURNS AND NATALIE ROBERTS

5 Global Health Security in Humanitarian Medicine: What Is the Greater Good? 96
MELISSA MCRAE

Zoom-in: The IFRC's Community-driven Approach in DRC's Ebola Outbreak 114
OMBRETTA BAGGIO

6 Caught in the Crossfire? International NGOs and Contemporary Forms of Protest and Resistance 116
MAELLE L'HOMME

Zoom-in: Protecting Humanitarian Action in an Age of Disinformation 129
SANDRINE TILLER

7 Speaking Out With, Not For: Rethinking Humanitarian Narratives 135
SOPHIE DÉSOULIÈRES AND JULIETTE GARMS

PART III
Challenging Adaptations 155

8 Liberal vs. Critical: Diverging Paths in Humanitarian Aid and Global Health 157
PATRICIA NAYNA SCHWERDTLE

Zoom-in: Reflecting on Diversity, Equity, and Inclusion in MSF 177
MEG ADHIAMBO OTIENO

9 Absorbed into the War Machine: What Is Independence When Everything Is Connected? 183
MARTIN SEARLE AND BEATRICE LAU

10 Without Borders, Within Boundaries: Learning How to Deliver Aid in Light of the Climate Emergency 203
BRUNO JOCHUM, DIKOLELA KALUBI, AND BÉATRICE GODEFROY

Epilogue: Negotiating Spaces, Defending Convictions 224
FRANÇOISE DUROCH

Appendix: The Charter of Médecins Sans Frontières 229
Index 231

Figures

7.1 Just-washed clothes drying in the trees. © Texas/Projet Calais Darkroom/MSF 144

7.2 Teolinda Castro heals the photograph of her community with a *resucito* flower, which she uses as an infusion to treat headaches and stomach aches. © Yazury Dumaza/Fernanda Pineda/MSF 144

Contributors

Thierry Allafort-Duverger has played a key role as a practitioner in major humanitarian crises. Former General Director of MSF France and President of ALIMA, he now focuses on field operations, research to enhance humanitarian practices, and knowledge transmission. He collaborates with various NGOs and academic institutions, including MSF, ALIMA, and the University of Manchester.

Mahamat Seid Arabi is a committed humanitarian professional with more than 16 years of experience, particularly with MSF. Throughout his career, he has undertaken diverse roles and contributed to numerous country programmes across Africa, the Middle East, and Asia. Since 2023, Seid has been MSF's Field Security Advisor based in Amsterdam.

Ombretta Baggio is an experienced humanitarian professional with over 20 years of expertise, including a decade in Africa. She is currently Senior Adviser for Community Engagement and Accountability at the IFRC, working on community engagement and accountability systems, including in public health emergencies.

Jacob Burns has worked for MSF in numerous roles in communication and operations, and for their centre of reflection, the CRASH. That work has taken him to Haiti, Palestine, Iraq, Jordan, Yemen, Turkey, and the Democratic Republic of Congo. Before MSF, he worked as a freelance journalist and in human rights research.

Stephen Cornish, General Director of MSF Switzerland since 2020, has over 25 years' experience with MSF, managing humanitarian interventions and negotiating access in conflict zones. He has held leadership roles with MSF Canada, the Canadian Red Cross, and CARE Canada, and holds advanced degrees in crisis management and conflict resolution.

Sophie Désoulières heads MSF Netherlands' humanitarian affairs, operational communications and advocacy department. She started working with MSF as a humanitarian affairs adviser supporting operations in Northeast Syria,

Iraq, Jordan, Pakistan, Afghanistan, Yemen, and Venezuela. Prior to joining MSF, Sophie was a senior analyst with the International Crisis Group.

Marc DuBois is an independent humanitarian consultant, a senior fellow at SOAS, University of London, and an elected member of MSF's International Board. Previously, Marc worked for fifteen years in MSF and was the General Director of MSF UK/IE.

Juliette Garms is a photo editor, writer, and project manager currently working as a Photography Project Manager for MSF.

Béatrice Godefroy is the former policy engagement director at Climate Action Accelerator. She worked for several years at MSF, and was most recently appointed as Deputy Director at DCAF, the Geneva Center for Security Sector Governance. Béatrice is a Sciences Po Paris graduate and holds a master's degree from Princeton University.

Bruno Jochum is the Executive Director of the Climate Action Accelerator, a non-profit initiative based in Geneva, launched in 2021. He was previously director general, director of operations, and programme manager for MSF Switzerland, after several years in the field, and holds a master's degree in political science and international law.

Dikolela Kalubi is a specialist in water and environmental management, with nearly 15 years of experience in the humanitarian sector. He joined MSF Switzerland in 2022 as the Climate, Environment, and Health Coordinator.

Marie-Hortense Koudika is a doctor specialising in gynaecology and obstetrics. She has worked with MSF for over 20 years and has held various positions of responsibility in many countries. She currently works at headquarters in Dakar as Deputy Manager in charge of medical issues for Burkina Faso, Mali, Niger, and Mauritania.

Maelle L'Homme holds a master's degree in public affairs and an MSc in health, population, and society. After several years' experience working with MSF in a variety of contexts (Democratic Republic of the Congo, Central African Republic, Chad, Yemen, Sudan, South Sudan), Maelle joined MSF's research unit in Geneva as Researcher in 2021.

Beatrice Lau is a humanitarian professional from Hong Kong with over 20 years at MSF. Formerly head of mission, she now serves as Legal Advisor on IHL and counterterrorism. Holding an LLB (England and Wales) and an advanced LLM in Public International Law, her publications to date focus on hostage diplomacy.

Melissa McRae is an Australian emergency medicine specialist and public health physician working with MSF. Over the last 20 years, she has worked in humanitarian and non-humanitarian emergencies due to conflict, disaster, forced displacement, and disease outbreaks in Australia, Haiti, the Philippines, Sierra Leone, and Yemen, amongst others.

Reem Mussa is a PhD candidate at the University of Bern and lecturer at Sciences Po, Paris, focused on migration, law, and violence. She was previously the head of the forced migration unit and a humanitarian advisor for MSF.

Patricia Nayna Schwerdtle is a Senior Researcher at Heidelberg University and leads a research group on climate change, migration, and health. She was formerly vice president of MSF Australia and advised the International Board on climate change and health. Her research also explores academic freedom, viewpoint diversity, and constructive dissent in research and education.

Karsten Emmanuel Noko works for MSF as Head of Mission and has previously worked in various programme management positions in countries that include Zimbabwe, Nigeria, Afghanistan, and South Sudan. He holds an LLB from the University of South Africa.

Meg Adhiambo Otieno is an organisational development and communication specialist with over a decade of experience embedding DEI strategies into global organisations. As the DEI Lead at MSF Switzerland, she drives inclusive workplace strategies across more than 20 countries. A former Oxfam leader, she champions cultural transformation and systemic equity.

Alejandro Pozo is Humanitarian Affairs Senior Researcher at MSF Spain and a member of the Centre for Applied Reflection on Humanitarian Practice. He joined MSF in 2002, working as adviser to the director of operations and in the field as head of mission, project coordinator, and researcher, mostly in armed conflict settings.

Natalie Roberts is an emergency doctor and Executive Director of MSF UK. She worked for MSF across the Middle East, Africa, and Asia before becoming head of emergency operations for MSF in Paris. Prior to her current role, she worked for the CRASH, one of MSF's reflection centres.

Martin Searle is Director of Analysis at MSF Hong Kong. He has spent ten years at MSF. He previously worked on new technologies' impact on humanitarian theory and practice while Associate Research Fellow at the S. Rajaratnam School of International Studies in Singapore, and while consulting for UNOCHA, ICRC, and the World Economic Forum.

Sandrine Tiller has been a humanitarian aid worker for over 20 years. She has worked in Venezuela, Eritrea, Tanzania, Israel, the Occupied Palestinian Territory, Lebanon, and Ukraine. She is currently the Humanitarian Access and Networking Team Coordinator at MSF.

Foreword

At the beginning of my work with Médecins Sans Frontières (MSF), I found myself facing an impossible decision: with only a few antifungal treatments left, I had to choose which of several patients should receive them. The infection, frequent among people living with HIV, would be fatal without medication. I remember the injustice I felt; the helplessness of having to determine who would get care, and who would not. It was not a clinical question – it was an ethical, emotional, and deeply disturbing one.

Humanitarian Myths and Hubris invites us to engage with these dilemmas more consciously. It challenges us to confront the distance between who we believe we are and how we operate in today's fragmented and complex world – a world in which humanitarian principles are put to the test, where the notion of international solidarity is questioned, and where the very legitimacy of aid actors is scrutinised, sometimes rightly so.

What makes this book especially important is that it does not seek to offer simple answers. Instead, it presents a mirror – unsettling at times, always thought-provoking – reflecting the contradictions, tensions, and aspirations within MSF. It raises questions about the principles we uphold, the evolution of our narratives, and the moral and operational limits we encounter on the ground. It asks whether our choices are guided by needs or by convenience; whether we are truly listening or simply replicating our own systems; and whether the people we aim to help are partners in our response, or still, too often, passive recipients.

At MSF, we often speak of bearing witness; of refusing to remain silent in the face of suffering. Bearing witness also means daring to look inward, to question not only the world around us, but the very foundations of our choices, our assumptions, and the systems we are part of.

Humanitarian Myths and Hubris proposes to undertake precisely that kind of examination. It confronts us with difficult, necessary questions: who decides which lives are prioritised? How do our internal frameworks – medical, operational, institutional – shape the image of the "victim" we are able or willing to help? Are we truly as independent, as neutral, as inclusive as we claim to be? How can we combat discriminations in the humanitarian sector? What challenges have been encountered in ensuring the safety of personnel? How does MSF respond when its colleagues are confronted with political repression?

Drawing on concrete examples from our history and present-day action, from the fight against HIV to the climate emergency, this book challenges us to reflect on the gap between our ideals and our practices. It does not offer comfortable conclusions. Instead, it reveals paradoxes that illustrate the tensions between technique and technicity; between liberal and critical visions of justice; between our commitment to humanity and the unequal structures in which we operate.

It also reminds us that emotion – often dismissed in the name of "rational" decision-making – is not a weakness but a compass. That the legitimacy of humanitarian action cannot be claimed; it must be earned. And that the credibility of MSF depends not only on our ability to act, but on our willingness to interrogate our role, to listen to the people we aim to assist, and to construct with them responses that respect their dignity, context, and agency.

In a moment marked by renewed challenges to science, rights, and solidarity, this conversation feels not only timely but essential. May it resonate within and beyond our movement, and contribute to a broader collective reflection on the ethics, politics, and legitimacy of humanitarian action in the world today.

Dr Micaela Serafini, President of MSF Switzerland

Acknowledgements

The editors would like to express their gratitude to all the authors, especially for having put up with our seemingly endless comments and questions. We also wish to thank the many valued first readers who contributed to the review and refinement of the texts – some of whom were harassed more frequently than we would have liked – notably members of the Centre de réflexion sur l'action et les savoirs humanitaires (CRASH) and the Sharing Incident Memory and Mitigation project (SIMM). MSF colleagues working in countries of intervention, and in headquarters, were likewise generous with their time in providing multiple reflections which helped feed the analysis, much appreciated; as was the guidance of MSF Switzerland's leadership. The timely translation services of Philippa Bowe, Derek Scoins, and Karen Stokes were essential. And beyond their individual contributions, a special thanks to the full Research Unit on Humanitarian Stakes and Practices (UREPH) team, who were heavily involved in all stages of the process; their support and input were invaluable. Finally, we would like to dedicate this book to all MSF project teams and patients; undeniably the reason we continue in this line of work.

Duncan McLean, Françoise Duroch, and Amy Mavor

Abbreviations

AI	Artificial Intelligence
AIDS	Acquired Immunodeficiency Syndrome
BLM	Black Lives Matter
CDC	Centers for Disease Control and Prevention
COVAX	COVID-19 Vaccines Global Access
CSJ	Critical Social Justice
DEI	Diversity, Equity and Inclusion
DII	Demographically Identifiable Information
EU	European Union
GAVI	Global Alliance for Vaccines and Immunization
HIV	Human Immunodeficiency Virus
IASC	Inter-Agency Standing Committee
ICC	International Criminal Court
ICJ	International Court of Justice
ICT	Information and Communications Technology
ICRC	International Committee of the Red Cross
IFRC	International Federation of Red Cross and Red Crescent Societies
IHL	International Humanitarian Law
IHR	International Health Regulations
IO	International Organisation
INGO	International Non-governmental Organisation
LGBTQI+	Lesbian, Gay, Bisexual, Transsexual, Questioning (or Queer), Intersex and other gender and/or sexual preference identity terms
LSJ	Liberal Social Justice
MoH	Ministry of Health
MSF	Médecins Sans Frontières
NATO	North Atlantic Treaty Organization
NGO	Non-governmental Organisation
NSAG	Non-state Armed Group
NTD	Neglected Tropical Disease
OCHA	Office for the Coordination of Humanitarian Affairs

P&I	Privileges and Immunities
PII	Personal Identifiable Information
UN	United Nations
UNDP	United Nations Development Programme
UNHCR	United Nations High Commissioner for Refugees
UNSC	United Nations Security Council
USAID	United States Agency for International Development
WHO	World Health Organization

Introduction

Humanitarianism in Retreat?

Duncan McLean

That the humanitarian enterprise is being brought into question can be read as both a perplexing development and a dramatic understatement. The former because it arrives at a time when a record number of vulnerable and crisis-affected populations depend on external assistance; the latter because it caricatures the depth and pace of change currently convulsing the aid sector.[1] At the sharp end, and certainly the most visible change, has been the dismantling of the US Agency for International Development, but this should not mask the retreat of major donors from across the political spectrum. Nor should the acceleration of other long-standing trends – notably a broader realignment of foreign assistance towards national security and economic interests – be ignored.

There is no shortage of singular events that provide insight into the wider challenges faced by humanitarian organisations today, as well as the retreat in global solidarity. The hoarding of vaccines during the COVID-19 pandemic reflected age-old perceptions of double standards as per the health priorities of high-income countries. The conscious dismissal of international humanitarian law (IHL) in Gaza might be one of the most egregious examples of Western hypocrisy, but it is far from alone when cataloguing transgressions from conflicts around the world. Anti-humanitarian narratives emerging in traditional funding countries, in addition to those where operations occur, amplify suspicion and distrust of assistance.

The above sit awkwardly with the high regard aid organisations have often had for their endeavours. The United Nations Refugee Agency's *Emergency Handbook* aptly describes the central motivation behind humanitarian action as being to *"save lives and alleviate suffering while upholding and restoring personal dignity"*.[2] Unlike seemingly more politicised development or bilateral assistance, this basic objective, structured around a supposedly shared common humanity, is fundamentally appealing. While the clichéd image of the heroic aid worker struggling against dark forces bent on destruction might be outdated, the premise of transforming good intentions into concrete action is still difficult to reproach.

Yet, in reality, there have always been critiques of the aid sector, many coming from within. The historian Michael Barnett memorably described humanitarianism as *"one part Trojan horse, one part opiate"*, a reference to both the potential instrumentalisation of aid for less-than-noble objectives and

DOI: 10.4324/9781003542247-1

a ready-made balm for guilty consciences.[3] Whether a convenient alibi to avoid addressing the root causes of human suffering or the unwitting co-opting of humanitarian semantics for other ends, aid organisations have often found themselves the collateral damage of realpolitik. And the historical baggage associated with a prolonged colonial hangover, accompanied by perceptions of prescriptive arrogance, is likewise difficult to dismiss, especially coming from regions that have long been subjected to the whims of external influence.

It is in the spirit of such criticisms that this collective work attempts to find its place. Contributing authors have all been, or continue to be, associated with Médecins Sans Frontières (MSF)[4] in different capacities. Founded in 1971 by a handful of doctors and journalists in Paris, MSF has grown to more than 67,000 people working in over 70 countries, with an annual budget in excess of 2 billion euros. With its own codes, language, and semiology, the organisation still imparts its mythology to newcomers: volunteer doctors rejecting the silence of the International Committee of the Red Cross during the Biafra conflict, priding themselves on their financial independence, or standing up to belligerents when their hospitals are attacked.

This iconography, including the principles enshrined in its Charter, which brings together neutrality, impartiality, independence, and the spirit of volunteerism, is now widely debated and challenged. A half-century later, MSF is a far different beast to the one that initially embarked on modest interventions of medical support; the scale and sophistication of its operations is incomparable to earlier incarnations. But if growth is interpreted as a sign of success, a degree of hubris – perhaps always necessary – can also be detected. While the courage to adapt and innovate in the provision of medical assistance holds tremendous value, notably for the patients treated, reconciling ambition and means can be a trickier balancing act.

The original premise of this book was to deconstruct a series of pressing humanitarian issues, both new and old, through a critical and uncompromising self-portrait of MSF. The current shocks infusing the aid sector gave the task greater urgency, and we hope the concerns raised will echo those of other humanitarian organisations. MSF's ability to adapt and reinvent itself is regularly questioned internally, especially in light of its own moral, political, and operational limits.

Three constants are taken for granted throughout the narrative. As stated from the outset, the existence of dramatic medical needs in multiple contexts is not under dispute, even as expectations on the part of recipients of humanitarian aid have changed; and such recipients are certainly not the passive beneficiaries of external largesse, as has periodically been portrayed. The highly visible wars in Ukraine and the Occupied Palestinian Territory are no more terrifying than the under-reported conflicts in Sudan, the Democratic Republic of the Congo, Myanmar, and elsewhere. All have contributed to levels of displacement, internally and across borders, that eclipse previous numbers on a yearly basis.[5] Whether directly related or the enduring consequences of poverty, debt, and the slow burn of climate change, the burden of disease weighs heavily.

Secondly, those needs are occurring just as the aid sector is undergoing a forced contraction, posing questions about where the priorities should lie, given the resources available, and, indeed, whether opportunities will emerge. It is far from the first time that circumstances have imposed reforms on the humanitarian system, such that it is, but the speed of events has raised the stakes and added a temporal factor. Already strained, response capacity to major crises is clearly at risk, as are less visible mechanisms such as disease surveillance. Global health and food security will experience similar knock-on effects. Meanwhile, socially and politically conservative agendas have expanded as demonstrably successful initiatives around reproductive rights and gender equality are in retreat, and LGBTQI+ individuals are targeted. Irrespective of status, migrants remain convenient scapegoats for society's ills.

Finally, the space carved out by aid organisations to run operations, always precarious, is in danger of being further reduced – a slippery slope that risks banalising transgressions. It is a historical truism that multilateralism depends on some semblance of a rules-based order, a necessary condition to restrain national self-interest and limit cycles of conflict and violence. Even if more aspirational than a reality, aid organisations rely on similar rules. As legal frameworks for humanitarian action are diluted or simply ignored through muscular projections of unilateral political and economic prerogatives, existing norms are bled of their legitimacy.

None of these problems are uniquely recent, even if their acceleration and scale are remarkable. Rather, for the purpose of this analysis, identifying and understanding longer-term trends is given precedence. With this in mind, the collective work is structured around historical points of continuity and change; prescient challenges and dilemmas; and factors not traditionally associated with humanitarian action. The focus is very much the twenty-first century, even if it is necessary to reach back further at times.

Taking a self-consciously historical perspective, the text begins with an exploration of the rationales for operational choices – essentially how priorities are set. While an objective determination of needs would seem most obvious, the authors provide valuable nuance in demonstrating how emotional, political, and economic factors also play a role. The labelling of so-called good and bad victims is particularly evident in the double standards around migrants, and is treated accordingly in a zoom-in. MSF's periodic ambiguity towards the broader aid sector is then broached through an analysis of humanitarian principles, accountability frameworks, and rights-based approaches over time, raising questions around power and responsibility. Security discourses hold significant sway in the aid sector today, frequently influencing what can and cannot be implemented operationally, and MSF is no different. In this contribution, the authors delve into hostility towards humanitarian actors – both its historical and its contemporary manifestations. A specific focus is provided on the evolving role and exposure of locally hired staff in security management.

Current challenges and dilemmas will be familiar to many humanitarian actors, and will be treated in Part II. This includes the difficulties of reconciling technical aspirations with the inherent limitations found in conflict areas or resource-poor settings, illustrated through the evolution of MSF's medical operations via a series of case studies. The concept of global health security in humanitarian medicine will likewise be examined, again raising the question of where intervention priorities should lie, given public health demands for the greater good, and MSF's own past emphasis on the health needs of vulnerable or excluded populations. Engagement with civil society in contexts of popular uprisings, and the resulting dilemmas, is another timely addition considering the near-impossible task of reconciling the expectations of opposition activists with the principles of neutrality and impartiality on the part of humanitarian actors like MSF. Challenges linked to disinformation in such contexts, and elsewhere, will be treated specifically. Changes in MSF's version of *témoignage* will also be explored, notably its continued relevance as the organisation struggles to make its voice heard in what has become the aid market while moving towards more collaborative attempts at bearing witness.

Emerging challenges to the aid sector make up the third and final part of the collection. The diverging philosophical underpinnings of humanitarian aid and global health are given a critical analysis, with decolonisation narratives featuring prominently. Diversity, equity, and inclusion initiatives, packaged as the saviour of structural racism, and now used as a rationale for cutting aid altogether, are likewise explored through individual experience. Vulnerabilities around digitalisation for humanitarian organisations like MSF, and the specific risks to independence, are examined in reference to the as yet still limited international legal frameworks that can be applied. And finally, the threat posed by climate change, insofar as humanitarian organisations retain a viable model of response, is analysed. Hardly a new phenomenon, the amplification of needs, many of which fall under the purview of actions traditionally associated with the humanitarian sector, is treated, including unwitting contributions from aid actors like MSF.

This thematic list is clearly far from exhaustive. A number of internal issues specific to MSF, such as the challenges of adapting its associative element to what has essentially become a multinational, and grappling with growth, are only considered indirectly. No dedicated chapter examines the long-term impact of the funding cuts, given the speed at which the situation is evolving; nor are there conflict-specific chapters, knowing that any assessment would be quickly out of date. And despite the MSF focus and lens of analysis, the authors are acutely aware that there is no monopoly on the interpretation of humanitarian action. While MSF's own funding model might provide a degree of resilience, the aspiration remains that the fundamental questions raised will resonate with other aid actors.

Ultimately, though, the purpose of this analysis is to reflect on how MSF can pursue its initial social mission of delivering independent medical care to the most vulnerable without compromising the distinctive identity and approach which established its reputation in the first place. Operating on the margins of society, taking care of forgotten populations, being on the front lines, and operating – alone, at times – in the world's most dangerous places make up part of this reputation – indeed, mythology. For all its periodic benefits, hubris contains its own pitfalls, opposing the advantages of staying nimble with the constant ambition to do more. Reconciling past aspirations with present expectations when humanitarian aid itself is under threat remains an essential concern.

Notes

1 OCHA, 2023.
2 UNHCR, 2025.
3 Barnett, 2011, p. 6.
4 Throughout the book, when Médecins Sans Frontières (MSF) is used, it is in reference to the MSF movement, meaning operational centres, partner sections, and so on. Country-specific sections (MSF Switzerland, MSF France, etc.) are used only when necessary for narrative clarity. Internal acronyms abound in MSF, a language unto itself, but are avoided as much as possible in this publication.
5 See UNHCR figures, available at https://www.unhcr.org/about-unhcr/overview/figures-glance.

References

Barnett, Michael N. (2011), *Empire of Humanity: A History of Humanitarianism*, Ithaca, NY: Cornell University Press. doi:10.7591/9780801460616.

OCHA (2023), 'Global Humanitarian Overview 2024'. [https://www.unocha.org/publications/report/world/global-humanitarian-overview-2024-enarfres].

UNHCR (2025), *Emergency Handbook*. [https://emergency.unhcr.org/protection/protection-principles/humanitarian-principles].

UNHCR, 'Figures at a glance'. [https://www.unhcr.org/about-unhcr/overview/figures-glance].

Part I

Elements of Change and Continuity

1 Good and Bad Victims?

A Matter of Choice

*Thierry Allafort-Duverger, Marie-Hortense Koudika, and Françoise Duroch**

> *Before individuals are triaged, those in charge of relief operations select the locations and situations – and therefore the groups of people – prioritised over others when allocating emergency assistance. Under these circumstances, the different ways in which people's misfortunes are portrayed in the public arena, as well as medical and health criteria, determine which populations will be assisted first and which will have to wait, or even resign themselves to not receiving the help they hope for.*[1]
>
> (Jean-Hervé Bradol)

This chapter seeks to examine the decisions that medical humanitarian organisations have to make in order to define the contexts, types of activities, and groups of people to care for, beyond any objective needs based on biomedical criteria, degree of urgency, or scarcity of resources, particularly human and financial.[2] As the above quote describes, every humanitarian response is the result of a selection process which, unlike medical triage, does not assess affected individuals solely based on the immediacy of their health needs.[3] Besides these mechanisms, organisations are subject to specific dynamics, while certain contexts attract more sustained attention than others. For instance, in 2015, an MSF emergency programme manager sent a message to his colleagues as part of an internal debate on rescue operations in the Mediterranean Sea:

> *For your information, Burundian refugees in Tanzania and Rwanda outnumber the migrants who have arrived in Europe over the past three months [...] I'm not saying we shouldn't make every effort to help migrants in Europe, but we also need to keep these forgotten refugees in Africa among our priorities.*[4]

He wanted to highlight a major crisis in Africa at a time when the organisation seemed to be suffering from a certain weariness towards events that appeared to be unending.

Operational decision-making in a medical emergency is influenced by a range of factors, including the severity of the crisis, the degree of personal identification felt by actors from the aid sector, media coverage, and the ability to raise

DOI: 10.4324/9781003542247-3

large funds for a particular region. Rivalries between different MSF sections can also emerge in some contexts, resulting in competing interests among decision-makers:

> *If we opt not to take action, the MSF movement is quick to ask questions. It's something we saw in recent years, in the aftermath of earthquakes in Turkey and Morocco. [...] What fuels this internal pressure? Competition between sections is a factor, the desire not to be seen as absent – all the more so when intense media interest arises. It's as if every section has to be associated with every major emergency.*[5]

The urge to bear witness and speak out can also shape choices about the context or group of people to assist, especially if no other actors are present. Social and political movements, as well as team diversity, are further variables influencing operational decisions. Strategic choices are sometimes the determining factor for entities, such as MSF Switzerland when it ran a series of evaluations in Southeast Asia. According to the director of operations, the region, where the Swiss section has rarely worked, will suffer disproportionately from the effects of the climate crisis in the coming years, making it a timely opportunity to find out more about the needs and ability to respond of the local population.[6] A desire to diversify the organisation's portfolio in terms of contexts and activities, or to ensure a presence in a particular region and plan ahead for responses to future crises, might likewise impact the selection process. Lastly, MSF may want to treat neglected pathologies or provide support to people marginalised for cultural or religious reasons or because of their sexual orientation, as well as to victims of violence and abuse, particularly in conflict situations. It is by making choices among these widely differing categories that MSF defines its operational policy.

The fact is that the quality and nature of assistance provided are always a product of these operational choices. In 1995, at a camp for displaced people in western Bosnia, a midwife raised questions about the distribution of menstrual items to women: "*It's the first time I've seen MSF distribute this type of product; oddly, to the best of my knowledge, this has never happened in other contexts, notably in Africa.*" In 1999, as war raged in Congo-Brazzaville, leading to severe infant malnutrition and large numbers of wounded and sexually assaulted women, a researcher and MSF board member analysed the lengthy delays in setting up care for rape victims:[7]

> *From the standpoint of the organisation's leaders who were involved in the central management of operations, it was not a matter of minimising the importance of providing care to children and the injured, but of questioning the more-or-less exclusive nature of a commitment to these categories of victims, which was detrimental to severely traumatised women at risk from HIV infection.*[8]

Furthermore, the emotions triggered by some crises, the scope of their media coverage, and the associated fundraising possibilities can, on occasion, lead to other tragedies being overlooked:

> *it's impossible to feel all the suffering in the same way. The extraordinary outpouring of emotion triggered by the Indian Ocean tsunami illustrates the variability of people's sensitivities, since other natural disasters, doubtless on a smaller scale, failed to arouse the same feelings.*[9]

MSF is not the only organisation that has to make these trade-offs: the World Health Organization (WHO) points out that the allocation of its resources is a process that has developed tentatively over the years.[10] Moreover, a study commissioned by Institut Bioforce notes that decisions relating to the opening and closing of projects incorporate emotional dimensions, as some operations can be closer to people's hearts.[11] The role of the emotional component as a driver for launching an activity is tricky to determine.[12] While it is understandable that public opinion, politicians, and the media pay closer attention to events occurring in a geographical or cultural space that feels more familiar, the core issue resides in the fact that MSF, as an entity independent from states and autonomous in its choices of aid provision, needs to keep a reasonable distance from these agendas in order to pursue its own aims. The analysis of a number of the dynamics described above will be based on case studies that are particularly emblematic of selection processes that apply within the organisation: Kosovo, Congo-Brazzaville, Ukraine, and the Southeast Asian tsunami.

I Different Perspectives on Competing Crises

The war in Kosovo (March 1998 to June 1999) opposed the Federal Republic of Yugoslavia and Kosovo Albanian separatists represented by the Kosovo Liberation Army. The majority Albanian population of Kosovo demanded independence in the face of determined opposition from the Serbian government. The conflict saw intense fighting, Serbian bombardments, and a riposte from the North Atlantic Treaty Organization (NATO). Some 860,000 Albanian Kosovars fled the repression,[13] with over 200,000 Serbs and non-Albanians also leaving the region.[14] Both sides committed acts of savagery, including rape and murder. Over 13,500 people were killed.[15] In March 1999, NATO launched air strikes without authority from the United Nations, finally compelling Serbian forces to withdraw.

Population movements triggered an emergency response to support refugees in neighbouring countries, such as Macedonia, Montenegro, and Albania. A large number of organisations became operational in Kosovo in the aftermath of the NATO intervention.

Almost a year after the withdrawal of Yugoslav troops from the territory, Philippe Biberson, then president of MSF France, noted in his annual report that "*what happened in Kosovo was more about redressing a profound injustice and 10 years of abandonment than a humanitarian emergency, in the strict sense*".[16] MSF's actions had a limited impact in the region, mainly because, during the conflict, functioning medical facilities had continued operating in Kosovo and in areas where refugees moved to. It was also due to the arrival of significant aid linked to the deployment of a major military–humanitarian effort in an easily accessible part of the world.[17]

Activities performed by the organisation included the distribution of medicines; training; psychological support; and assistance to displaced people, particularly in Montenegro. MSF teams also responded to unusual requests, such as retrieving corpses dumped in wells by federal troops, in collaboration with the International Criminal Tribunal for the former Yugoslavia, in order to document war crimes and allow families to mourn.[18] With a severe winter approaching and a large number of houses having burned down, MSF completed the UN shelter construction programmes that had not yet been implemented. It launched a project called "1,000 roofs for Kosovo", despite internal debate regarding its appropriateness when set against other situations requiring emergency action, such as Brazzaville in the Republic of the Congo, where fierce fighting was ongoing.[19]

The president of MSF France, at the time, later mentioned that the organisation should possibly have declined to take action, citing the role played by NATO:

> *we failed to respond in the proper manner and oppose the humanitarian label forced on us by NATO. [...] Our position as Europeans, and thus parties to the conflict, was inevitably ambiguous. [...] In future we should be extremely vigilant and determined to ensure MSF remains distinct [...] even if it comes at the price of keeping our distance.*[20]

In the Republic of the Congo, in October 1997, former president Denis Sassou-Nguesso returned to power after four months of intense fighting in the capital. In December 1998, while hostile militias had entered areas of Brazzaville, government forces conducted a systematic sweep to clear the Bakongo and Makélékélé districts, supported by groups loyal to the regime, and foreign troops (Angolan, Chadian, and Rwandan Hutus). The conflict forced approximately 20,000 people to flee the southern districts of Brazzaville, mostly heading to the Pool region and the neighbouring Democratic Republic of the Congo. The refugees spent months living in the forest, suffering from hunger and ongoing violence, before they began to return to Brazzaville along the only access route, the so-called "corridor of death" controlled by militias and the military.[21] The precise number of women raped and men executed arbitrarily during this period remains unknown.

Between May and September 1999, over 170,000 refugees and displaced persons returned to Brazzaville, with as many as 10,000 people sometimes arriving in a single day. The state of these abused, exhausted, starved, and injured human beings bore witness to the scale of the tragedy. Starting in May 1999, MSF teams working at the sports centre, a former airport serving as a transit camp, began the task of providing first aid and transferring patients. Ten or more ambulances criss-crossed the city to deliver victims and the sick to hospitals and nutrition units. MSF set up four nutrition centres that treated thousands of children, teenagers, and adults (more than 9,000 children received inpatient care over a six-month period), while Action contre la Faim and other organisations tended to the needs of countless other patients. MSF also reopened the emergency and surgical services at Makélékélé Hospital. Almost 1,600 cases of rape were identified, but victims of sexual violence did not receive appropriate care, owing in particular to the lack of abortion access and HIV prevention treatment. It should, likewise, be noted that activities relating to social support and legal assistance were not seen as priorities during decision-making at that time.

Writing in the 2000 *Annual Report*, the president of MSF France said, "*This is a medical emergency on a scale Médecins Sans Frontières has rarely encountered.*" He also highlighted the imbalance in terms of media coverage: "*The contrast with Kosovo [...] is striking. Far from the cameras [...], the Congolese only had themselves and a small handful of organisations to count on.*"[22] MSF itself was far more invested in the aftermath of the war in Kosovo. In 1999, the crisis attracted a budget of 18.6 million euros, with a massive deployment of international staff and many visits from HQ teams from various sections. On the other hand, also in 1999, MSF France was the only section with a presence in Brazzaville, operating with a budget of 3 million euros and a small-scale team.

The level of danger in Brazzaville meant that the teams were scaled back and operated under the strict supervision of the Paris-based programme manager. But the needs remained immense, leading to tensions when personnel on-site demanded greater resources, whereas HQ, concerned with safety issues, preferred to limit staff numbers. On the other hand, Kosovo witnessed a major operational deployment. When NATO bombing provided air support for the recapture of the town of Peć, the president, programme manager, head of emergency response, and a communications manager from MSF France all took considerable risks, not unlike many other actors, so that they would be the first to arrive as soon as hostilities ceased – despite a limited impact on the medical situation.

Leaving aside the help afforded to victims, competition between different MSF sections and a desire to play a part in history as it unfolded seemed to drive this risk-taking. Humanitarian actors are often guided by a twofold aspiration: providing immediate assistance and participating in major events. The duality of their motivations adds an extra dimension to the role they play, establishing them not only as aid providers but also as active observers of era-defining crises.

In 2022, MSF invested 49.7 million euros in funding for medical activities during the conflict in Ukraine, resulting in around 90,000 consultations, 235 hospitalisations, and 161 surgical operations. In comparison, teams in Afghanistan with an almost identical budget (48.7 million euros) carried out 185,000 consultations, 88,000 hospitalisations, and 13,600 surgical interventions.[23]

In March 2022, two managers from the French MSF section wrote an article highlighting the need to concentrate efforts on vulnerable groups, particularly the elderly and people suffering from mental disorders, given the strength of the Ukrainian medical system and the groundswell of international support.[24] They insisted on the importance of ensuring that other crises did not go unnoticed, in view of the probable repercussions of the war on food security around the world. Additionally, a former operational manager takes a harsh view of the analysis of the activities put in place, especially at the start of the conflict:

> *I think that initially we forgot to say, let's stop and think. [...] We were also heavily influenced by the desire to be visible with actions considered as "noble", such as surgical interventions. We let ourselves get completely swept up in a whirlwind and lost our ability to stay objective; I'm part and parcel of this failure to think it through.*[25]

While some MSF sections chose to remain in Ukraine, others left the country, feeling that the MSF presence was disproportionate to the assessed needs. Questions remained, essentially around the risks involved and the nature of aid provision. Assistance seemed somewhat irrelevant given local capacities, the roll-out of emergency relief, and the number of humanitarian actors already responding.[26] During a visit to Ukraine, a surgeon said to MSF France's director of operations, "*How can I explain to my daughter that I'm risking my life just to provide training?*"[27] Eventually, the various MSF sections renounced most of their surgical activities near combat zones, continuing to offer mental health services and organise medical referrals.

Similar dynamics to those seen in the 1999 Kosovo response emerged, i.e. the allocation of important resources in a particularly high-profile context, with limited relevance to the local population. In this respect, the organisation observed that certain events generate significant fundraising, depending on the nature of the crisis and the type of people needing aid. The waves of generosity that drive humanitarian operations also tend to favour certain categories of victims, particularly during responses to natural disasters.[28] The case of the 2004 tsunami in the Indian Ocean, for example, offers food for thought in terms of MSF's choice to resist the excessive exploitation of an unusual level of worldwide financial solidarity.

On 26 December 2004, an earthquake measuring 9.1 to 9.3 on the Richter scale struck off the coast of Indonesia. It triggered a tsunami, with waves as high as 35 metres in some areas. Killing at least 250,000 people, it was one of the deadliest earthquakes in history, with around 170,000 fatalities in Indonesia, 31,000 in Sri Lanka, 16,400 in India, and 5,400 in Thailand.

The disaster prompted an unprecedented outpouring of solidarity, with individuals, trusts, foundations, and businesses contributing 40% of the 13.5 billion dollars in donations.[29] No other humanitarian response has elicited such a large amount of private funding.[30] Several factors explain the groundswell of generosity: the event happened during the festive season, European tourists were among the victims, and it was the sort of crisis that usually arouses more empathy than conflicts, given the political nature of their causes. It is easy to perceive victims of a natural disaster as having no responsibility at all for the tragedy that has struck them, especially since these events, often on a very large scale, occur suddenly. The tsunami garnered more media exposure over two months than any of the ten major "forgotten" crises of 2003, including the start of the war in Darfur and the earthquake in Bam, Iran, which resulted in the deaths of over 25,000 people.[31]

At the time, MSF made what proved to be a highly controversial statement when it called for a halt to tsunami-related fundraising, as it had collected enough money for its operations. The MSF leadership asked donors for permission to reassign the excess donations to other, overlooked causes.[32] Initially seen as suspicious, this approach was later adopted by other non-governmental organisations. After receiving 40 million euros in one week, MSF stopped appealing for donations, recognising that it would be impossible to spend the funds raised on this single crisis. MSF ultimately collected 110 million euros of donations and allocated 25 million euros to activities related to the tsunami while exploring alternative initiatives, such as building boats and providing the people affected with cash payments.[33] Rebuilding soon emerged as the priority, since most victims had already died and healthcare structures only required limited support. Additionally, the massive presence of international medical teams created a situation where multiple actors found themselves on the ground without always having any concrete tasks. Nevertheless, some organisations, including WHO, doubled down on the disaster by highlighting the risk of an epidemic that could multiply the number of deaths twofold – a risk questioned by several scientists.[34]

It is interesting to note that many foreign humanitarian workers could have left the damaged areas three months after the earthquake without their departure having any significant impact on the health of the people affected. However, the desire to be active on the ground, motivated in particular by the need to justify money provided by donors, took precedence over the relevance of the programmes put in place.[35] Years later, the French Court of Auditors carried out an analysis showing that the funds collected exceeded the various organisations' capacity to use them immediately, and advised the recipient bodies to learn lessons from this situation and inform their donors with complete transparency.[36]

While certain groups of people can find themselves in the media spotlight due to the nature of the disaster that has hit them, others attract little public attention: the wrong gender, an illness seen as shameful, or a lack of political or economic interest on the part of countries to a specific context. The wave of generosity triggered by a tragedy such as the tsunami should not overshadow all the silent crises that occur against a background of widespread indifference.

II From Ideal Victims to Those Ignored by Humanitarian Action

The process of selecting which people to help naturally highlights a moral and political economy,[37] often underestimated by many stakeholders, but sometimes knowingly employed. We should not forget how slowly patients in the Global

South[38] received access to therapies to combat tuberculosis and HIV. Suspicions persisted that they would not be capable of regularly taking their treatment,[39] along with concerns over protecting the patents and economic interests of the pharmaceutical industry.[40] This discrimination in access to antiretroviral drugs led to an alarming mortality rate in patients with HIV, particularly in sub-Saharan Africa.

The pressure to act during natural disasters, such as after the tsunami, or to try and provide aid to the wounded without access to the combat zone, which occurred in Ukraine, highlights a persistent paradox. This distinction between priority victims and those overlooked by humanitarian action remains a reality for many different categories of people. For instance, certain pathologies, particularly those that are infectious, are especially lethal, and nevertheless remain on the margins of political and media agendas:

> *War is not the only circumstance where the death of a swathe of humanity is at stake. According to the WHO's latest estimates, several million people die from AIDS every year while conflicts kill a few hundred thousand. In other words, AIDS kills ten times more people than war.*[41]

The emblematic figure of the wounded, namely in conflict situations, is central to humanitarian iconography, no doubt echoing the origins and history of the Red Cross.[42] However, providing surgical care in wartime is not risk-free and sometimes takes place at the expense of other patients. These complex dilemmas caused a deputy director of operations in the MSF French section to exclaim in the 2000s: "*That's enough of your wounded in Afghanistan, it's women in labour who are dying.*"[43] The organisation's directors have cited reflexes that need to be suppressed within MSF if the aim is primarily to reduce mortality rates. For example, a former director of operations for the Swiss section denounced "*instinctive actions we need to avoid. Do we systematically need to provide wartime surgery in a country at war? Not necessarily. It would probably be better to provide post-operative treatment and maternity care.*"[44] Selecting which people to help and which activity to implement is also influenced by gender-related concepts and more or less implicit cultural considerations, often analysed after aid has been delivered. For instance, in the case of the people of Brazzaville and the Pool region during the 1998 conflict, the image of starving children overshadowed that of raped women,[45] although the consequences of sexual violence became clear as soon as people returned to the capital. Nevertheless, MSF personnel continued to underestimate the need to develop specific assistance: "*one does not die of rape.*"[46] The MSF teams referred, surely justifiably, to a work overload which prevented them from properly assessing which activities were necessary.[47]

Medical care, social assistance, and legal aid were thus not fully rolled out until 2000, when the situation stabilised. Thanks to the criticism that followed the Brazzaville operation, as well as the media scandal in the wake of the United Nations High Commissioner for Refugees report on abuse in the Mano

River region,[48] MSF now routinely includes medical care for victims of sexual violence in most of its activities.

While pregnant women, and children under five, are often given priority as part of humanitarian medical aid due to their heightened exposure to specific pathologies, these choices still raise ethical and practical questions, particularly over the monitoring of this type of patient:

> *with changing demographics, we have to adapt our decision-making criteria. The frequently used approach of "saving mothers and babies" can lead to carrying out neonatal activities in situations where we are not even capable of anticipating the social consequences in the medium term of a disabled child.*[49]

The organisation's definition of priority patients can also be contested by the people receiving aid, highlighting the need for a better understanding of the social dynamics in contexts of intervention.

Political representatives and members of the local community have often expressed their discontent with aid that specifically targets children under five. Examples include Niger in 2005 (Keita and Tahoua) and 2017 (Maine Sora), and Burkina Faso in 2022 (Boucle du Mouhoun). Negotiations with armed non-state actors in Nigeria in 2022 led to a ban from the territory if only children were treated.[50] In 2021, in Nouna in Burkina Faso, a father whose sick child was receiving care asked for medical aid for himself. He feared that, without treatment, he would no longer be able to work and provide for his family.[51]

Specific requests relating to the nature of the aid to be delivered have also been formulated: in Pakistan in 2008 (Peshawar), regional managers insisted on the provision of non-food items, while in Nigeria in 2020 (Maiduguri), food aid was distributed to families to improve the nutritional status of children. In these contexts, aid recipients become part of the decision-making process concerning what type of assistance to provide, and who should receive it first. However, it is important to maintain a balance between the legitimate demands of local communities and the organisation's freedom to make its own choices, given that it needs to keep its distance from social and political dynamics which could be too partisan or prescriptive.

III Opportunities

Humanitarian responses entail making choices that can be standardised or marked by moral considerations that are often implicit. On the other hand, the changes resulting from widely publicised interventions with a smaller operational scope have driven improvements in humanitarian practices. These situations offer opportunities for valuable introspection, leading to a process of in-depth questioning and discussions that are key to continuously strengthening MSF's impact when operating in emergency conditions. They attract closer attention from within the organisation, as well as from the media and academic spheres. And they sometimes serve to stimulate innovation, encouraging the development of approaches with the potential to become norms for future humanitarian practices, as well as for some overall policies. These operations thus seem to have helped to consolidate reflection on MSF's financial autonomy and independence:

> *It is very difficult to resist the urge to intervene in major crises. What we managed to do with the tsunami was to use the money to care for tens of thousands of children suffering from severe malnutrition in Niger. [...] Our financial resources play a crucial role in this process, as demonstrated by our response in Chechnya, despite Europe's refusal to provide funding since it was seen as an internal Russian crisis. We also refused further money from the European Union after the agreement between Turkey and the EU on managing migration. What I mean to say is that the construction of MSF's culture of financial autonomy was particularly concentrated during these episodes. The tsunami was a major event in this regard, and our decision left its mark.*[52]

The tsunami served to better define the MSF emergency fund,[53] making it possible to avoid allocating excessive resources to a single context, as happened with other widely publicised crises (Armenia, 1988; Romania, 1989; and Hurricane Mitch in South America, 1999).[54] As a result of this initiative, MSF can now redirect certain donations, with the donors' prior agreement, when needs have been covered or operational constraints arise, guaranteeing efficient distribution of resources. This also calls for accountability, and MSF publishes an annual report on the use of the funds.[55]

Furthermore, the Kosovo crisis marked the beginning of financial resources being shared between the different MSF sections: a number of them with fewer funds threatened to resort to European state funding so they could expand their activities in a wartime context when NATO was involved as a belligerent, endangering the organisation's image of independence.[56] This initiative laid the foundations for a system which continued to develop over time. Today, collected donations are distributed between operational sections, which rarely need to call on institutional funds.[57]

Noteworthy developments also include the changes observed in Armenia in 1988. At the time, MSF paid close attention to operations due to the groundswell of solidarity and emotion and the extraordinary amount of funding received in response to the earthquake in a country with strong ties to France. This clearly encouraged MSF, in the absence of other needs such as surgical care, to introduce mental health services for the first time.[58] The earthquake in Armenia was also the first time Médecins du Monde ran a psychological care programme.[59]

Similarly, discussion about the roofs of houses in Kosovo triggered the reassessment of standards for refugees, with the creation of adequate shelter in camps in Guinea-Conakry, as well as the revision of existing practices.

IV An Element of Subjectivity

While choices made by MSF are, to some extent, arbitrary and subjective, this is part and parcel of work that remains profoundly human, where emotions clearly have their place. These choices also lie at a nexus of internal and external constraints that MSF struggles to extricate itself from. Nevertheless, the standardisation of approaches, particularly the priority given to the mother–child dyad, is still open to debate, whether by social and political movements that criticise culturally normative practices, or by the people the organisation assists. The so-called "ideal" victim is not, therefore, always the victim as imagined by MSF. The goal should eventually be a co-construction that takes into account the organisation's objectives and the choices of the people concerned, linked to the sociocultural specificities of the places affected by crises. The part played by emotions in establishing priorities is also one of the many fields still to be explored. Rarely mentioned by the people in charge of operational policies, the emotional component remains overlooked despite its role as one of the factors motivating the choices made. Identification with a specific form of distress, a political event that resonates with an aid worker's convictions, or a staff member's attachment to a region related to a past experience in the same context: emotions are underpinned by multiple elements that are no doubt necessary when confronted with the responsibility of deciding where to send aid and to whom. However, regardless of the choice made, there is a duty to justify the allocation of resources and correlated risk-taking. This applies even when the decision is the fruit of an opportunity rather than a conventional consultation process generally involving several actors. Racial and gender-based discrimination can further hinder access to care: according to a recent study in the *European Journal of Emergency Medicine*, pain is taken more seriously depending on whether the person experiencing it is a man or a woman, Caucasian or African.[60] Further studies in the gynaecological field corroborate this observation, highlighting that women seen as coming from sub-Saharan Africa are more likely to give birth via Caesarean section.[61] From the MSF standpoint, exploring the question of the possible stereotypes at play in deciding which people to assist would certainly be useful, especially since sociocultural diversity among the people working within the organisation continues to grow.[62]

Notes

* Translated from French by Philippa Bowe.

1 Bradol, 2014, pp. 103–23.

2 Lachenal, Lefève, and Nguyen, 2014, pp. 1–25.

3 *"This series of choices is what constitutes humanitarian triage. A major difference between medical triage and humanitarian triage is that candidates for assistance, who are too numerous, are not examined prior to selection."*: Péchayre, 2014, p. 6. Translated from French by Philippa Bowe.

4 Hugues Robert, emergency programme manager with MSF Switzerland, referring to the mass arrival of refugees following post-electoral violence in Burundi.

5 Interview with Kenneth Lavelle, director of operations, MSF Switzerland, 2024.

6 *Ibid.*
7 The distinction between "victim" and "survivor" is particularly sensitive in relation to sexual violence. Many prefer the term "survivor", as it presents the person in a more empowering way. However, the notion of survival is a social and personal one. In MSF, the terms "survivor", "patient", and "victim" are used interchangeably in relation to sexual violence. The same applies throughout this book.
8 Le Pape, 2004. Translated from French by Philippa Bowe.
9 *"A few months later, after the very powerful earthquake in Kashmir (70,000 dead, 40,000 injured), things were different. There was no massive humanitarian support, no TV specials, no national collections. Doubtlessly because this part of the world is influenced by fundamentalist Islam and associated with terrorism. But also because, in the meantime, the headlines had been dominated by a hurricane that struck New Orleans, a global bird flu epidemic and another earthquake, this time in Java. Unsurprisingly, after so many physically threatening events, a degree of emotional fatigue became apparent."*: Brauman, 2009, pp. 9–19. Translated from French by Philippa Bowe.
10 Seabright, 1993, p. 347.
11 Bioforce, 2003.
12 *"For example, the degree of urgency or outrage felt by experienced aid workers might be the best way for NGOs with limited resources to gauge the degree of need in a particular place."*: Rubenstein, 2008, p. 230.
13 UNHCR Standing Committee, 2000.
14 UNHCR, 1999.
15 Kosovo Memory Book 1998–2000.
16 Biberson, 2000. Translated from French by Philippa Bowe.
17 Weissman, 2000.
18 MSF, 2013, p. 276.
19 Biberson, 2000.
20 *Ibid.* Translated from French by Philippa Bowe.
21 Le Pape et al. (eds), 2001.
22 Biberson, 2000. Translated from French by Philippa Bowe.
23 MSF, 2024a.
24 Neuman and Allafort-Duverger, 2022.
25 Interview with Christine Jamet, former director of operations, MSF Switzerland, 2024. Translated from French by Philippa Bowe.
26 Interview with William Hennequin, director of operations, MSF France, 2024. Translated from French by Philippa Bowe.
27 *Ibid.*
28 Brauman and Vidal, 2011, p. 291.
29 Oxfam, 2014b.
30 Oxfam, 2014a.
31 Oxfam, 2014b.
32 Hofnung, 2005.
33 Data provided by Rémi Obert, former financial coordinator, MSF International.
34 Watson, Gayer, and Connolly, 2007.
35 Werly, 2005.
36 Cour des Comptes (France), 2011.
37 *"We will consider moral economy to be the production, distribution, circulation, and use of moral sentiments, emotions and values, and norms and obligations in social space."*: Fassin, 2009, p. 1257. Translated from French by Philippa Bowe.
38 For a definition of the notion of the Global South, see https://www.globalsouthstudies.org/what-is-the-global-south.
39 In 2001, Andrew Natsios, head of the US Agency for International Development (USAID), told the US Congress that it was difficult to distribute antiretroviral

therapy to people living with HIV in Africa due to weak infrastructure and patients' inability to take the drugs at the right time, since they did not have watches.
40 Eboko, 2005, pp. 789–98.
41 Weissman, 2003.
42 ICRC, 2017.
43 Pierre Pascal Vandini, deputy director of operations for MSF France, during an operations meeting in Paris.
44 Interview with Christine Jamet, former director of operations, MSF Switzerland, 2024. Translated from French by Philippa Bowe.
45 Le Pape et al. (eds), 2001.
46 Dr J. Liu, in charge of medical activities in Congo-Brazzaville at the time: Duroch and Schulte-Hillen, 2015.
47 Le Pape et al. (eds), 2001.
48 The report accused dozens of NGOs of providing aid in exchange for sexual favours in the refugee camps of Guinea, Sierra Leone, and Liberia: UNHCR, 2002.
49 Interview with Christine Jamet, former director of operations, MSF Switzerland, 2024. Translated from French by Philippa Bowe.
50 Interview with Issiaka Abou, former emergency coordinator and programme manager, MSF France, July 2024.
51 Reported by Marie-Hortense Koudika, medical manager and co-author of this chapter.
52 Interview with Jean-Hervé Bradol, former president, MSF France, January 2024. Translated from French by Philippa Bowe.
53 See https://www.msf.fr/agir/soutenir-nos-actions/fonds-d-urgence.
54 Interview with Jean-Hervé Bradol, former president, MSF France, January 2024.
55 See https://www.msf.fr/agir/soutenir-nos-actions/fonds-d-urgence.
56 MSF, 2013.
57 See https://www.msf.fr/decouvrir-msf/transparence-financiere.
58 Wolmark, 2023.
59 Martin, 2020.
60 Coisy et al., 2024, pp. 188–94.
61 Sauvegrain, 2012, pp. 81–100.
62 In 2023, for the second year in a row, MSF internationally mobile staff from countries on the continent of Africa outnumbered those from Europe (44% vs 30%). MSF, 2024b.

References

Biberson, Philippe (2000), 'Annual Report', 30th General Assembly, MSF France.

Bioforce (2003), 'Governance in European International Humanitarian Aid Organizations: The Decision-Making Process for Starting and Ending Humanitarian Field Missions'.

Bradol, Jean-Hervé (2014), 'En Situation de Catastrophe: S'orienter, Trier et Agir', *Les Cahiers du Centre Georges Canguilhem*, vol. 6, n° 1, pp. 103–123. doi:10.3917/ccgc.006.0103.

Brauman, Rony (2009), 'Emotion et Action Humanitaire', *Études*, t. 410, n° 1, pp. 9–19. doi:10.3917/etu.101.0009.

Brauman, Rony, and Claudine Vidal (2011), 'Natural disasters: "Do something!"', in Claire Magone, Michaël Neuman, and Fabrice Weissman (eds), *Humanitarian Negotiations Revealed: the MSF experience*, London: Hurst & Co. [https://msf-crash.org/en/natural-disasters/natural-disasters-do-something].

Coisy, Fabien, Guillaume Olivier, François-Xavier Ageron, Hugo Guillermou, Mélanie Roussel, Frédéric Balen, Laura Grau-Mercier, and Xavier Bobbia (2024), 'Do

Emergency Medicine Health Care Workers Rate Triage Level of Chest Pain Differently Based upon Appearance in Simulated Patients?', *European Journal of Emergency Medicine*, vol. 31, n° 3, pp. 188–194. doi:10.1097/MEJ.0000000000001113.

Cour des Comptes (2011), 'Synthèse du rapport sur les organismes faisant appel à la générosité publique'.

Duroch, Françoise, and Catrin Schulte-Hillen (2015), 'Care for victims of sexual violence, an organization pushed to its limits: The case of Médecins Sans Frontières', *International Review of the Red Cross*, vol. 96, n° 894. [https://international-review.icrc.org/articles/care-victims-sexual-violence-organization-pushed-its-limits-case-medecins-sans-frontieres].

Eboko, Fred (2005), 'Le Droit Contre La Morale? L'accès Aux Médicaments Contre Le Sida En Afrique', *Revue internationale des sciences sociales*, vol. 186, n° 4, pp. 789–798. doi:10.3917/riss.186.0789.

Fassin, Didier (2009), 'Les Économies Morales Revisitées', *Annales. Histoire, Sciences Sociales*, vol. 64, n° 6, pp. 1235–1266. doi:10.1017/S0395264900027499.

Hofnung, Thomas (2005), 'Tsunami: les dons ont-ils fait recette?', *Libération*, 26 December. [https://www.liberation.fr/evenement/2005/12/26/tsunami-les-dons-ont-ils-fait-recette_542815/].

ICRC (2017), 'History of the ICRC'. [https://www.icrc.org/en/document/history-icrc].

'Kosovo Memory Book 1998–2000'. [http://www.kosovskaknjigapamcenja.org/?page_id=29&lang=de].

Lachenal, Guillaume, Céline Lefève, and Vinh-Kim Nguyen (2014), 'Le Triage En Médecine, Une Routine d'exception', *Les Cahiers du Centre Georges Canguilhem*, vol. 6, n° 1, pp. 1–25. doi:10.3917/ccgc.006.0001.

Le Pape, Marc (2004), 'Guerre et viols au Congo: des urgentistes à Brazzaville', Conference: Guerre et Médecine: quel champ de recherche?', Université Paris Cité. [https://msf-crash.org/fr/guerre-et-humanitaire/guerre-et-viols-au-congo-des-urgentistes-brazzaville].

Le Pape, Marc, Rémy Bazenguissa-Ganga, François Guillemot, Dieudonné N'Gaba, and Pierre Salignon (eds) (2001), *Une guerre contre les civils: réflexions sur les pratiques humanitaires au Congo Brazzaville (1998–2000)*. Paris: Karthala.

Martin, Boris (2020), 'Médecins Du Monde, La Belle Histoire 1980–2020', Médecins du Monde. [https://issuu.com/medecinsdumonde/docs/medecin_du_monde-la_belle_histoire_1980-2020_boris].

MSF, 'Fonds d'urgence | Médecins sans frontières'. [https://www.msf.fr/agir/soutenir-nos-actions/fonds-d-urgence].

MSF, 'Transparence financière | Médecins sans frontières'. [https://www.msf.fr/decouvrir-msf/transparence-financiere].

MSF (2013), 'Violence against Kosovar Albanians, NATO's intervention 1998–1999', MSF Speaking Out case study. [https://www.msf.org/sites/default/files/2019-04/SOCSKosovoEnglish.pdf].

MSF (2024a), 'Typology 2023 Report', MSF Internal Report.

MSF (2024b), '2023 Staff Data and Trends Report', MSF Internal Report.

Neuman, Michaël, and Thierry Allafort-Duverger (2022), 'Medical aid in the time of war'. [https://msf-crash.org/en/blog/war-and-humanitarianism/medical-aid-time-war].

Oxfam International (2014a), 'Ten years on, the Indian Ocean Tsunami response reveals how people in crises can be helped by timely funding', 18 December. [https://www.oxfam.org/en/press-releases/ten-years-indian-ocean-tsunami-response-reveals-how-people-crises-can-be-helped].

Oxfam International (2014b), 'The Indian Ocean Tsunami, 10 Years On'. [https://www.oxfam.org/en/research/indian-ocean-tsunami-10-years].

Péchayre, Marion (2014), 'Impartialité et Pratiques de Triage En Milieu Humanitaire. Le Cas de Médecins sans Frontières Au Pakistan', *Les Cahiers du Centre Georges Canguilhem*, vol. 6, n° 1, pp. 125–142. doi:10.3917/ccgc.006.0125.

Rubenstein, Jennifer C. (2008), 'The Distributive Commitments of International NGOs', in Michael Barnett and Thomas G.Weiss (eds), *Humanitarianism in Question*, Ithaca: Cornell University Press, pp. 215–234. doi:10.7591/9780801461538–011.

Sauvegrain, Priscille (2012), 'La santé maternelle des « Africaines » en Île-de-France: racisation des patientes et trajectoires de soins', *Revue européenne des migrations internationals*, vol. 28, n° 2, pp. 81–100. doi:10.4000/remi.5902.

Seabright, Paul (1993), 'John Roemer: Distributing Health: The Allocation of Resources by an International Agency', in Martha Nussbaum and Amartya Sen (eds), *The Quality of Life*, Oxford: Oxford University Press, pp. 358–361. doi:10.1093/0198287976.003.0026.

UNHCR (1999), 'Kosovo: One Last Chance', *Refugees Magazine*, vol. 3, n° 116. [https://www.unhcr.org/media/refugees-magazine-issue-116-kosovo-one-last-chance].

UNHCR (2002), 'Note for Implementing and Operational Partners by UNHCR and Save the Children-UK on Sexual Violence & Exploitation: The Experience of Refugee Children in Guinea, Liberia and Sierra Leone'. [https://www.unhcr.org/media/note-implementing-and-operational-partners-unhcr-and-save-children-uk-sexual-violence].

UNHCR Standing Committee (2000), 'The Kosovo Refugee Crisis: An Independent Evaluation of UNHCR's Emergency Preparedness and Response'. [https://www.unhcr.org/publications/kosovo-refugee-crisis-independent-evaluation-unhcrs-emergency-preparedness-and].

Watson, John T., Michelle Gayer, and Maire A. Connolly (2007), 'Epidemics after Natural Disasters', *Emerging Infectious Diseases*, vol. 13, n° 1, pp. 1–5. doi:10.3201/eid1301.060779.

Weissman, Fabrice (2000), 'Kosovo, L'humanitaire, enjeu politique marginal', *Centre de réflexion sur l'action et les savoirs humanitaires*. [https://msf-crash.org/fr/guerre-et-humanitaire/kosovo-lhumanitaire-enjeu-politique-marginal].

Weissman, Fabrice (ed.) (2003), *À l'ombre des guerres justes: l'ordre international cannibale et l'action humanitaire*, Paris: Flammarion.

Werly, Richard (2005), *Tsunami: la vérité humanitaire*, Paris: Éd. du Jubilé.

Wolmark, Laure (2023), '"We don't do mental health": a review of Médecins Sans Frontières' first "psy" mission', *Humanitarian Alternatives*, no 22, pp. 8–19. [https://www.alternatives-humanitaires.org/en/2023/03/21/we-dont-do-mental-health-a-review-of-medecins-sans-frontieres-first-psy-mission/].

Zoom-in: Healthcare without Borders

Navigating Securitisation and Exclusion of Migrants

Reem Mussa

Borders, migration, and refugee policies are not merely physical demarcations and administrative tools. They are also active sites of power, control, and inequality. While globalisation has intensified mobility and migration, it has been coupled with increased militarised borders worldwide, including walls, checkpoints, detention centres, and discriminatory policing, along with a reduction in access to asylum – all common mechanisms of migration governance disproportionally targeting racialised migrants from the Global South.[1]

As migration securitisation grows, so, in turn, has the response of humanitarian actors. MSF, among others, has developed interventions which aim to address the health consequences of these policies. However, whilst these interventions have the potential to mitigate harm, they may also reinforce notions of "deservingness" and "undeservingness". Humanitarian action is often based on implicit assumptions and operationalised assessments of needs and vulnerability. Research on migrant and refugee deservingness identifies multiple dimensions, including those shaped by human rights and humanitarian logics.[2] Human rights-based deservingness relies on legal criteria, as outlined in the 1951 Geneva Refugee Convention, which defines eligibility for international protection. In contrast, humanitarian deservingness focuses on a *"politics of compassion"*, evaluating the needs of migrants based on their vulnerabilities and suffering.[3]

However, within the context of securitisation, both human rights and humanitarian logics are simultaneously merged with and superseded by security concerns.[4] Migrants, especially those that move irregularly or without documents, are deemed as threats. Migration security agendas often intersect with other security interests, such as counterterrorism, anti-trafficking, and global health security.[5] Recent examples include the 2017 US "Muslim Ban", which blocked refugees and migrants from Iraq, Iran, Sudan, and Syria under the guise of national security, and the closure of borders during the COVID-19 pandemic, which was used to further restrict migration and access to asylum.[6]

Meanwhile, humanitarian and migration governance frameworks frequently operationalise predefined categories of vulnerability, such as gender, age, disability, sexual orientation, nationality, and ethnicity. For instance, women and children are seen as more exposed, whereas men – especially young men – are viewed with suspicion unless they demonstrate their vulnerability.[7] Gendered,

DOI: 10.4324/9781003542247-4

xenophobic, and racist tropes reinforce the criminalisation of migration, fuelling cycles of exclusion, stigmatisation, and violence against migrants.[8]

Whilst humanitarians often try to draw attention to crises to mobilise assistance, such narratives have also been used to justify restrictive policies against migrants. During the so-called EU migration crisis, European states enforced extraordinary measures, including the EU–Turkey Deal, which fast-tracked asylum and return procedures, and intensified border control practices. These practices are now institutionalised in national and EU laws.[9] It is well demonstrated that these policies drive migrants into more dangerous routes, leading to increased precarity, injury, and deaths. Yet, states continue to respond with harsher control, containment, and criminalisation measures, all while shifting responsibility on to migrants for taking risks as they seek safety.[10]

This phenomenon is encompassed by the Australian response to the sea rescue of 433 asylum seekers, mainly from Afghanistan, by Norwegian vessel MV *Tampa* in 2001. The government accused the asylum seekers of putting themselves in danger and refused to let the boat enter Australian ports, despite the captain's request for assistance due to the medical condition of those on board. Amidst the stand-off, the Australian Prime Minister John Howard asserted, *"we will decide who comes into this country and the circumstances in which they come"*,[11] and infamously established the Pacific Solution, which outsourced detention and asylum processing to centres in Nauru and Papua New Guinea. While the psychological and physical harm of this policy has been well documented, other states, such as the United Kingdom and Italy, have now followed suit by pursuing similar deals with Rwanda and Albania.[12]

This hostile migration context has forced humanitarians to adapt their practices and assumptions, while also considering the limits, dilemmas, and potential blind spots of their interventions.

MSF's Response to the Securitised Migration Landscape

As a medical humanitarian organisation, MSF frames its migration projects as needs-based, prioritising access to health and well-being over the legal labels of "migrant" or "refugee". In a 2009 paper, two senior MSF analysts stated, *"for MSF there is no concept of 'illegal people' or 'illegal patients'. MSF interventions are a response to human beings in need of assistance."*[13] MSF migration projects often respond to health needs which emerge from living conditions, exclusion, and a lack of access to medical care impacting on people's physical and mental health. These activities require the organisation to adopt a multifaceted approach that combines biomedical understanding of needs with advocacy, and social and legal support components.

While MSF has worked in refugee and displacement settings since its inception, projects addressing the needs of people on the move and people without legal status became more visible in the 1990s and 2000s, with early programmes in France and Belgium which supported *sans-papiers* (undocumented migrants) who were left out of the healthcare system and faced hostile policing practices and deportation. As well as providing access to medical care, MSF projects have successfully advocated for a "humanitarian clause" to prevent the deportation of sick people unable to receive adequate healthcare in their home country.[14]

Since then, MSF's migration-focused operations have spanned diverse regions and contexts, aiming to improve healthcare access and address migration-related vulnerabilities. These efforts target the physical and mental health impacts of precarious living conditions, xenophobic violence, lack of care continuity, detention, violence, and torture affecting migrants, including those in transit, migrant workers, returnees, and other vulnerable groups in countries like Italy, South Africa, Egypt, Yemen, Malaysia, Panama, and Brazil. MSF has also launched targeted initiatives, such as search and rescue (SAR) operations in the Central Mediterranean, addressing the gap left by the suspension of Italy's Mare Nostrum mission.

As restrictive migration policies have intensified, MSF projects have tried to address the escalating forms of direct and structural violence impacting on patients, humanitarian operations, and the broader protection landscape. The 2016 EU–Turkey Deal illustrates many of the challenges. Ostensibly justified as a measure to "save lives" by preventing dangerous crossings, the agreement was accompanied by the establishment of containment hotspots on Greek islands to screen arrivals and facilitate deportations. MSF stopped accepting EU funding, to oppose the instrumentalisation of humanitarian aid for migration control, and suspended its operations inside the hotspot centres on the island of Lesvos, preferring to provide medical assistance in an independent space.

The organisation's approach to migration was formalised in 2017 with a framework that underscored key elements that MSF activities should address. This involved documenting and denouncing the health consequences of migration policies based on containment, deportation, and deterrence, and developing new models of support that go beyond medical response to include protection and resistance against the criminalisation of solidarity.[15]

Beyond Greece, MSF projects in other contexts, such as the Balkan route, Libya, Mexico, and Niger, often tried to reach migrants who were excluded. Among them are many young men who, according to studies conducted by MSF projects, frequently experience various forms of state-perpetrated violence, including physical violence in detention centres and during pushbacks.[16]

The racial and gendered hierarchy of suffering usually sees black and brown men as not vulnerable, allowing for greater permissibility to cause them harm.[17] This dichotomy is all the clearer when comparing EU states' response to and narratives surrounding displacement from Ukraine in 2022 with their hostile reception of asylum seekers from the Middle East and Africa – exposing the geopolitical underpinnings of border and migration policies, also described as *"selective solidarity"*.[18]

Furthermore, criminalisation has become a central tool in the enforcement of the "good" and "bad" migrant dichotomy, wherein those deemed unworthy of protection are subjected to punitive measures. Across the EU and beyond, policies targeting irregular migration increasingly lean on criminal law to sanction both migrants and those who assist them. For example, in Italy, charges against humanitarian organisations conducting rescue operations at sea, including MSF, were used to portray civil SAR organisations as people smugglers and criminal networks enabling irregular migration. Although these charges were eventually dropped, the prolonged legal battles had a chilling effect on humanitarian space, disrupted life-saving missions, and stigmatised people providing aid, all the while further isolating those in need of assistance.[19]

Navigating Humanitarian Borders – Challenges and Limits

William Walters coined the term "humanitarian border" to describe the entanglement of the politics of care and rescue with policing and control.[20] Despite MSF's attempts to challenge and denounce the harmful impact of migrant securitisation, it is impossible for humanitarian organisations to fully extricate themselves from criteria of inclusion and exclusion, as well as mechanisms of migration governance.

Humanitarian interventions at borders can mask states' responsibilities to protect populations, as NGOs take on the "care" work while authorities focus on "control". The EU's externalisation policies and funding for migration management in countries like Libya, Egypt, and Turkey exemplify the intersection of humanitarian and security agendas. This funding is also disproportionately directed towards enforcement actors for "border management" – police, coastguards, border guards, and military known for widespread abuses and violence, as seen in Libya, Tunisia, Sudan, or Egypt. This landscape not only has knock-on effects for migrants, but for the population as a whole.[21]

While MSF often uses its advocacy and public statements to counter the potential instrumentalisation of humanitarianism for security-based objectives, humanitarian organisations, MSF included, must continually reflect on the implications of their presence in perpetuating harmful practices and mitigate their impact. This should inform the design of interventions and the approach to negotiations, ensuring as much independence as possible, and a course of action which prioritises the agency of migrants themselves. These decisions must be made on a case-by-case basis, taking into account the environment, the risks, and capacity to reach people in a safe and effective way.

Additionally, although MSF does not limit its interventions to legal categories of "migrant" or "refugee", scholars such as Ticktin argue that health can also be used to establish hierarchies between the deserving and undeserving, leading to a form of exclusion.[22] Notions of medical vulnerability have been exploited by states to further limit categories of vulnerability and protection. For example, in the Greek hotspots, health screenings are used to determine vulnerability status, which should be supported by safeguards within fast-track border and asylum procedures; however, in practice, often these screenings are rushed and do not adequately ascertain people's health condition. Furthermore, in 2020 the Greek government passed laws that exclude several mental health issues, including post-traumatic stress disorder.[23] MSF has advocated for better implementation of health and vulnerability screenings in Greece, whilst in other contexts, such as in Italy, it has supported local authorities to conduct such screenings on disembarkation from SAR vessels.[24] As border security and health procedures are more closely intertwined, it is important for MSF and other health actors to interrogate how medical notions of triage and care are instrumentalised to justify exclusion.

Finally, humanitarian organisations, including MSF, must continue to challenge their own geopolitical and regional blind spots. Border securitisation has intensified globally. Walls, more commonly imagined at the US–Mexico border, can be found between Pakistan and Afghanistan or Turkey and Iran, where pushbacks also occur. The displacement crisis caused by the conflict in Sudan exposed the militarised southern border of Egypt, where fleeing Sudanese refugees faced entry restrictions in harsh desert environments. Bangladesh's containment of Rohingya refugees in mega-camps in Cox's Bazar demonstrates that "containment" and "border violence", often denounced by NGOs in the EU or North American contexts, are rife globally, with effects that are just as significant.[25] As geopolitical tensions, anti-migration sentiment, and crises related to climate change, health, or conflicts intensify, we can expect an increase in migration securitisation. MSF and the humanitarian system at large must challenge themselves to avoid normalising practices of exclusion and control, and instead continue to leverage a principled response based on solidarity with affected migrants.

Notes

1 Walia, 2021; Jones and Johnson, 2016, pp. 187–200.
2 Welfens, 2022, pp. 1103–24.
3 Fassin, 2012.
4 Walters, 2011.
5 Guild, 2021, pp. 385–404.
6 Cainkar, 2020; Guild, 2021.
7 Sözer, 2019.
8 Fekete, 2001.
9 MSF, 2021.
10 Fine and Lindemann, 2024.
11 See University of South Wales, 2018.
12 Shachar and Ghezelbash, 2024.
13 Derderian and Schockaert, 2009.
14 Ticktin, 2007, pp. 116–35; Izambert, 2014, pp. 199–215.
15 MSF, 2017a and 2017b.
16 Arsenijević et al., 2018, pp. 86–94.
17 Fekete, 2001.
18 Duroch and Ponthieu, 2022.
19 MSF, 2024; PICUM, 2024.
20 Walters, 2011.
21 Barfuss, 2023.
22 Ticktin, 2007.
23 Amnesty International, 2019.
24 MSF, 2024.
25 L'Homme, 2021.

References

Amnesty International (2019), 'Greece: Proposed Bill on Asylum Downgrades EU and International Law Standards on Refugees' Protection', 23 October. [https://www.amnesty.org/en/documents/eur25/1278/2019/en/].

Arsenijević, Jovana, Doris Burtscher, Aurelie Ponthieu, Nathalie Severy, Andrea Contenta, Stephane Moissaing, Stefano Argenziano, *et al.* (2018), '"I Feel like I Am Less than Other People": Health-Related Vulnerabilities of Male Migrants Travelling Alone on Their Journey to Europe', *Social Science & Medicine*, vol. 209, pp. 86–94. doi:10.1016/j.socscimed.2018.05.038.

Barfuss, Reta (2023), 'How the European Union Finances Oppression', *Migration Control.* [https://migration-control.info/en/blog/how-the-european-union-finances-oppression/].

Cainkar, Louise (2020), 'The Muslim Ban and Trump's War on Immigration', *Middle East Report*, n° 294. [https://merip.org/2020/06/the-muslim-ban-and-trumps-war-on-immigration-2/].

Derderian, Katharine A., and Liesbeth Shockaert (2009), 'Responding to "Mixed" Migration Flows: A Humanitarian Perspective', *Sur International Journal on Human Rights*, vol. 6, n° 10, pp. 105–114.

Duroch, Françoise, and Aurélie Ponthieu (2022), 'Solidarité sélective?', *Le Courrier*, 8 May. [https://lecourrier.ch/2022/05/08/solidarite-selective/].

Fassin, Didier (2012), *Humanitarian Reason: A Moral History of the Present*, translated by Rachel Gomme, Oakland, CA: University of California Press.

Fekete, Liz (2001), 'The Emergence of Xeno-Racism', *Institute of Race Relations.* [https://irr.org.uk/article/the-emergence-of-xeno-racism/].

Fine, Shoshana, and Thomas Lindemann (2024), 'Migrant Deaths in the Name of Law', *Security Dialogue*, vol. 55, n° 3, pp. 237–256.

Guild, Elspeth (2021), 'Schengen Borders and Multiple National States of Emergency: From Refugees to Terrorism to COVID-19', *European Journal of Migration and Law*, vol. 23, n° 4, pp. 385–404. doi:10.1163/15718166–12340111.

Izambert, Caroline (2014), 'Les limites de l'universel. L'accès des sans-papiers à une couverture maladie en France depuis 1999', *Les Cahiers du Centre Georges Canguilhem*, vol. 6, n° 1, pp. 199–215. doi:10.3917/ccgc.006.0199.

Jones, Reece, and Corey Johnson (2016), 'Border Militarisation and the Re-Articulation of Sovereignty', *Transactions of the Institute of British Geographers*, vol. 41, n° 2, pp. 187–200.

L'Homme, Maelle (2021), 'Humanitarian Discourse and the Challenges of Migration: The European Exception?', *Humanitarian Alternatives*, n° 18, pp. 59–67. [https://www.alternatives-humanitaires.org/en/2021/11/10/humanitarian-discourse-and-the-challenges-of-migration-the-european-exception/].

MSF (2017a), 'Framing MSF's response to contemporary displacement and migration: Fights to pick, blind spots, how to go about it', MSF internal document.

MSF (2017b), 'EXCOM-driven workshop on displacement and migration – Outcomes Report', MSF internal document.

MSF (2021), 'Constructing Crisis at Europe's Border – Migration Report'. [https://www.msf.org/constructing-crisis-europe-border-migration-report].

MSF (2024), 'Charges in Case against Rescues at Sea Dropped in Italy', 19 April. [https://www.msf.org/charges-case-against-rescues-sea-dropped-italy].

PICUM (2024), 'Cases of Criminalisation of Migration and Solidarity in the EU in 2023'. [https://picum.org/wp-content/uploads/2024/04/Cases-of-criminalisation-of-migration-and-solidarity-in-the-EU-in-2023.pdf].

Shachar, Ayelet, and Daniel Ghezelbash (2024), 'How and Why "Ideas Travel" in Migration Law and Policy', forthcoming in Kevin Cope, Stella Burch Elias, and Jill Goldenziel (eds), *The Oxford Handbook of Comparative Immigration Law*, Oxford: Oxford University Press. [https://papers.ssrn.com/abstract=4842136].

Sözer, Hande (2019), 'Humanitarianism with a Neo-Liberal Face: Vulnerability Intervention as Vulnerability Redistribution', *Journal of Ethnic and Migration Studies*, n° 46, pp. 1–18.

Ticktin, Miriam (2007), 'Medical Humanitarianism in and Beyond France: Breaking Down or Patrolling Borders?', in Alison Bashford (ed.), *Medicine at the Border: Disease, Globalization and Security, 1850 to the Present*, London: Palgrave Macmillan UK, pp. 116–135. doi:10.1057/9780230288904_7.

University of South Wales (2018), 'The Tampa Controversy', *Howard Library*. [https://www.howardlibrary.unsw.edu.au/explore/tampa-controversy].

Walia, Harsha (2021), *Border & Rule: Global Migration, Capitalism, and the Rise of Racist Nationalism*, Chicago (Ill.): Haymarket Books.

Walters, William (2011), 'Foucault and Frontiers: Notes on the Birth of the Humanitarian Border', in Ulrich Bröckling, Susanne Krasmann, and Thomas Lemke (eds), *Governmentality: Current Issues and Future Challenges*, Abingdon/New York: Routledge, pp. 138–164.

Welfens, Natalie (2022), '"Promising Victimhood": Contrasting Deservingness Requirements in Refugee Resettlement', *Journal of Ethnic and Migration Studies*, vol. 49, n° 5, pp. 1103–1124. doi:10.1080/1369183X.2022.2117686.

2 The Evolution of How MSF Treats People

Karsten Emmanuel Noko and Marc DuBois

Organisational *esprit de corps* runs deep in Médecins Sans Frontières (MSF). Is this useful self-confidence? The glue behind MSF's laudable operational commitments? Does this faith in its uniqueness, along with an independence from what it sees as an ineffective and politically corrupted system, not only instil a sense of pride, but also cloak MSF's debts and contributions to, or embeddedness in, the aid sector?

The authors approach this question through the formative years of the formal humanitarian sector, and specifically the period of the 1990s and early twenty-first century. This period is remembered for its brutal post-Cold War conflicts – Angola, Sudan, Somalia, the First Gulf War, Sierra Leone, Chechnya, Liberia, ex-Yugoslavia, Rwanda and the Great Lakes – yet also saw the foundational growth of a more structured humanitarian sector, of a conviction in global governance within an internationalist and interventionist template, and then of the securitisation of aid within the rubric of a global war on terror.

This chapter probes two axes of the modern humanitarian enterprise that contributed to the building of today's MSF or were influenced by it in return. The first axis follows the "head" of humanitarianism: the command-level institutionalisation of the sector along three strands – the development of principles, accountability (the birth of standards and intentions of accountability to crisis-affected people), and the rights-based approach – and follows these same strands as they shaped more recent ambitions of the sector. How did MSF embrace, reject, adapt, or influence these developments? The second axis begins in the "body" of humanitarianism: in the clinics and hospitals of MSF projects in places like Mozambique, the Great Lakes region, and Thailand, where MSF teams staring HIV in the face tossed aside the dogmatic insistence that treating people with HIV was not within the scope of humanitarian action. Perceived as an issue requiring a system-building response,[1] the scale of mortality due to AIDS among populations in MSF crisis contexts, combined with the insufficiencies of either state or global agencies' actions, quietly revolutionised MSF's approach to people and to development, though without verbalising it in those terms.

Following the discussion of these two axes in sections I and II, section III analyses how the challenges and sectoral fervour of the 1990s and early 2000s helped build MSF's current operational ideology – as well as certain operational myths.

DOI: 10.4324/9781003542247-5

I The "Head" of Humanitarian Action: the 1990s and the Building of the Modern Humanitarian Sector

In essence, the 1990s saw various actors coalesce into today's humanitarian sector. Leaving Cold War politics behind, the brutal first half of the 1990s spurred a steep rise in agencies, funding mechanisms, aid workers, and programmatic areas. The decade also brought internal sectoral developments to strengthen normative coherence and build institutional support. This section explores MSF's relationship to the sector's growth across three themes – principles, accountability, and the rights-based framework – that remain cross-cutting, and which heavily influence how humanitarians engage with crisis-affected people and communities.

Principles for All

A Plethora of Principles

The diversity of actors led to an expanding diversity of thinking on humanitarianism, prompting multiple projects to set guiding principles. In 1992, the United Nations (UN) General Assembly created the Office for the Coordination of Humanitarian Affairs (OCHA) and endorsed three core principles of humanitarian action: humanity, impartiality, and neutrality.[2] In 1994, the Red Cross and Red Crescent Movement codified its highly influential Code of Conduct for the International Red Cross and Red Crescent Movement and Non-Governmental Organisations (NGOs) in Disaster Relief, signed/adopted by over 600 organisations, including one MSF section (Belgium).[3] In its own words, the Code of Conduct (CoC) is *"not about operational details"* but *"maintaining high standards of independence, effectiveness, and impact"*.[4]

A similar emphasis on principles can be found in the Sphere Project, better known for establishing sector-wide performance standards (see section below, "The Rise of Accountability"). Its Humanitarian Charter provides higher reference points to guide action, opening the original *Sphere Handbook* with, *"Sphere is not just a manual of humanitarian good practice: it is a statement about rights and duties."*[5] Tellingly, the Humanitarian Charter has long remained virtually invisible.

These initiatives shared a common aim: to delineate the ethical duties and legal principles that would shape and direct humanitarian action,[6] thus framing a collection of independent agencies into a more structured sector – one that continues to proclaim its devotion to "the" humanitarian principles.

MSF Establishes Its Principles

Founded in 1971, MSF authored a simple Charter of four paragraphs. Twenty years later, after intense debate on neutrality and the practice of speaking out, MSF adopted a new Charter which shifted away from a strict neutrality (as interpreted by the International Committee of the Red Cross – ICRC), removing obstacles to speaking out or public denunciation and committing to full financial independence.[7] Otherwise, MSF's 1991 Charter largely echoed ICRC's delineation of the principles, and similarly defined impartiality and neutrality without further spelling out their practical application. In the early 2000s, MSF again debated neutrality's removal but ultimately retained it.

Separate from the Charter, in 1995 an expanding MSF formally outlined its institutional principles at the Chantilly meetings, which served to define the organisation's identity following a wave of office openings in different parts of the world. This relatively concise explanation of MSF's "mandate" (complemented by the 2006 La Mancha Agreement) opens with an existential declaration: *"Who Are the Médecins Sans Frontières"*. Still in force today, the Chantilly Principles effectively codified MSF's identity (its "community and practice"), prioritising *"medical action first"* and then *témoignage* (speaking out) as modes of action, and enunciating commitments to impartiality, neutrality, independence, transparency, and accountability.[8] Uncommon among aid agencies at the time, MSF reinforced its independence by rejecting reliance on institutional donors, agreeing on a strategic objective to secure maximum private funding – a stance that continues to set MSF apart.

The Rise of Accountability

The discussion on accountability came tellingly late to humanitarian action, illustrating one detrimental effect of unchallenged self-belief. As Hilhorst et al. observe: *"Until the adoption of the code of conduct for humanitarian agencies in 1994, accountability was of little concern to humanitarians, who organised their domain around the idea that saving lives could never be wrong."*[9] The spectacle of the humanitarian response to the crises in Rwanda and the Great Lakes – where an estimated 42,000 refugees died in a cholera outbreak[10] while aid agencies fumbled to mount effective support – provoked a reckoning in the evolving sector,[11] and marked an *"end to the age of innocence"*.[12] The March 1996 publication of the Joint Evaluation of Emergency Assistance to Rwanda (JEEAR) solidified this assessment: good intentions proved insufficient, with principledness and aid effectiveness proving particularly weak.[13]

Amid media critique and public pressure on government donors to show results, internal discussion among agencies led to calls for humanitarian practice standards, and for an independent ombudsman to assess compliance. This wellspring of activity sparked the establishment of the Sphere Project, People in Aid,[14] and think tanks intent on performance, learning, and accountability.

Progress on accountability – especially "downward" accountability to beneficiary communities, in contrast to "upward" accountability to donors and headquarters – remains underwhelming. This chapter focuses on accountability to people and being held to account by them,[15] examining two key early initiatives: the Sphere Project and accountability to affected populations (AAP – the 'P' also refers to People).

The Drive for Programmatic Standards

The Sphere Project became synonymous with the establishment of technical standards for key areas of humanitarian intervention. Hosted by the Steering Committee for Humanitarian Response (SCHR), conceived and then spearheaded by Oxfam's Nick Stockton and the IFRC's Peter Walker, it aimed to create standards based on the rights of crisis-affected populations rather than agency priorities. The fundamental question was, what responsibility did humanitarians have in relation to the people who required assistance? Stockton and Walker saw the establishment of the Code of Conduct and core humanitarian principles as important yet incomplete progress towards answering that question, and the Sphere standards intended to correct the sector's haphazard quality of programming.

Rather than being about what agencies should do, the standards were about *"what people in crisis had a right to expect"*,[16] and thus supported a Copernican realignment of the sector, placing crisis-affected populations at the heart of the accountability matrix.[17]

Accountability to People

Founded in 2003, the Humanitarian Accountability Partnership (HAP, later HAP-I(nternational)) promoted accountability to disaster-affected populations through seven principles, including transparency on standards and rights, and meaningful beneficiary involvement in planning, implementation, and evaluation. Greater accountability to people intended to strengthen three objectives: (i) aid quality, impact, and efficiency; (ii) protection of dignity;[18] and (iii) aid worker security and satisfaction.[19]

HAP was not alone. As the 2000s progressed, the humanitarian sector increasingly recognised its weak performance on accountability to affected people. Despite numerous policy (re)formulations and a drumbeat of collective foot-stamping from the top (e.g. OCHA, Inter-Agency Standing Committee), this goal remains elusive. In 2005, OCHA launched the UN coordination reform, introducing the cluster system to enhance response coordination and quality within each subsector (e.g. health, protection, water/sanitation). A half-decade later, the UN's 2011 Transformative Agenda sought to strengthen humanitarian coordination, leadership, and AAP,[20] and was explicitly linked to HAP.[21]

UN-led reform efforts coalesced around the 2016 World Humanitarian Summit (WHS) in Istanbul, bringing together states, donors, UN agencies, and (I)NGOs to reaffirm broad goals: preventing/ending conflict and violence against civilians, reducing vulnerability and suffering, and expanding local/national roles in crisis response. UN Secretary-General Ban Ki-moon declared a new standard: humanitarian assistance should be *"as local as possible and as international as necessary"*.[22] Programmatically, the WHS prioritised: (i) greater support for local humanitarian actors (via the Grand Bargain agreement); and (ii) addressing relief, development, and peace in protracted crises through improved complementarity and collaboration among the various sectors. Thus, in 2017, OCHA launched its New Way of Working,[23] soon absorbed by the Triple Nexus or Humanitarian-Development-Peace (HDP) Nexus, to reduce vulnerability and unmet needs, strengthen risk management capacities, and address root causes of conflict.[24]

While political interests undeniably shaped the WHS agenda, these shifts responded to people's expressed needs. Pre-WHS consultations were extensive; in one survey, 71% of beneficiaries felt the aid they had received was either not relevant (25%) or only partially relevant (46%) to their needs.[25] In effect, this dissatisfaction signalled a structural disconnect: humanitarians were failing at the most basic level of accountability – listening to people.

MSF's Disengagement from the Sphere Project, HAP, and Sectoral Accountability

According to Sphere insiders Walker and Purdin, "*MSF played a challenging role in the work that eventually became the Sphere standards.*"[26] The organisation shared concerns over industry performance in the Great Lakes region and had already been developing internal standards for MSF action.[27] MSF supported Sphere and contributed substantially to its health standards, nonetheless pulling away from further involvement with the project, formally declaring that "*MSF believes that [the] answer to the problem Sphere tries to tackle is political and not technical.*"[28]

In a series of articles, MSF criticised sectoral efforts to establish standards,[29] citing both technical issues (e.g. the scourge of quantification, burdensome processes)[30] and political objections. As MSF Netherlands General Director Austen Davis explained, this was less about accountability itself than how differing views on the concept reflected divergent interpretations of humanitarian action. MSF rejected the charity model where aid alleviates pain without challenging the status quo.[31] Instead, MSF viewed aid as a "*radical response*" rather than a technical exercise.[32] While maintaining neutrality towards the conflict itself, MSF believed that its presence "*demonstrates (rather than substitutes for) political failure*",[33] a fundamentally political stance.

In service to such a humanitarian project, independence is a pillar of MSF's identity, reinforced by its rare degree of financial autonomy. MSF feared that rising government donor funding "*changed the original function of non-governmental organisations and merged their purpose with that of their funders*".[34] Its rejection of Sphere reflected its opposition to an international community – political donors, UN agencies, NGOs – increasingly devoted to the establishment of a singular benevolent purpose.[35] The Global War on Terror further revived state ambitions of merging political, military, development, and humanitarian efforts, prompting MSF to denounce the "*blurring [of] the lines*" – humanitarianism's subsumption into Western political and military objectives.[36]

MSF also feared losing independence from "below", vis-à-vis people or national authorities. Intrinsic to the Sphere standards is the potential to be held to account. MSF was concerned that, within the rights-based approach (see dedicated section below), shifting power to crisis-affected populations allowed people to make legal claims against aid agencies.[37]

The MSF Charter does not directly reference accountability. However, the Chantilly Principles commit to accountability, emphasising quality, effectiveness, and direct control over aid distribution. While significant, this pledge leaves MSF to hold itself accountable. A decade later, the 2006 La Mancha Agreement moved closer to a higher standard by declaring MSF *"accountable and actively transparent to those we assist, our donors, and the wider public"*.[38] Still, MSF has only just begun to practice active accountability towards communities for programme choices and implementation, most visibly through a decade of planning and debate on patient-centred care (PCC). Even there, MSF consistently placed greater attention on accountability in relation to individual patients.[39] Despite *"significant efforts"* and PCC's designation as a strategic operational priority, it remains under-implemented. MSF's 2021–24 movement-wide consultation, "The MSF We Want to Be", identified this shortfall, and PCC was selected as one of four collective priorities, moving forward.[40]

MSF's Distance from the Sector

Amid concerns over the Global War on Terror-enhanced blurring of humanitarian, political, and military lines, MSF avoided the 2005 UN reform, rejecting "coordination by" the donor-driven cluster system, and resisted engagement with bureaucracy, coordination meetings, and other forms of perceived inaction. As the sector grew closer to Western donors, MSF further distanced itself, and the Transformative Agenda sparked little debate within MSF.

MSF's muted, if any, significant involvement with AAP contrasts with its well-publicised decision to disengage from the WHS. Just three weeks before the event, the organisation delivered a withering critique. First, it bore witness to states' staggering disregard for the protections of international law and a *"shocking lack of humanity"*, accusing the summit of being transformed into a *"fig-leaf of good intentions"*. Second, it criticised the WHS for incorporating *"humanitarian assistance into a broader development and resilience agenda"* along with peacebuilding and other political agendas.[41] Later, this latter critique was redeployed as a sweeping dismissal of the HDP Nexus, seeing it as an existential threat to humanitarian action that seeks to subsume neutral and independent humanitarianism into the political aspirations of development and peace.[42]

The Rights-based Approach

Developments within the Sector

In the mid-1990s, the rights-based approach (RBA) gained renewed traction within the humanitarian sector. In essence, the drive was to centre human rights as a key pillar in the delivery of assistance to populations in need. Often referred to as the human rights agenda, the idea was that humanitarian relief needed to go further than providing "passive" assistance, regarding recipients of assistance as holders of rights and members of the humanitarian sector as advocates of these rights. The Rwanda genocide served as a wake-up call to the failures of the international protection system and, as a consequence, human rights and protection gradually became cornerstones of humanitarian policy and humanitarian programming.

One could trace, as James Darcy does, the roots of this agenda to the fall of the Berlin Wall, and the end of the stiff polarisation of the world that consumed international politics in the 1990s.[43]

In an attempt to define the scope of the human rights agenda with the humanitarian sector, Benelli contends that, *"Human rights-based approaches generally anchored the plans, policies and processes of development (and humanitarian) aid in a system of rights and corresponding obligations established by a series of international treaties."*[44]

Practitioners questioned the notion that RBAs could deliver real change for international development. Tsikata contended that RBAs were not able to redefine development practices because they do not challenge economic models. In addition, RBAs could be seen as yet another form of donor conditionalities at a time of increasing wariness of new obligations by many recipient governments and communities, who argue that development aid should not seek to transform their societies to model Western donor countries.[45]

Developments within MSF

Some authors have traced MSF's interaction with the human rights agenda to its very formation, describing that the *"emergence of Médecins Sans Frontières (MSF) as an organisation was precisely a response to the desire to incorporate advocacy and the defence of human rights after the crisis in Biafra"*.[46]

Inside MSF, a specific focus on the human rights agenda was topical in the 1990s, just as it was developing in the sector. In section 4 of the Chantilly Principles, entitled "Defence of human rights", MSF committed itself to the human rights agenda. This included the internal functioning of the organisation, the rights of "victims" to receive assistance, and the right of humanitarian organisations to provide assistance.

The human rights approach faced scrutiny within MSF, notably by Rony Brauman, former president of MSF France, in relation to a World Health Organization (WHO) programme conceived in the 1990s to eradicate tuberculosis (TB).[47] As per WHO guidance, TB patients were to be excluded from care if an 80% rate of compliance from the population they belonged to was unlikely. For Brauman, a human rights-based approach posed a conflicting body of rights that is neither *"consistent"* nor *"coherent"*, and is thus unable to assist medical practitioners to adjudicate difficult decisions in a morally and medically acceptable manner.[48]

Following the La Mancha consultation process, MSF again reaffirmed its distance from human rights: "*MSF does not take responsibility for the development of international justice and MSF's social mission is not the promotion of human rights but humanitarian medical action.*"[49] In MSF Netherlands, however, there was an interest in taking this on board, not least because of the creation of the Humanitarian Affairs Department in Amsterdam, mostly made up of human rights lawyers[50] who recognised the limits of medical action and sought to centre protection in the delivery of humanitarian assistance.

Thus, despite an initial dalliance with human rights and earlier attempts to engage with the human rights corpus, in the mid-2000s MSF thinking came full circle with a clear rejection of a role in human rights-based approaches, in favour of medical humanitarian action. In spite of this clarion position, MSF has found itself denouncing certain human rights abuses, such as the European Union's migration policies that put people in danger while crossing the Mediterranean Sea.

II From the Ground Up: Humanitarianism and the HIV/AIDS Pandemic

In the mid-1990s, MSF teams started to witness a growing number of patients infected with HIV, and for which there was little medical care to give. In clinics in the Democratic Republic of the Congo, Mozambique, Kenya, and Thailand, doctors and medical cadres were confronted with feelings of helplessness and despair due to the inaction from states and development organisations. These frustrations pushed some inside MSF to reject the status quo and seek a new and different solution to try to bring care to these patients.[51] Unbeknownst to them, MSF's involvement in HIV care was to change the organisation in a way no other disease had done in its past.

At the time, MSF had emerged with a renewed and invigorated sense as a financially independent organisation, often wary of instrumentalisation by political movements and various state authorities.[52] MSF internal debates during that period highlight anxieties about accepting funding from the European Commission and the risk of being controlled. However, providing HIV treatment required, if not demanded, for MSF to put aside, or at the very least reinterpret, its understanding of independence.

MSF Responds to the HIV Pandemic

When MSF teams arrived in South Africa in 1999, the state authorities initially rejected the proposal of offering treatment to pregnant women to help prevent their unborn children from contracting the virus.[53] Needless to say, part of the reason was that MSF was perceived as a group of foreigners with suspicious motives. This was in addition to the already disturbing position of President Thabo Mbeki's government, which argued for what has been described as an African solution to the disease. As the national spokesperson of the governing

African National Congress party remarked, "*MSF was fomenting biological warfare in South Africa by experimenting with toxic drugs on black people.*"[54] The fact that MSF teams were seen as propagating the same theory – approaching HIV from a biomedical lens – that Mbeki had clearly rejected did not help their cause.

The antidote to this identity "dis-ease", which denied legitimacy to MSF teams, was for the organisation to partner with the Treatment Action Campaign (TAC), a grass-roots organisation made up mostly by people living with HIV.[55] Similarly, relationships were developed with the Provincial Department of Health and a local university:

> *At a time when the country had just rid itself of white power, MSF could hardly draw legitimacy from its identity as an organisation from the global North. Thus, the alliances built by MSF were a means of gaining the space it needed to develop its activity and advocate for access to treatment.*[56]

In one fell swoop, MSF was able to leverage the political standing of TAC and secure the space needed to run programmes, even amidst a clear rejection of MSF-supported access to antiretrovirals (ARVs), and a lack of legitimacy. However, MSF was less enthusiastic about joining TAC's court action against the South African government, anxious about potential reputational risks that would make it more difficult to work in other contexts.

Another dilemma faced by MSF was the financial sustainability of offering mass HIV treatment,[57] given that ARVs were a lifetime commitment and far too expensive to deliver at scale, costing between $10,000 and $15,000 per patient per year. How could an entity modelled as an emergency organisation, with annual planning and budgeting cycles and plans revised every six months, be able to provide and sustain lifelong treatment? How could the organisation pay for this? Would MSF's budget be consumed to the extent that it would hinder its ability to respond to emergencies – its *raison d'être*? All these were practical questions and yet they did not reduce the pressure that MSF HQs were facing from project teams.

While the organisation grappled with the operational and financial implications of engaging in the provision of lifelong ARV treatment, the simple fact that HIV could not be cured inevitably demanded system changes for MSF teams, both at HQ and project level. MSF had to find ways to rationalise its own systems beyond financial and operational adaptability, especially for an entity that took pride in being an emergency response organisation, operating on a "first in, first out" basis.

Confronting a Pandemic and Associated Dilemmas

It is important to recall that, as these discussions and operational decisions were being made, the organisation continued to reflect on a common identity and common rules regarding operational and financial independence.[58] This coincided with the complexities that MSF suddenly found itself in because of the War on Terror post-9/11. MSF was once again reminded of the practical and operational value of operational and financial independence, as the War on Terror successfully co-opted a vast number of humanitarian actors as "force multipliers" in Afghanistan.[59]

In the early 1990s, the choices before the organisation were stark. While MSF project teams pushed for more to be done as they witnessed staff and communities succumb to the virus, the treatment options were considered by some in HQ as impossible. As a former General Director remarked, "*In the first part of the 90s, we just rejected the possibility of doing anything.*"[60] Perhaps more than with any other disease, the response to the HIV epidemic has been described as "atypical", one of the reasons being that MSF was confronted by pressure from "below" – medical staff whose focus was the patients in front of them. Unlike other interventions where project teams put pressure to respond to a particular epidemic or humanitarian crisis, HIV went further because it demanded a system rethink from an organisation whose systems were designed for emergency interventions. A striking illustration of how HIV programming and related perceptions had changed by the late 2010s was that a patient could also be a member of staff and a member of the association, attending a General Assembly and participating in governance processes and decision-making!

At the end of the first decade of the twenty-first century, MSF emerged with a rather differentiated model in its understanding and interpretation of independence, where funding and programme design were not straitjacketed by the emergency response logic of the organisation. There is little doubt that the work and programming in HIV played a key role in this model, where up to 35% of some MSF sections' budget was committed to HIV activities.

On the one hand, in countries like South Africa, Zimbabwe, and Malawi that formed the bulk of HIV programmes for the organisation, MSF accepted institutional funding from states and used it to scale up treatment, quickly becoming one of the leading organisations in HIV care. This increased its political capital to take on big pharma regarding the prices of ARVs, which completed the circle for an even bigger scale-up of access to treatment. This differentiated model was more palatable to MSF, partly because the Southern African region was not experiencing conflict (the war in Angola had ended in 2002), and being associated with states through institutional funding posed a lesser risk as compared to the contexts confronted with the Global War on Terror. This way, MSF found itself interacting with several ministries of health and donor countries on HIV programming and scaling-up of treatment. Similarly, collaborations were formed with the Joint UN Programme on HIV/AIDS (UNAIDS) and patient groups, and investments were made in research and development.[61] Suddenly, MSF was a player on the global stage of policy-making, providing technical guidance to states and intergovernmental bodies.

On the other hand, in conflict areas like Afghanistan, Somalia, and Iraq, MSF stuck to its guns and refused institutional funding due to the greater risk of being associated with governments and being put in the same basket as other perceived "force multipliers".[62]

It can indeed be argued that engaging in HIV treatment compelled MSF to review and reinterpret the meaning of financial and operational independence. This shift marked a move away from the almost sacrosanct model of thinking towards a more nuanced approach that sought to understand the local dynamics of a conflict. Once the institutional capacity and experience in HIV programmes were developed, they could then be used across other contexts where MSF was confronted by different sets of complexities, not least conflict settings.

HIV Response in the Sector

As early as 1988, WHO began responding to the HIV pandemic in countries where MSF teams would later see a significant rise in cases. WHO programmes started to include components of HIV prevention as well as to mobilise national and international efforts to fight the virus. The historical account of the founding of UNAIDS indicates that initial endeavours did not recognise AIDS as a medical problem, but as a *"social, economic, demographic, cultural and political"* issue, partly owing to the lack of medical treatment.[63] The reluctance to acknowledge the medical nature of AIDS was so great that, by 1991, donors to the WHO's Global AIDS Program (GAP) expressed reservations that the GAP was taking an overly medical approach to AIDS instead of the above, seemingly preferred, approach.

By 1996, when UNAIDS was officially formed, a major breakthrough had come with the announcement of antiretroviral therapy, albeit at an astronomically high cost. It was only in 1999 that generic companies started to enter the market and produce medicines that were more affordable. However, UNAIDS was reluctant to work with these manufacturers, leading to criticism from NGOs that UNAIDS had become hostage to big pharma, intellectual property, and World Trade Organization rules.

In the decade to come, entities like UNAIDS, the US President's Emergency Plan for AIDS Relief (PEPFAR), and the Global Fund drove the bulk of their funding towards ministries of health to treat patients with HIV, often providing technical support and ensuring the availability of medicines. NGOs (Save the Children and the International Rescue Committee, among others) generally limited their role to prevention work, including social education and the distribution of condoms, despite maintaining large medical programmes within their portfolios.

III Analysis: The Treatment of People

From the Top Down – The Treatment of People Across Principles, Accountability, and the Rights-based Agenda

The relationship between MSF and the humanitarian sector evolved with significant mutual influence during the 1990s and early twenty-first century, a seminal period of organisational growth and ideological consolidation in the sector. Examining MSF's interactions with the development of humanitarian principles, accountability initiatives, and the rights-based agenda reveals four key lessons on the treatment of people.

First, MSF's hard-nosed defence of its independence – political, financial, and operational (with neutrality) – has been vital for accessing conflict zones and crisis areas.[64] Perhaps less trumpeted, this detachment from mainstream sector initiatives also helped MSF avoid bogging down in ineffective self-improvement schemes.[65] MSF has largely shielded itself from external pressures that distance other humanitarian actors from the fundamental moral necessity of reaching and treating people in crisis. Further, the independence of MSF serves its "rebel humanitarian" commitment to bearing witness and speaking out to the causes of displacement, trauma, and death. Its *témoignage* exists to hold world powers, state authorities, and warring parties accountable to their responsibilities and obligations.

Second, and arguably a fertile breeding pool for hubris, this independence can shield MSF from meaningful external accountability, a risk exacerbated by its internal governance structures largely composed of former staff. In part, MSF rejected "merging" with the sector and opposed sectoral norms that could empower affected populations to hold humanitarians (including MSF!) accountable. For example, MSF's dismissal of Sphere standards was not primarily about contesting standards themselves – indeed, its operations are highly standardised.

More generally, MSF has struggled to engage with La Mancha's directive to be *"accountable and actively transparent to those we assist"*, as shown by the challenges in adopting patient-centred care (PCC). Despite much discussion, MSF has centred PCC within the rubric of quality of care, an instrumental logic of engagement with patients to improve programming results[66] rather than a transformative participation rooted in the (higher) principle of people's agency, autonomy, and right to hold MSF accountable. Notably, MSF Netherlands' recent power dynamics study identified an *"implementation gap"* in PCC, including issues of paternalism, a rejection of patient criticism, and concerns from the programme's PCC ambassadors.[67] Beyond this low level of engagement with, or accountability to, its patients, there is also still a long way to go in terms of systematically involving communities in programme choices and strategic decision-making, let alone being accountable to them.

Third, MSF's Chantilly document highlights the principle of humanity, affirming MSF's commitment to act out of *"respect for human dignity"*. Yet MSF's culture of treating people as "mere" patients with urgent needs often collides with treating people as autonomous, or recognising the long-term health needs of communities. As Sphere co-founder Stockton explained, accountability reconciles charity with human dignity, because humanity demands *"'respect for the individual' as an essential moral value"*, and accountability is the *"necessary expression of that value"*.[68] However, MSF's emergency-focused mandate has often been treated as incompatible with long-term development approaches: as Tong analysed the Sphere standards debate, MSF regarded the participation of people as a development issue, associating it with threats to neutrality and impartiality.[69]

Fourth, the HDP Nexus requires nuanced engagement rather than over-simplification and dismissal. While MSF rightly prioritises its humanitarian response to immediate needs, and rightly highlights how these are not being met, it mistakenly juxtaposes these emergencies against longer-term efforts in development or peace; or it dismisses the HDP Nexus as a danger to MSF's independence or neutrality.[70] Globally, protracted crises result in prodigious structural human suffering, including institutional collapse and service erosion. Given the weight of protracted crises – over 90% of the global humanitarian budget in 2022[71] – MSF should strengthen its assessment of the limitations and negative consequences of short-term approaches when deployed for decades. At a minimum, an HDP Nexus approach would allow MSF to recognise and mitigate the cumulative or long-term damage of its short-term approaches.

Communities in crisis consistently express a desire for long-term stability alongside immediate relief. Surveys of aid recipients regularly show that people in protracted crises rate unemployment and poverty as their greatest problems, or the need for peace and security.[72] Insights gathered by the Collaborative Learning Projects found that people appreciate relief assistance, yet also voice concern that it can undermine dignity and self-reliance over time.[73] Further research reveals the complexity of aid in the eyes of its recipients, as they experience both relief and *"feelings that they are not self-reliant"*.[74] Effective crisis response thus defies sequestering people's needs into the siloed sectors of international intervention – human needs exist in a nexus. Can MSF identify where its brand of humanitarian relief is unfit for purpose over decades in a protracted crisis? What does MSF's observance of humanity and impartiality mean if, over years of intervention, it remains ignorant of or ignores people's most important needs, and does not involve them in decision-making? These are the sorts of questions that arise with nexus thinking and with treating people as people, ensuring that they participate meaningfully in the selection, design, and accountability of programming.

From the Bottom Up – The Treatment of People through the Lens of HIV/AIDS

While there was a lot of talk in the 1990s about centring human rights in policy circles, there were huge limitations in how this was operationalised in the delivery of assistance.

Inside MSF, and notwithstanding the aforementioned differences between the two versions of the Chantilly Principles, the overwhelming interpretation of the opening clauses means that MSF is, first and foremost, an organisation that places medical action first, and has thereafter sought to "protect" this identity against the suggestion of it being on an equal footing with *témoignage*. Such a debate was not unique to MSF. As Benelli writes, there were considerable discussions on what people understood to be the core business of humanitarian action, thus seeing the rights-based approach as an "agenda" that served as a distraction from saving lives.[75]

HIV programming also had a profound impact on the evolution of how MSF treated people. From the civil society organisations that MSF sought to partner with to forge its own operational space, to ministries of health, and global development organisations like UNAIDS and Global Fund, MSF needed to build alliances with others, despite the common perception that MSF's claim of independence means working as an island.

Furthermore, the HIV pandemic exposed MSF HQs to a ground-up rejection of the accepted thinking that providing access to HIV treatment was not a job for humanitarians. In this way, project teams inspired MSF to leverage the weight of its operational volume to bear on policymakers, which catalysed access to treatment. Patients and front-line medical staff used the organisation as a platform not only to confront governments that denied them access to care, as was the case in South Africa, but also to challenge pharmaceutical companies and the trade policies enforced by the World Trade Organization.

IV Conclusion

The humanitarian handwringing following the Rwanda genocide and Great Lakes crisis marked the end of the *"unquestioning acceptance"* of agencies' *"good work"*.[76] While frameworks like the Red Cross CoC or the Sphere standards generated debate, these sector-wide agreements proved to be less about negotiating standards, accountability, or rights than about forging institutional answers to the question of what it meant to be humanitarian. MSF actively engaged in that existential discussion, and on paper mirrored the sector's emphasis on human dignity as the ultimate purpose of aid. Treating people as people, over time, though, can conflict with treating people to save their lives today.

Much like others in the sector, MSF's humanitarian action has struggled with: (i) direct involvement of people in project design; (ii) responsiveness to how people understand their needs; and (iii) enabling people and communities to hold the organisation to account. Central to these challenges lies power imbalance. The idealism of sectoral principles, the rights-based agenda, and the many accountability initiatives offer testament to the lofty intentions of the sector in regard to dignity, and to the need to transcend charity models that treat people as passive, desperate victims. A brutal reckoning: MSF's political independence from the mainstream sector has not resulted in ideological independence from these historically paternalistic and inequitably balanced relationships of power.[77] Decades of interventions have compounded systemic inequities, raising the troubling possibility of inhumanity within MSF's work of "saving lives".

A different MSF is not hypothetical. The early evolution of MSF's response to HIV, driven by community collaboration and ground-up engagement, led to more inclusive care models where patient treatment rested upon an agency that was essential to health, dignity, and successful programme development.

MSF's history reveals an organisation both principled and prescient in its resistance to joining the humanitarian herd, yet unaccountable and self-serving in operationalising its commitment to humanity and dignity. MSF's political and financial independence from institutional donors and its formidable capacity to reach and treat those most in crisis make MSF exceptional in its treatment of patients. MSF's treatment thus delineates a dual identity: a politically maverick, talented emergency health responder, yet also an organisation that nonetheless remained a product of modern humanitarianism, deeply invested in the hierarchical dynamic of foreign deliverer superiority over local receivers of treatment.

Notes

1 In part because the fight against HIV fitted poorly within the emergency mentality – high numbers of patients who could not be discharged (due to the lack of a cure) and hence would remain MSF's responsibility for years to come. HIV thus more directly called for the building of a system and an approach that addressed root causes.
2 UN General Assembly, 1991. A later resolution added independence to this threesome: UN General Assembly, 2004.
3 International Federation of Red Cross and Red Crescent Societies, 1994.
4 International Federation of Red Cross and Red Crescent Societies, 1994, p. 1. The first four principles of the Red Cross Code of Conduct track the four core humanitarian principles of humanity, impartiality, neutrality, and independence.
5 Darcy, 2011, p. 2.
6 Buchanan-Smith and ODI, 2003; Walker and Purdin, 2004.
7 See the MSF Charter Factsheet, n.d. for a record of the evolution of the MSF Charter.
8 MSF, 1997.
9 Hilhorst et al., 2021, p. 364.
10 Shannon et al., 2019.
11 Buchanan-Smith and ODI, 2003.
12 Stockton and Walker, 2015.
13 Walker and Purdin point out that, prior to the actual JEEAR's publication, eight similar initiatives were working to address standards, including MSF taking a lead role in developing response packages (the "kit system"): Walker and Purdin, 2004, p. 101.
14 Non-governmental organisation created in 1995 and focused on the quality of people management in the humanitarian and development sectors.
15 Hilhorst et al., 2021, p. 366.
16 Stockton and Walker, 2015.
17 Humanitarian Quality Assurance Initiative, 2019, p. 3.
18 While improved aid quality clearly supports human dignity, the authors emphasise the criticality of dignity as an ethical undertaking within the ambit of the humanitarian principle of humanity.
19 HAP International, 2008.
20 Inter-Agency Standing Committee, n.d.
21 Inter-Agency Standing Committee, 2014.
22 UN Secretary-General, 2016, p. 30.
23 OCHA, 2017.
24 OECD, 2019, p. 6.
25 World Humanitarian Summit Secretariat, 2015, pp. 16–8.
26 Walker and Purdin, 2004, p. 106.

27 Orbinski, 1998.
28 Tong, 2004, p. 186, quoting a March 2003 letter to the field from MSF Secretary-General Rafa Vila San Juan.
29 See, e.g. Tong, 2004; Davis, 2003 and 2007.
30 MSF and some of the French INGOs held a vision of humanitarian action being slowed by a mounting bureaucracy. On this count, the opponents to Sphere seem somewhat prescient, with a stifling *"culture of compliance and risk aversion"* that has emerged from intentions to improve accountability: Buchanan-Smith, 2011, p. 19.
31 Davis, 2003, p. 17.
32 Davis, 2007.
33 Davis, 2003, p. 17.
34 Davis, 2007, p. 7.
35 Davis, 2003, p. 16.
36 de Torrenté, 2002.
37 Tong, 2004; Davis, 2003.
38 MSF, 25 June 2006, para. 2.3. Explanation of the commitment continues, *"Accountability to those we assist may be difficult to achieve in certain situations, but the minimum requirement is that we are actively transparent about the choices made [and our limits]."*
39 Many practical reasons might impede the establishment of accountability to people in crisis during the early stages of an emergency response, but such a justification falls short over years and decades.
40 MSF WWTB Team, 2024.
41 MSF, 2016b.
42 Christou, 2020.
43 Darcy, 2004.
44 Benelli, 2013.
45 Tsikata, 2004.
46 Benelli, 2013.
47 Brauman, 2003.
48 *Ibid.*
49 Binet and Saulnier, 2019, p. 15. Also noteworthy in this regard is paragraph 1.12 of the La Mancha Agreement (MSF, 2006), where MSF clarifies that it *"differs from justice organisations by not taking on the responsibility for the development of international justice and does not gather evidence for the specific purpose of international courts or tribunals"*.
50 Somewhat shockingly, the Dutch section of MSF maintains an official version of the Chantilly Principles (MSF Netherlands, 1997) that differs significantly from the Chantilly document used by the rest of the movement, instructing that MSF action should be *"protecting human dignity"* and placing medical aid and witnessing on a seemingly equal footing.
51 Neuman, 2011, p. 163.
52 Binet and Saulnier, 2019, p. 149.
53 Interview with Eric Goemaere, who led the MSF Belgium team to South Africa.
54 Darder, McGregor, and Devine, 2014.
55 *Ibid.*
56 Neuman, 2011, p. 166.
57 Calmy, 2005.
58 Binet and Saulnier, 2019, p. 149.
59 See Donini, 2009, where he highlights the dangers of the conflation of humanitarian response with the conduct of hostilities in a counterterrorism context and restates the importance of principled humanitarian action that responds to the needs of affected communities and not the state-building agenda of the International Security Assistance Force in Afghanistan.

60 Darder, McGregor, and Devine, 2014.
61 See the Drugs for Neglected Diseases initiative (https://dndi.org/) and the MSF Access Campaign (https://msfaccess.org/).
62 Donini, 2009.
63 Knight, 2008.
64 In one way, MSF has become less independent, as it now collaborates with ministries of health in well over half of its projects. Yet despite this significant partnership with health ministries, research has revealed the persistent myth of MSF as a *"Lone Ranger, the heroic actor and leader"*; or how, even within ministry of health structures, MSF often operates not in collaborative support but more as *"islands of substitution"*, maintaining full control over its operations: Healy et al., 2020.
65 Davey, Espada, and Scriven, 2024.
66 See, e.g. MSF WWTB Team, 2024.
67 Davey et al., 2023, p. 160.
68 Stockton, 2005.
69 Tong, 2004, p. 180.
70 To understand MSF's position, see its Call for Action: MSF, 2016a.
71 Development Initiatives, 2023. For a more thorough discussion on why humanitarian engagement with the HDP Nexus is not a contradiction of humanitarian principles, see DuBois, 2020.
72 World Humanitarian Summit Secretariat, 2015, p. 55.
73 Anderson, Brown, and Jean, 2012.
74 Mosel and Holloway, 2019, p. 18.
75 *Ibid.*
76 Buchanan-Smith, 2003, p. 14.
77 ALNAP's 2022 report found that, despite increased attention to accountability to affected people, the conclusion of its 2015 and 2018 editions still held true: such efforts *"have not yet delivered greater accountability or participation"* (ALNAP, 2022, p. 303).

References

ALNAP (2022), "The State of the Humanitarian System", ALNAP/ODI. [https://alnap.org/help-library/resources/2022-the-state-of-the-humanitarian-system-sohs–full-report/].

Anderson, Mary B., Dayna Brown, and Isabella Jean (2012), *Time to Listen: Hearing People on the Receiving End of International Aid*, Cambridge, MA: CDA Collaborative Learning Projects. [https://www.cdacollaborative.org/publication/time-to-listen-hearing-people-on-the-receiving-end-of-international-aid/].

Benelli, Prisca (2013), 'Human Rights in Humanitarian Action and Development Cooperation and the Implications of Rights-Based Approaches in the Field', Advanced Training Program on Humanitarian Action. [https://reliefweb.int/report/world/human-rights-humanitarian-action-and-development-cooperation-and-implications-rights].

Binet, Laurence, and Martin Saulnier (2019), 'MSF, Evolution of an International Movement: Associative History 1971–2011', Médecins Sans Frontières. [https://www.msf.org/associativehistory].

Brauman, Rony (2003), 'Health and Human Rights', *Centre de réflexion sur l'action et les savoirs humanitaires*. [https://msf-crash.org/en/medicine-and-public-health/health-and-human-rights].

Buchanan-Smith, Margie (2011), 'Humanitarian Leadership and Accountability: Contribution or Contradiction?', *Humanitarian Exchange*, n° 52, pp. 18–20.

Buchanan-Smith, Margie and Overseas Development Institute (eds) (2003), *How the Sphere Project Came into Being: A Case Study of Policy-Making in the Humanitarian Aid Sector and the Relative Influence of Research*, London: ODI.

Calmy, Alexandra (2005), 'AIDS, MSF in Question', MSF internal forum.

Christou, Christos (2020), 'MSF International President's Moral Report 2019–2020', Médecins Sans Frontières.

Darcy, James (2004), 'Human Rights and Humanitarian Action: A Review of the Issues', Workshop on Human Rights and Humanitarian Action convened by the IASC Sub-Working Group: HPG background paper. [https://odi.org/en/publications/human-rights-and-humanitarian-action-a-review-of-the-issues/].

Darcy, James (2011), 'User Guidance and Commentary on the Humanitarian Charter', *The Sphere Project*.

Darder, Marta, Liz McGregor, and Carol Devine (2014), 'No Valley Without Shadows: MSF and the Fight for Affordable ARVs in South Africa', *MSF Belgium*.

Davey, Eleanor, Fernando Espada, and Kim Scriven (2024), 'Humanitarian Reform beyond the Mega-Crisis', *Humanitarian Practice Network*. [https://odihpn.org/publication/humanitarian-reform-beyond-the-mega-crisis/].

Davey, Eleanor, Lioba Hirsch, Myfanwy James, and Molly Naisanga (2023), 'In Service of Emergency: Understanding Power and Inequality in MSF', Médecins Sans Frontières. [https://msfuk.unbounddocs.com/wp-content/uploads/2024/02/Understanding-Power-Inequality-in-MSF-UK-FINAL-Full-Research-1.pdf].

Davis, Austen (2003), 'Accountability and Humanitarian Actors: Speculations and Questions', *Humanitarian Exchange*, n° 24, pp. 16–18.

Davis, Austen (2007), 'Concerning Accountability of Humanitarian Action', *Humanitarian Practice Network*, n° 58. [https://odihpn.org/wp-content/uploads/2007/04/networkpaper058.pdf].

Development Initiatives (2023), 'Global Humanitarian Assistance Report 2023', Bristol. [https://devinit.org/resources/global-humanitarian-assistance-report-2023/].

Donini, Antonio (2009), 'Afghanistan: Humanitarianism under Threat', *Feinstein International Center*.

DuBois, Marc (2020), 'Triple Nexus – Threat or Opportunity for the Humanitarian Principles?', Centre for Humanitarian Action. [https://www.chaberlin.org/en/publications/triple-nexus-threat-or-opportunity-for-the-humanitarian-principles-2/].

HAP International (2008), *The Guide to the HAP Standard: Humanitarian Accountability and Quality Management*, Cowley, UK/Herndon, VA: Practical Action Publishing. [https://www.jstor.org/stable/j.ctt1hj58r2].

Healy, Sean, Urvashi Aneja, Marc DuBois, and Paul Harvey (2020), 'Lone Ranger No Longer: MSF's Engagement with Ministries of Health', MSF Reflection and Analysis Network.

Hilhorst, Dorothea, Samantha Melis, Rodrigo Mena, and Roanne van Voorst (2021), 'Accountability in Humanitarian Action', *Refugee Survey Quarterly*, vol. 40, n° 4, pp. 363–389. doi:10.1093/rsq/hdab015.

Humanitarian Quality Assurance Initiative (2019), 'Independent Quality Assurance and the Humanitarian Sector: A History'. [https://hqai.contentfiles.net/media/documents/history-of-hqai_web.pdf].

Inter-Agency Standing Committee, 'Key Messages: IASC Transformative Agenda'. [https://interagencystandingcommittee.org/iasc-transformative-agenda].

Inter-Agency Standing Committee (2014), 'Accountability to Affected Populations Operational Framework'. [https://interagencystandingcommittee.org/sites/default/files/migrated/2014–2010/AAP%20Operational%20Framework%20Final%20Revision.pdf].

International Federation of Red Cross and Red Crescent Societies (1994), 'The Code of Conduct for the International Red Cross and Red Crescent Movement and Non-Governmental Organisations (NGOs) in Disaster Relief'. [https://www.ifrc.org/sites/default/files/2021–2007/code-of-conduct-movement-ngos-english.pdf].

Knight, Lindsay (2008), 'UNAIDS: The First 10 Years', UNAIDS. [https://www.unaids.org/en/resources/presscentre/featurestories/2008/november/20081103tfty].

Mosel, Irina, and Kerrie Holloway (2019), 'Dignity and Humanitarian Action in Displacement', HPG report. [https://odi.org/en/publications/dignity-and-humanitarian-action-in-displacement/].

MSF, 'MSF Charter Factsheet'. [https://www.msf.org/sites/default/files/2022-06/MSF%20Charter.pdf].

MSF (1997), 'Chantilly Principles'. [https://www.msf.org/sites/default/files/Principles%20Chantilly%20EN.pdf].

MSF (2006), 25 June. 'La Mancha Agreement'. [https://www.msf.org/sites/default/files/La%20Mancha%20Agreement%20EN.pdf].

MSF (2016a), 'EMERGENCY NOW: A Call for Action beyond Summits. MSF's Reflections on the World Humanitarian Summit'. [https://www.aerzte-ohne-grenzen.at/sites/default/files/attachments/whs-report-msf-2015.pdf].

MSF (2016b), 'MSF to Pull out of World Humanitarian Summit – Statement', 5 May. [https://www.msf.org/msf-pull-out-world-humanitarian-summit].

MSF Netherlands (1997), 'Chantilly Principles, MSF Holland Version'.

MSF WWTB Team (2024), 'MSF We Want To Be: Final Project Report', MSF internal document.

Neuman, Michaël (2011), 'South Africa: MSF, an African NGO?', in Claire Magone, Michaël Neuman, and Fabrice Weissman (eds), *Humanitarian Negotiations Revealed: The MSF Experience*, London: Hurst & Co.

OCHA (2017), 'New Way of Working'. [https://agendaforhumanity.org/sites/default/files/20170228%20NWoW%2013%20high%20res.pdf].

OECD (2019), 'DAC Recommendation on the Humanitarian-Development-Peace Nexus'. [https://legalinstruments.oecd.org/public/doc/643/643.en.pdf].

Orbinski, James (1998), 'On the Meaning of SPHERE Standards to States and Other Humanitarian Actors', London. [https://www.msf.fr/sites/default/files/1998–1912–03-Orbinski.pdf].

Shannon, Kerry, Marisa Hast, Andrew S. Azman, Dominique Legros, Heather McKay, and Justin Lessler (2019), 'Cholera Prevention and Control in Refugee Settings: Successes and Continued Challenges', *PLoS Neglected Tropical Diseases*, vol. 13, n° 6. doi:10.1371/journal.pntd.0007347.

Stockton, Nicholas (2005), 'The Accountable Humanitarian', Luce Lecture, Tufts University.

Stockton, Nicholas, and Peter Walker (2015), 'The Sphere Story, a Video Documentary'. [https://www.spherestandards.org/the-sphere-story-a-video-documentary/].

Tong, Jacqui (2004), 'Questionable Accountability: MSF and Sphere in 2003', *Disasters*, vol. 28, n° 2, pp. 176–189. doi:10.1111/j.0361–3666.2004.00251.x.

Torrenté, Nicolas de (2002), 'The War on Terror's Challenges to Humanitarian Action'. [https://www.msf.fr/sites/default/files/2002–2009–19-Torrente.pdf].

Tsikata, Dzodzi (2004), 'The Rights-Based Approach to Development: Potential for Change or More of the Same?', *IDS Bulletin*, vol. 35, n° 4, pp. 130–133. doi:10.1111/j.1759–5436.2004.tb00167.x.

UN Secretary-General Ban Ki-moon (2016), 'One Humanity: Shared Responsibility. Report of the Secretary-General for the World Humanitarian Summit', United Nations. [https://digitallibrary.un.org/record/822154].

UN General Assembly (1991), 'UN Resolution 46/182: Strengthening of the Coordination of Humanitarian Emergency Assistance of the United Nations'.

UN General Assembly (2004), 'UN Resolution 58/114: Strengthening of the Coordination of Emergency Humanitarian Assistance of the United Nations'.

Walker, Peter, and Susan Purdin (2004), 'Birthing Sphere', *Disasters*, vol. 28, n° 2, pp. 100–111. doi:10.1111/j.0361–3666.2004.00246.x.

World Humanitarian Summit Secretariat (2015), *Restoring Humanity: Global Voices Calling for Action. Synthesis of the Consultation Process for the World Humanitarian Summit*, New York: United Nations. [https://agendaforhumanity.org/sites/default/files/resources/2017/Jul/Restoring_Humanity_Synthesis_of_the_Consultation_Process_for_the_World_Humanitarian_Summit.pdf].

3 Hostility to Aid Actors

Normalising Transgression?

Stephen Cornish, Alejandro Pozo, and Duncan McLean

A cursory look at the fate of aid and healthcare workers in major conflicts in 2025 makes for sombre reading. On 6 May, Médecins Sans Frontières (MSF) condemned the *"deliberate bombing"* of its hospital in Old Fangak, South Sudan by helicopter gunships.[1] The previous month, a Rapid Support Forces (RSF) attack on Zamzam displacement camp in North Darfur, Sudan resulted in hundreds of deaths, amongst them 11 employees of Relief International who were running a health clinic.[2] Less than two weeks earlier, the bodies of 15 paramedics and civil emergency responders were discovered in southern Gaza, including eight members of the Palestinian Red Crescent Society, hastily buried after their ambulances had come under fire from Israeli forces.[3] MSF has regularly denounced Russia's large-scale bombardments of civilian areas in Ukraine, sparing none of *"hospitals, residential buildings, humanitarian workers, and patients"*.[4]

These forms of violence are among the most visible and dramatic types of hostility directed against humanitarian action. Sadly, there have been peaks and troughs in such attacks throughout history; repeated patterns often focused on a limited number of highly violent contexts. The degree to which this has been normalised is a perpetual concern, particularly in moments of acceleration, as is the failure of the parties to international humanitarian law (IHL) to dissuade or hold accountable those responsible.

The term "hostility" has been described as *"relating to an enemy"*, *"marked by malevolence: having or showing unfriendly feelings"*, and *"having an intimidating, antagonistic, or offensive nature"*.[5] However, these definitions address the meaning of hostility rather than how it is projected. For the International Committee of the Red Cross (ICRC), violence against healthcare structures includes *"bombing, shelling, looting, forced entry, shooting into, encircling or other forceful interference with the running of health-care facilities (such as depriving them of electricity and water)"*. For personnel and patients, this could involve intimidation, injuring threats, and killing, while freedom deprivation events by both states and non-state armed groups (NSAGs) are likewise on the list.[6] Other forms of hostility, subtle but effective, can also be mentioned, such as non-violent obstruction through bureaucratic and administrative restrictions, or further examples of state sovereignty being asserted in ways that may conflict

DOI: 10.4324/9781003542247-6

with *"the self-declared moral primacy of the humanitarian model"* and international laws that impose obligations – and limits – to such sovereignty.[7]

A legitimate question is, how representative are events such as those described of the broader humanitarian sector? Despite the horrors visited on the inhabitants of all four countries mentioned above, the answer is probably "not very". 2023 marked the highest number of aid workers' deaths ever recorded but *"62% of all victims were in just three contexts, Gaza, Sudan and South Sudan."* Nevertheless, major attacks impacting on aid workers that same year were reported in 30 other countries.[8] IHL *"specifically proscribes violence against humanitarian organizations and accords protected status to their facilities and activities during armed conflict"*.[9] In 2016, the United Nations Security Council (UNSC) adopted Resolution 2286, *"strongly condemning attacks on medical personnel in conflict situations today"*, and unanimously demanded an *"end to impunity for those responsible"*.[10]

The passage of this resolution can be seen retrospectively as one of partial optimism, and was followed by a surge in initiatives aimed at reporting and monitoring attacks on medical and humanitarian missions. However, lofty language was not accompanied by concrete measures to strengthen the protection of medical facilities. And despite world leaders appearing united over the protection of healthcare, states failed to endorse the practical recommendations needed to operationalise the resolution. The degree to which attacks on health facilities are part of a systematic and intentional war strategy is difficult to prove irrefutably, but this perception certainly applies to a number of armed conflicts. This chapter aims to review and analyse the alleged rise in hostility towards humanitarian actors, as well as the structural changes and shifting concerns this has brought about in the aid sector.

I Historical Tensions

The contemporary humanitarian system has been described as fundamentally shaped by the liberal order that emerged after the Second World War, which itself was a descendant of *"the imperial world of the nineteenth and early twentieth centuries and the global political and economic system the European empires created"*.[11] The subsequent period of Cold War rivalry saw humanitarianism constrained by limited room for manoeuvre in the internal affairs of states, with sovereignty expressed through rigid ideological lines. Often perceived or, indeed, behaving in a partisan manner, aid agencies benefited from broad support from Western states and the general public, notably when aligned with anti-communist movements.[12] A direct consequence of this was humanitarian action focused on the periphery of major armed conflicts, where access to refugee populations was comparatively easier.

There were, of course, multiple contradictions and exceptions, such as the Nigerian Civil War and the contested status of Biafra in the late 1960s. Deeply ingrained in the founding mythology of the *sans frontières* movement, many of the challenges and dilemmas faced during this period were eventually echoed in post-Cold War crises. These included the propaganda value of televised images depicting large-scale human suffering and the unintended negative impact of humanitarian action in armed conflict settings, the latter evident in the taxation of aid agencies by the Biafran leadership and their refusal to countenance a "land corridor" for delivering assistance in the place of more dramatic night flights. The downing of the Swedish Red Cross plane by Nigerian forces in June 1969 was emblematic of frictions with the state over the conditions of providing relief.[13]

The 1983–85 famine in northern Ethiopia likewise stands out for the tensions generated with aid agencies. Given Addis Ababa's alignment with the Soviet Union, the consequences of a two-year drought, forced collectivisation, and secessionist rebellions in Tigre and Eritrea were largely ignored; that is, until the region captured media attention in late 1984, bringing images of starving children into people's homes. Now remembered for the well-intentioned but deeply paternalistic Band Aid concerts the following year, humanitarian relief was portrayed as an apolitical necessity to halt the mounting death toll.[14] The forced transfer of suspect populations was an inconvenient narrative, both for the Ethiopian government and the many agencies that remained silent. Accusations on the misuse of aid eventually resulted in the expulsion of MSF's French section for making *"politically motivated false allegations"*.[15]

There is no shortage of examples, both preceding the end of the Cold War and afterwards, that demonstrate a latent hostility to aid actors when they are deemed inconvenient. Claims of a gradual degradation in operating environments or diminishing respect for the protected status of humanitarian organisations can be challenged. Each incident is context-specific, and the threat typology is manifested differently over time. Nevertheless, even if often grouped around a limited number of extremely violent conflicts, there is a risk of normalising the unacceptable. A key element contributing to the perception of increased insecurity is the dramatic growth in the number of aid actors, notably non-governmental organisations. This was especially apparent in the 1990s, but also includes established organisations like MSF, whose operating budget and staffing have grown exponentially over the last 30 years.[16]

It is not only private charities and UN agencies that operate under the humanitarian label; states have likewise appropriated the term when useful. The 1990s saw unilateral military interventions carried out under the banner of humanitarianism in contexts as varied as Somalia and Kosovo. The 1999 bombing of the latter was described as the *"high point of the post-Cold War humanitarian international"*, with the bypassing of international law later justified as *"illegal but legitimate"*.[17] But if actions over the previous decade seemed to suggest that traditional interpretations of state sovereignty were on the wane, the 11 September 2001 attacks on the US brought internal security concerns to the forefront, including a *"with us or against us"* refrain essentially rejecting neutrality. The widespread labelling of armed opposition groups as terrorists, regardless of their grievances or actions, provided a convenient rationale for limiting humanitarian access to inconvenient populations, much like past embargoes imposed on insurgent-controlled areas.

The logic of counterterrorism, also with counter-insurgency roots from earlier periods, was arguably taken to a new extreme in some cases, with efforts to render aid itself illegal. In Syria, laws issued on 2 July 2012 criminalised medical aid *"to anyone injured by pro-government forces in protest marches against the government"*.[18] A broad practice of criminalising humanitarian and medical assistance was applied to populations in areas no longer controlled by the government. Bashar al-Jaafari, the Syrian Permanent Representative to the UN, referred to MSF in this way at the UNSC on 17 April 2018: *"Just like Da'esh, it entered Syria without the Government's approval. Doctors Without Borders can be compared to smugglers without borders, criminals without borders, opposition without borders, foreign agents without borders, aggressors without borders and terrorists without borders."*[19]

While the developments outlined above have reinforced the centrality of state-driven aid, they are not simply the result of security factors. The paradigms pushing state-building or peacebuilding initiatives, to name just a few, have a long history under different guises, inevitably challenging the autonomy of aid organisations. Driven by concepts such as integration (building synergies with political goals) and stabilisation (helping governments to rule), there has been no shortage of attempts at co-opting the humanitarian system for seemingly lofty political objectives.[20] Working closely with recognised governments has obvious appeal when framed around national stability and development; less so when those same governments are parties to a conflict.

The inverse relation is, likewise, relevant to engagement with NSAGs. MSF has sometimes been perceived as working on the side of the rebels. Far from an ideological stand, MSF's frequent interventions in opposition-controlled areas are driven in part by the imperative to respond where medical needs are most acute, which often coincides with regions where the ministries of health – part of the government – are either dysfunctional or non-existent in practice, but also where access is feasible. Cross-border operations without a host country's authorisation can be seen as a consequence of being denied access through more formal channels, but also the conscious decision to *"set up illegal medical services"* where support is most relevant.[21]

Accessing areas where territorial control is contested or fragmented through armed conflict obliges negotiation with armed actors irrespective of their designation, in essence a *de facto* form of sovereignty.[22] This is a striking point of continuity with past epochs as concerns humanitarian access and the protections outlined in the Geneva Conventions. Attempts to define who is not covered by IHL included similar exclusions, be they *"barbarians, uncivilized natives or those responsible for seditious rebellion"*.[23] A relevant concern today is whether the IHL framework remains sufficiently robust to assert the legitimacy of humanitarian work wherever there are needs, including in areas outside the purview of state control.[24]

Any shift from suspicion to outright hostility from states or NSAGs towards humanitarian actors naturally requires a great deal of nuance. The aid sector has never been static, and the brief historical comments above must also account for changes within the sector itself, such as the noted increase in the number of humanitarian organisations active – currently estimated at over 4,000 – as well as the scope of support provided.[25] Moving well beyond life-saving activities, broad interventions that touch on everything from economic livelihoods to peacebuilding, gender equality, or justice can bring tension when perceived as encroaching on the traditional preserve of states. Misgivings on the part of recipient countries are likewise understandable, given the degree to which Western aid policy has been intertwined with political and economic interests that threaten their hold on national power and resources.[26]

It is also important to note that it remains exceptional for the described hostility to manifest itself violently – the reality is often far more banal. In this regard, one obvious change in almost all contexts in which humanitarian action occurs is the domestic regulatory environment that oversees how aid agencies operate. Common issues for humanitarian organisations have included long custom delays for imported supplies; the banning of goods essential to assistance, due to their potential dual use; restrictions on movements; and the imposition of armed escorts. Whether driven by malice, opportunism, inefficient bureaucracy, or genuine concerns in the administration of a sovereign territory, these restrictions can be onerous, irrespective of the justifications employed. The consequences include limitations on the quality, quantity, and timeliness of the support that aid agencies are able to provide.[27]

II New and Old Patterns

If tensions between either state or non-state actors and humanitarian organisations are not a recent development, it is still reasonable to ask how such tensions manifest themselves today, and what novel trends, if any, can be identified. Radically different perspectives on migratory questions in the Global North have become notably more pronounced as measures ostensibly designed to ensure border protection have resulted in the *"deaths of thousands and a multiplication of indefensible violence"*.[28] Aid agencies have not ingratiated themselves to populist leaders in this regard, either through their actions or their speaking out. But other aspects are hardly new; economic incentives that motivate plunder, or simply being seen as an obstacle to military necessity, all have a chequered past.

Returning to the numbers available, it is difficult to determine whether reports of increasing violence impacting on healthcare are due to a rapid deterioration, improved reporting, or broader strategies of exhaustion that go far beyond the medical sector. A comparative analysis on overall trends is also complex, if not impossible. Figures vary significantly across different databases, case definitions are not uniform, and denominators such as the scale of a humanitarian presence are generally not obtainable. Projects are constantly shifting, including downsizing operations due to perceived risks, leading to erroneous conclusions over the lack of security incidents. The actual number of attacks may also go under-reported, either due to the normalisation of insecurity or intentional under-reporting, as organisations may hesitate to openly acknowledge an incident, given the potential sensitivity or victims involved.[29]

Nevertheless, some conclusions can be drawn. In reviewing the Aid Worker Security Database figures from 2023, the Global Interagency Security Forum and Humanitarian Outcomes noted a slight reduction in the risks posed to humanitarians by the Islamic State and similar groups, replaced by *"the challenges of operating in both new, large-scale major conflicts and disintegrating, lawless environments"*.[30] The shift from low-intensity civil wars to major armed conflicts in countries such as Syria, Yemen, Myanmar, Ethiopia, and Ukraine over the past decade now also applies to the Occupied Palestinian Territory and Sudan. Questions over security are intrinsically linked to the individual conflict dynamics. Both humanitarian access and staff safety have been fraught, with significant areas and populations *"functionally inaccessible for aid organizations, due either to the intensity of hostilities and risk to staff, restrictions by the controlling authorities, or both"*.[31]

From a legal perspective, the framework that humanitarians and health workers generally refer to for protection and legitimacy has frequently been challenged. Given that history is littered with examples of transgressions, comparing epochs can be a frustrating and ultimately futile exercise, knowing that there can be political interest in underestimating or exaggerating levels of violence.[32] And, regardless, perpetrators are unlikely to hold themselves accountable, *"preferring to deflect blame and question the legitimacy of medical action"*. IHL itself is also divisive in other aspects. Detractors have noted that limiting belligerents to what cannot be done to non-combatants and related structures *"legitimizes the brutality of war rather than curtailing it"*. Meanwhile, supporters emphasise the need to reinforce the only internationally agreed framework that aid organisations can use to *"justify their own presence in war zones and make demands for access and protection"*.[33]

It is certainly undeniable that health facilities continue to be *"bombed, looted, occupied, raided, and vandalized"*, with nearly half of all reported incidents attributed to state actors.[34] Obligations of *"precautions and proportionality"* are highly susceptible to the self-serving interpretations of the aggressor, *"drain[ing] the law of its protective function"*.[35] The 2015 US and Afghan targeting of the MSF hospital in Kunduz is an obvious example, with the public narrative of the perpetrators shifting from collateral damage and self-defence to an accident in the days and weeks that followed. The deaths of 42 people, including staff members, patients, and caretakers, occurred in a clearly marked medical structure with all belligerents notified of its location. In a context where a coalition of military actors utilised overlapping legal frameworks of IHL and counterterrorism, a confused patchwork fostered an *"environment conducive to mistakes"*.[36]

So-called mistakes that result in the bombing of healthcare facilities are hardly reassuring. However, the recent military operations in Gaza indicate a shift in narratives, with Israeli forces arguing that the medical facilities *"lost their protection under IHL*", making them legitimate targets for direct attack. Hospitals have been attacked or rendered inoperable at a dramatic rate. Despite the very different dynamics in the current incarnation of Sudan's civil war, hospital neutrality has been regularly and violently challenged. As the ICRC has rightly pointed out, "*the basic principle that a health facility is of civilian character today is questioned*". Rather than a default protected status, "*a population or a health facility has to prove that it is not of military character*".[37]

Hospitals can lose their protection from direct attack if they are used to commit "*acts harmful to the enemy*" outside of their humanitarian function, such as sheltering able-bodied fighters or serving as a weapons depot. IHL provides a general rule: "*if in doubt, presume civilian*". This protective presumption of civilian status has been interpreted to extend to medical facilities and transports.[38] Moreover, the specific protection afforded to healthcare ceases only after a warning has been issued, whenever feasible, with a reasonable time limit.[39] Even in cases where a medical facility loses its protected status, this does not amount to a carte blanche to attack the facility, despite what was initially claimed after the destruction in Kunduz.[40]

An additional dynamic should also be highlighted, distinct from the logic of mistake and deliberate attacks, whether intended to cause harm or as an instrumental use of violence. This involves subordinating the protected character of humanitarian action to political, economic, or military objectives. In fact, this is how IHL works: it does not prohibit harm to civilians, but conditions it based on the concept of military advantage. This balance of proportionality is determined not by the civilian population or those who represent it, but by military and political strategists. Drawing parallels, humanitarians are sometimes viewed as obstacles, for which IHL requires unwanted prudence, caution, and proportionality in military operations. When certain actions are prioritised, everything else can be subordinated.

The balance of proportionality has shifted for a number of reasons: the rise of anti-terrorism rhetoric and legislation exacerbates the risk posed by perceived threats; the association of populations with armed groups, which deprives them of protection – while IHL distinguishes between civilians and combatants, counterterrorism measures and public opinion sometimes draw a distinction between the innocent and the non-innocent, which can be arbitrary. The non-innocent may include not only those who take up arms, but also those who do not resist "sufficiently", simply remain passive, or comply as a survival strategy. This category may also include humanitarians, whose innocence is questioned by accusations that they are complicit with suspects, or unwelcome witnesses who could force accountability.

Impunity likewise plays a role. In a depressing constant as concerns legal accountability, it can also be argued that the political cost of transgressions has weakened. In 2018, former Israeli minister of defence Avigdor Liberman stated, "*There are no innocent people in the Gaza Strip. Everyone has a connection to Hamas.*"[41] Collective punishment and ethnic cleansing are now being publicly defended, so far without political or judicial consequences. It is difficult not to be sceptical that the perpetrators will ever be held accountable or that the provisions of IHL will be applied evenly. However, this is not only the case with the US and Israel. The unrestrained actions of Rwanda in the Democratic Republic of the Congo in 2025, Russia in Ukraine since 2014, and various parties to ongoing conflicts in Sudan and Myanmar, among many others, are challenging not only international law but also an international relations architecture that once assigned humanitarian action a role in alleviating the system's excesses.

None of the above should downplay the challenges and risks also posed by armed groups. The kidnapping and killing of aid workers are still widespread, as are the looting of medical supplies and general obstruction of populations attempting to access healthcare.[42] From massacres and hostage-taking to indiscriminate rocket fire, Hamas has demonstrated a *"disdain for the law"* that states are similarly accused of breaching.[43] The Taliban, prior to retaking power, and Ansar Allah, in Yemen, have fared little better.[44] The massacre of 24 people, including 16 mothers and an MSF midwife, by armed men at the Dasht-e-Barchi maternity ward in Kabul remains a particularly traumatic episode.[45] Elsewhere, negative perceptions of humanitarians – especially those associated with the West, due to political, ideological, religious, or historical animosities – create specific risks, as aid workers become easy, accessible proxy targets in the place of a perceived enemy.[46] Suspicions have hardly been allayed by the occasional use of health facades to undertake military operations, as during the fake poliomyelitis vaccination campaign to track Osama bin Laden in Pakistan.[47]

Access to crisis-affected populations requires negotiations with self-declared *"enemies of liberal democracies"*, who may have little tolerance for humanitarian actors unless deemed particularly useful.[48] Aid organisations may be reluctant to engage with them, and donors may even prohibit such engagement when armed groups are designated as terrorist organisations. However, it is often not up to the humanitarians to decide. While some armed groups may be looking for legitimacy, others may refuse direct dialogue and only tolerate aid under specific conditions. These conditions – such as banning or imposing severe restrictions on female staff (like in Afghanistan or Yemen) or non-Muslim staff (in areas with Islamic State-affiliated groups), or prohibiting certain services, like sexual and reproductive health – challenge the very foundation of principled humanitarian action.

In contrast to armed groups with extreme political or religious ambitions, dealing with criminal groups or banditry presents an equally daunting challenge. In place of a structured hierarchy with a clear ideology, brutal as it might be, the fragmentation of armed opposition into factions focused on economic gain blurs the line between politically motivated violence and criminal activities. Mapping their movements and levels of threat, let alone identifying interlocutors in highly unstable environments, poses its own risks.[49]

Finally, the fluctuating state use of private military and security contractors is similarly difficult to categorise. While operating with important resources and a high degree of impunity, *"there are obvious inconsistencies with a mix of economic motivations influenced by their political connections*". The practice of hiring these companies for various purposes is not new; their expansion and increasing legitimacy are. Afghanistan and Iraq saw a boom in the early years of the so-called War on Terror, while Wagner is reportedly backed by the Russian state and has a significant presence in Mali, the Central African Republic, and elsewhere.[50] Today, these groups can be considered military actors; some purport to become humanitarian partners, such as through armed escorts or other initiatives, and certain governments may support this shift.

III Some Responses from the Aid Sector

Risk exposure may have increased as aid operations have shifted from the periphery to the centre of armed conflict zones, but a narrative has also emerged which acknowledges "*the danger faced by aid workers in the context of the changing nature of conflicts and the declining status of humanitarian personnel*".[51] The historical challenges and more recent developments outlined above may explain some of the fluctuating hostility aid workers have faced, whether from states or armed groups. However, these changes did not occur in a vacuum. It is worth pausing to see how security concerns have evolved over time and whether the current architecture is sufficiently adapted to mitigate present-day risks.

While there have been multiple historic incidents where humanitarian organisations or their staff were targeted intentionally, it has also been argued that "*many severe incidents resulted from misunderstanding, mistakes, errors of judgment, negligence, individual initiatives, or a faulty chain of command*".[52] Simplistic explanations hardly cover all cases and ignore context; genuine malice, outright hostility, and specific acts of cruelty stand out. Examples include the "*execution-style murder of ICRC workers in Chechnya in 1996*", the bombing of the UN's Baghdad headquarters in 2003, or the killing of 17 aid workers from Action Against Hunger in their offices in Muttur, Sri Lanka, in 2006.[53] Also significantly, concerns over duty of care and liability came to the fore, especially after a former employee of the Norwegian Refugee Council (NRC) won a court ruling claiming gross negligence over a 2012 kidnapping on the Kenyan–Somali border.[54]

Risk is determined by both threat and exposure. Regarding exposure, for those that can afford them, it is now common to find security professionals in prominent roles in humanitarian organisations.[55] Security risk management, essentially "*measures aimed at mitigating risk as far as possible*" to maintain operations, has become widespread. While some have credited this development with facilitating relief in extreme circumstances, it has also been criticised for fostering "*risk aversion and bureaucratization*".[56] The latter is perhaps unsurprising, given that the perception of risk has been demonstrated to rise with each related experience. Be it "*an attack on a compound, lawsuit, forensic audit, or media scandal*", the resulting vigilance to a specific risk can be expected to increase accordingly.[57] But more worrying is a concern raised by another

MSF publication, portraying humanitarian security *"as a technical problem requiring technical solutions"*, at the cost of rationalising losses incurred.[58]

One element that has continually re-emerged since 2000 is the concept of acceptance: the basic precept that *"humanitarians can enhance their security by actively seeking to cultivate familiar relationships and goodwill among the communities they serve and gaining the tolerance of armed actors."*[59] A seemingly reasonable approach, many aid agencies have *"resolutely and deliberately"* integrated its use *"as a core element of their security management strategy"*, a low-cost initiative *"consistent with their values, missions and mandates"*.[60] The problem lies not so much with what is arguably a common-sense way to engage with different stakeholders, but the false sense of security this can promote. Being accepted or even tolerated is difficult to qualify, let alone quantify, and is inconsistent. Indeed, while being perceived as valuable to those benefiting from assistance might seem relatively straightforward, at least in theory, those same actions could alienate or undermine other influential actors and interests with the means to retaliate.

The reality is that not many aid workers wander around a conflict zone with a copy of the Geneva Conventions tucked into their back pocket, hoping to negotiate acceptance. This is not a dismissal of IHL either; far from it. The point is that access and protection do not depend exclusively on laws and principles; power dynamics and interests must also be accounted for. To operate with a reasonable degree of safety, repeated transactions must occur, resulting in value in the eyes of the forces at play, be it through services provided, the money spent, the credibility gained, or even the image projected.[61] In the words of an MSF analyst, *"instrumentalization is the condition inherent for action"*; the problem arises in situations where *"we are more useful dead than alive, as hostages rather than caregivers"*.[62]

A cursory overview of security incidents affecting humanitarian organisations reveals an obvious truth: securing acceptance, let alone tolerance, is hardly a magical elixir to resolving all challenges related to reducing risk and managing operations safely. Much like deconfliction measures (which aim to *"prevent mistaken attacks"*), protection initiatives such as "bunkering" or fortifying bases also have their limits.[63] A certain degree of residual risk invariably remains, linked to the nature of the exercise itself. Even advocating more forcefully for the security and protection of aid workers can lead to the so-called security paradox, resulting in *"resentment, reprisals, and even violence"*, the very outcomes they sought to avoid.[64]

IV Gaps Between Rhetoric and Reality

It is difficult to avoid the conclusion that even the most adroit combination of security measures and practices will not suffice. Numerous historic examples demonstrate that *"there has never been a golden age of protection of the wounded, the sick, and their caregivers from violence"*.[65] The "humanitarian space" – a space of relative freedom in which humanitarians are able to independently assess needs, monitor the distribution and use of aid, and engage in dialogue with the population – has always, strictly speaking, been an objective rather than a reality in armed conflicts, as the restriction of such freedom is inherent to these environments.

The uniqueness of each era and context makes it difficult to conduct a comparative analysis that determines whether we are living in a time of greater hostility towards humanitarian action. However, in certain environments this deterioration is evident, and conclusions can be drawn regarding basic variables, such as the respect for rules, impunity for perpetrators, and the acceptance of aid.

The oft-repeated claim that "*even war has rules*" is not difficult to challenge – power often eclipses the law.[66] Even while IHL infractions are easier to document than diligent compliance, IHL is disregarded by too many armed groups and its precepts ignored by too many armies that prioritise their own rules of engagement, domestic manuals, and military doctrines, even when they conflict with international standards. Former UN Secretary-General Kofi Annan stated in 2005: "*Nowhere is the gap between rhetoric and reality – between declarations and deeds – so stark and so deadly as in the field of international humanitarian law.*"[67] The violation of IHL is intrinsic to war; once again, while complete compliance is unrealistic, its observance is challenged far too often.

While impunity has gained ground in the recognition of transgressions, the concept itself is hardly a new development. As Leonard Rubenstein pointed out, "*since the creation of international criminal tribunals in the 1990s, no international prosecution has focused on attacks on healthcare infrastructure and their staff, no matter how open and vicious*".[68] It is necessary to return to the Leipzig war crime trials of 1921 to find an example of perpetrators being punished for attacks on healthcare, in this case the sinking of a hospital ship by a German submarine.[69] Mechanisms such as the International Humanitarian Fact-Finding Commission (IHFFC) are also ineffective, as it can only operate with the authorisation of the states involved. MSF unsuccessfully turned to this mechanism three times between October 2015 and February 2016 to address attacks in Afghanistan, Yemen, and Syria, respectively.[70]

Acceptance has its uses so long as it is not taken in isolation in security management. IHL might be aspirational at times but continues to be a point of reference for aid actors. The humanitarian endeavour is rejected in certain contexts and remains challenged in others. Direct engagement with armed actors is a prerequisite for humanitarian work in the areas they control, but this dialogue has been partially discredited with designated terrorist organisations and is further demonised by other interlocutors, including opposition rebel groups, pro-government militias, private security actors, *de facto* governments, and even states. In these cases, indirect dialogue through locally hired staff or community leaders may involve the transfer of risk, explored in the following zoom-in. The above-mentioned actors may associate humanitarian workers with neocolonial, abusive, or self-serving practices, or perceive them as instruments in broader economic, political, or military strategies that affect their interests.

At the outset of this chapter, reference was made to peaks and troughs when documenting attacks on aid workers, essentially emphasising the need for caution before drawing grand conclusions applicable beyond a limited number of contexts of extreme behaviour. This is not to negate the impact or repetitive nature of violence employed or, indeed, the normalisation of abuse. Be it through the periodic dismissal of IHL, the rationales provided, or indeed the resulting human cost, the gap between rhetoric and reality has arguably grown, while the political cost of transgressions has diminished. We may be at the end of a cycle: a kind of naive hypocrisy that for a long time involved believing that states should act with diligence in their relations with others, while ignoring the historical power dynamics that shaped the development of these norms in the first place.

Notes

1 MSF, 2025b.
2 Relief International, 2025.
3 IFRC, 2025.
4 Since the escalation of the war in Ukraine, *"around 2,000 medical facilities have been damaged or destroyed"*: MSF, 2025a.
5 *Merriam-Webster Dictionary*, available at https://www.merriam-webster.com/dictionary/hostility.
6 ICRC, 2011.
7 McLean and Hofman, 2023.
8 Humanitarian Outcomes, 2024.
9 Stoddard et al., 2017. pp. 1–25.
10 UN, 2016.
11 Hopgood, 2019.
12 Neuman, 2024.
13 Foley, 2010, pp. 17–9.
14 Barnett, 2011, pp. 156–7.
15 Letter from the Relief and Rehabilitation Commission (Provisional Government of Socialist Ethiopia) to Bertrand Desmoulins, Coordinator, MSF France, 2 December 1985 (in English): MSF, 2005–2013, p. 78.
16 Alexander and Parker, 2020.
17 Hopgood, 2019.
18 Fouad et al., 2017, pp. 2517–8.
19 UNSC, 2018.
20 Donini, 2011, pp. 141–57.
21 Brauman, 2012.
22 Hopgood, 2019.
23 McLean, 2019, pp. 771–803.
24 Routeau and Abou El Ghayt-Huart, 2024.
25 This includes *"international non-governmental organisations (grouped by federation), national NGOs that deliver aid within their own borders, UN humanitarian agencies, and the International Red Cross and Red Crescent Movement."*: Global Database of Humanitarian Organisations, available at https://humanitarianoutcomes.org/projects/gdho.
26 Hopgood, 2019.
27 IASC, 2022.
28 Neuman, 2024.
29 Blanchet et al., 2023.

30 Global Interagency Security Forum and Humanitarian Outcomes, 2024.
31 *Ibid.*
32 McLean, 2019, pp. 771–803.
33 Hofman, 2021, p. 204.
34 Safeguarding Health in Conflict and Security Insights, 2024.
35 Rubenstein, 2024.
36 Bouchet-Saulnier and Whittall, 2018, pp. 337–72.
37 Praz Dessimoz, 2024.
38 ICRC, 2023.
39 Additional Protocol I of the Geneva Conventions, art. 13, para. 1; Customary IHL Rule 28.
40 Pozo, Richards, and Sax, 2024.
41 Lazaroff, 2018.
42 Safeguarding Health in Conflict and Security Insights, 2024.
43 Rubenstein, 2024.
44 See MSF's public communications on Yemen and Afghanistan at https://www.msf.org/yemen and https://www.msf.org/afghanistan, by filtering by "attacks on medical care".
45 Segoni, 2020.
46 Global Interagency Security Forum, 2021.
47 Shah, 2012.
48 Neuman, 2024.
49 Global Interagency Security Forum and Humanitarian Outcomes, 2024.
50 Ladd, Nsaibia, and Gurcov, 2023.
51 Neuman, 2016, pp. 26–7.
52 Global Interagency Security Forum, 2021.
53 The Baghdad attack led to an overhaul of the UN's security set-up and the creation of the UN Department of Safety and Security (UNDSS): Global Interagency Security Forum and Humanitarian Outcomes, 2024.
54 Young, 2015.
55 Norman, 2023.
56 Global Interagency Security Forum and Humanitarian Outcomes, 2024.
57 Stoddard, Haver, and Czwarno, 2016.
58 Neuman and Weissman, 2016, pp. 10–1.
59 Global Interagency Security Forum and Humanitarian Outcomes, 2024.
60 Fast and O'Neill, 2010.
61 Magone, Neuman, and Weissman, 2011.
62 Fabrice Weissman, director of studies at the Centre de Réflexion sur l'Action et les Savoirs Humanitaires, written exchange with one of the authors, 24 April 2025.
63 Bebbington, et al., 2022.
64 Humanitarian Outcomes, 2024.
65 Rubenstein, 2021, p. 277.
66 UN, 2023.
67 Report of the UN Secretary-General, 2005.
68 Rubenstein, 2024.
69 McGreal, 2008, pp. 220–1.
70 Pozo, 2017, p. 32.

References

Alexander, Jessica, and Ben Parker (2020), '25 Years of Humanitarian Action – in Graphics', *The New Humanitarian*, 9 September. [https://www.thenewhumanitarian.org/maps-and-graphics/2020/09/09/25-years-of-humanitarian-data].

Barnett, Michael N. (2011), *Empire of Humanity: A History of Humanitarianism*, Ithaca, NY: Cornell University Press. doi:10.7591/9780801460616.

Bebbington, Carmen, Sierra Fang-Horvath, Georgia Harrington, David Polatty, and Jonathan Robinson (2022), 'Reviewing Guidance and Perspectives on Humanitarian Notification Systems for Deconfliction', Brown University: Center for Human Rights and Humanitarian Studies Watson Institute for International and Public Affairs and Humanitarian Response Program College of Maritime Operational Warfare US Naval War College.

Blanchet, Karl, Leonard Rubenstein, Bertrand Taithe, and Larissa Fast (2023), 'Have Attacks on Healthcare Become the New Normal? A Public Health Call to Action for Armed Conflicts before It Is Too Late', *Conflict and Health*, vol. 17, n° 1, p. 56. doi:10.1186/s13031–13023–00555–00554.

Bouchet-Saulnier, Françoise, and Jonathan Whittall (2018), 'An Environment Conducive to Mistakes? Lessons Learnt from the Attack on the Médecins Sans Frontières Hospital in Kunduz, Afghanistan', *International Review of the Red Cross*, vol. 100, n° 907–09, pp. 337–372. doi:10.1017/S1816383118000619.

Brauman, Rony (2012), 'Médecins Sans Frontières and the ICRC: Matters of Principle', *International Review of the Red Cross*, vol. 94, n° 888, pp. 1523–1535. doi:10.1017/S1816383113000283.

Donini, Antonio (2011), 'Between a Rock and a Hard Place: Integration or Independence of Humanitarian Action?', *International Review of the Red Cross*, vol. 93, n° 881, pp. 141–157.

Fast, Larissa, and Michael O'Neill (2010), 'A Closer Look at Acceptance', *Humanitarian Practice Network*, n° 47. [https://odihpn.org/publication/a-closer-look-at-acceptance/].

Foley, Conor (2010), *The Thin Blue Line: How Humanitarianism Went to War*, London: Verso.

Fouad, Fouad M., Annie Sparrow, Ahmad Tarakji, Mohamad Alameddine, Fadi El-Jardali, Adam P. Coutts, Nour El Arnaout, et al. (2017), 'Health Workers and the Weaponisation of Health Care in Syria: A Preliminary Inquiry for The Lancet–American University of Beirut Commission on Syria', *The Lancet*, vol. 390, n° 10111, pp. 2516–2526. doi:10.1016/S0140–6736(17)30741–30749.

Global Interagency Security Forum (2021), 'Achieving Safe Operations through Acceptance: Challenges and Opportunities for Security Risk Management'. [https://gisf.ngo/resource/achieving-safe-operations-through-acceptance/].

Global Interagency Security Forum, and Humanitarian Outcomes (2024), 'State of Practice: The Evolution of Security Risk Management in the Humanitarian Space'. [https://humanitarianoutcomes.org/security_risk_mgmt_humanitarian_space_2024].

Hofman, Michiel (2021), 'Naming and Shaming the Bombers', in Jehan Bseiso, Michiel Hofman, and Jonathan Whittall (eds), *Everybody's War: The Politics of Aid in the Syria Crisis*, New York: Oxford University Press. doi:10.1093/oso/9780197514641.003.0009.

Hopgood, Stephen (2019), 'When the Music Stops: Humanitarianism in a Post-Liberal World Order', *Journal of Humanitarian Affairs*, vol. 1, n° 1, pp. 4–14. doi:10.7227/JHA.002.

Humanitarian Outcomes, 'Global Database of Humanitarian Organisations (GDHO)'. [https://humanitarianoutcomes.org/projects/gdho].

Humanitarian Outcomes (2024), 'Aid Worker Security Report 2024: Balancing Advocacy and Security in Humanitarian Action'. [https://humanitarianoutcomes.org/AWSR_2024].

IASC (2022), 'IASC Guidance Understanding and Addressing Bureaucratic and Administrative Impediments to Humanitarian Action: Framework for a System-Wide

Approach'. [https://interagencystandingcommittee.org/operational-response/iasc-guidance-understanding-and-addressing-bureaucratic-and-administrative-impediments-humanitarian].

ICRC, 'Customary IHL Rules'. [https://ihl-databases.icrc.org/en/customary-ihl/v1].

ICRC (2011), 'Health Care in Danger: Making the Case'. [https://www.icrc.org/en/publication/4072-health-care-danger-making-case].

ICRC (2023), 'The Protection of Hospitals during Armed Conflicts: What the Law Says'. [https://www.icrc.org/en/document/protection-hospitals-during-armed-conflicts-what-law-says].

IFRC (2025), 'IFRC Condemns the Killing of Eight Palestine Red Crescent Medics in Gaza', 30 March. [https://www.ifrc.org/press-release/ifrc-condemns-killing-eight-palestine-red-crescent-medics-gaza].

Ladd, Serwat, Héni Nsaibia, and Nichita Gurcov (2023), 'Moving Out of the Shadows: Shifts in Wagner Group Operations Around the World', Armed Conflict Location & Event Data Project (ACLED). [https://acleddata.com/2023/08/02/moving-out-of-the-shadows-shifts-in-wagner-group-operations-around-the-world/].

Lazaroff, Tovah (2018), '"There Are No Innocents in Gaza," Says Israeli Defense Minister', *The Jerusalem Post*, 8 April. [https://www.jpost.com/arab-israeli-conflict/there-are-no-innocents-in-gaza-says-israeli-defense-minister-549173].

McGreal, Stephen (2008), *The War on the Hospital Ships, 1914–1918*, Barnsley: Pen & Sword.

McLean, Duncan (2019), 'Medical Care in Armed Conflict: Perpetrator Discourse in Historical Perspective', *International Review of the Red Cross*, vol. 101, n° 911, pp. 771–803.

McLean, Duncan, and Michiel Hofman (2023), 'International Humanitarian Law, State Sovereignty and the Erosion of the Humanitarian Consensus: The End of Humanitarianism?', *Humanitarian Alternatives*, n° 23. [https://www.alternatives-humanitaires.org/en/2023/07/22/international-humanitarian-law-state-sovereignty-and-the-erosion-of-the-humanitarian-consensus-the-end-of-humanitarianism/].

Magone, Claire, Michaël Neuman, and Fabrice Weissman (eds) (2011), *Humanitarian Negotiations Revealed: The MSF Experience*, London: Hurst & Co.

MSF (2005–2013), 'Famine and Forced Relocations in Ethiopia 1984–1986', Speaking Out Case Studies, Médecins Sans Frontières. [https://www.msf.org/speakingout/famine-and-forced-relocations-ethiopia-1984-1986].

MSF (2025a), 'The Relentless and Indiscriminate Bombing in Ukraine Must Cease', 24 April. [https://www.msf.org/relentless-and-indiscriminate-bombing-ukraine-must-cease].

MSF (2025b), 'South Sudan: MSF Strongly Condemns Deliberate Bombing of Its Hospital', 6 May. [https://msf.org.uk/article/south-sudan-msf-strongly-condemns-deliberate-bombing-its-hospital].

Neuman, Michaël (2016), 'On Danger, Sacrifice and Professionalisation: MSF and the Security Debate', in Michaël Neuman and Fabrice Weissman (eds), *Saving Lives and Staying Alive: Humanitarian Security in the Age of Risk Management*, London: Hurst & Co, pp. 26–27.

Neuman, Michaël (2024), 'Humanitaire et démocraties libérales', *AOC media*, 10 April. [https://aoc.media/opinion/2024/04/09/humanitaire-et-democraties-liberales/].

Neuman, Michaël, and Fabrice Weissman (2016), 'Humanitarian Security in the Age of Risk Management', in Michaël Neuman and Fabrice Weissman (eds), *Saving Lives and Staying Alive: Humanitarian Security in the Age of Risk Management*, London: Hurst & Co, pp. 10–11.

Norman, Jethro (2023), 'Security Professionals Are Changing How Humanitarian Organisations Operate', *Danish Institute for International Studies*, 21 March. [https://www.diis.dk/en/research/security-professionals-are-changing-how-humanitarian-organisations-operate].

Pozo, Alejandro (2017), 'The Moral Relativism of Subordinating Civilians to Terrorists: MSF Reflections after a Tragic Year of Hospitals Bombings', Centre for Applied Reflection on Humanitarian Practice, Médecins Sans Frontières. [https://arhp.msf.es/resource/the-moral-relativism-of-subordinating-civilians-to-terrorists/].

Pozo, Alejandro, Helena Richards, and Natasha Sax (2024), 'Medical Care under Fire; the New Normal? MSF's Experience in Gaza, Sudan & Ukraine', Humanitarian Action 2023–2024 report, IECAH-MSF. [https://arhp.msf.es/wp-content/uploads/2024/12/Medical-Care-Under-Fire.pdf].

Praz Dessimoz, Yasmine (2024), 'EVENT: Contemporary Armed Conflicts: Realities and How IHL Addresses Them', ICRC. [https://www.icrc.org/en/event/event-contemporary-armed-conflicts-realities-and-how-ihl-addresses-them].

Relief International (2025), 'Zamzam Camp, Sudan: A Profound Tragedy for Relief International', 13 April. [https://www.ri.org/zamzam-camp-sudan-a-profound-tragedy-for-relief-international/].

Report of the UN Secretary-General (2005), 'In Larger Freedom: Towards Development, Security and Human Rights for All', Ref. A/59/2005, 21 March. [https://digitallibrary.un.org/record/550204].

Routeau, Olivier, and Amal Abou El Ghayt-Huart (2024), 'Ukraine-Gaza: Why Is the Zone of Legitimate Humanitarian Applicability Shrinking so Fast?', *Humanitarian Alternatives*, n° 27. [https://www.alternatives-humanitaires.org/en/2024/11/27/ukraine-gaza-why-is-the-zone-of-legitimate-humanitarian-applicability-shrinking-so-fast/].

Rubenstein, Leonard (2021), *Perilous Medicine: The Struggle to Protect Health Care from the Violence of War*, New York: Columbia University Press.

Rubenstein, Leonard (2024), 'Threats to International Humanitarian Law in Ukraine and Gaza', *Humanitarian Alternatives*, n° 27. [https://www.alternatives-humanitaires.org/en/2024/11/27/threats-to-international-humanitarian-law-in-ukraine-and-gaza/].

Safeguarding Health in Conflict, and Security Insights (2024), 'Critical Condition: Violence Against Healthcare in Conflict 2023'.

Segoni, Francesco (2020), 'Dasht-e-Barchi: An Attack on Hazara Mothers', MSF International Activity Report 2020. [https://www.msf.org/international-activity-report-2020/dasht-e-barchi-attack-hazara-mothers].

Shah, Saeed (2012), 'CIA Tactics to Trap Bin Laden Linked with Polio Crisis, Say Aid Groups', *The Guardian*, 2 March. [https://www.theguardian.com/world/2012/mar/02/aid-groups-cia-osama-bin-laden-polio-crisis].

Stoddard, Abby, Katherine Haver, and Monica Czwarno (2016), 'NGOs and Risk: How International Humanitarian Actors Manage Uncertainty', Humanitarian Outcomes. [https://humanitarianoutcomes.org/publications/ngos-and-risk-how-international-humanitarian-actors-manage-uncertainty].

Stoddard, Abby, Shoaib Jillani, John Caccavale, Peyton Cooke, David Guillemois, and Vassily Klimentov (2017), 'Out of Reach: How Insecurity Prevents Humanitarian Aid from Accessing the Neediest', *Stability: International Journal of Security and Development*, vol. 6, n° 1, pp. 1–25. doi:10.5334/sta.506.

UN (2016), 'Security Council Adopts Resolution 2286 (2016), Strongly Condemning Attacks against Medical Facilities, Personnel in Conflict Situations', 3 May. [https://press.un.org/en/2016/sc12347.doc.htm].

UN (2023), 'Secretary-General's Remarks to the Press on the Situation in the Middle East', 13 October. [https://www.un.org/sg/en/content/sg/speeches/2023-10-13/secretary-generals-remarks-the-press-the-situation-the-middle-east].

UN Security Council (2018), 'The situation in the Middle East', 8236th Meeting, S/PV.8236, 17 April. [https://documents.un.org/doc/undoc/pro/n18/111/53/pdf/n1811153.pdf].

Young, Holly (2015), 'Steve Dennis and the Court Case That Sent Waves through the Aid Industry', *The Guardian*, 5 December. [https://www.theguardian.com/global-development-professionals-network/2015/dec/05/steve-dennis-court-case-waves-aid-industry].

Zoom-in: Security Management with Locally Hired Staff

A Collaboration with Gaps?

*Mahamat Seid Arabi**

Locally hired humanitarian workers, who account for over 90% of Médecins Sans Frontières (MSF) staff in the countries where the organisation operates,[1] have often been excluded from decision-making processes, particularly in matters of security management. It should be stressed, however, that this approach can sometimes be justified, given the challenges these professionals face in maintaining a distance from unfolding events. This was the case in Haiti, where the violence perpetrated by organised crime groups led some Haitian team members of MSF to openly oppose the organisation's operational policy of providing medical care to all, including gang members. Another common reason for this choice of strategy is the desire to ensure the safety of locally hired staff and the continuity of operations. Sometimes, the reluctance to include them in security-related decisions is rooted in other factors, such as their place in the organisation's management structure, the legal ramifications of an incident, or the degree of trust they enjoy when handling sensitive events.

Until recently, the duty of some locally hired staff was limited to purely administrative support. They generally acted as relays and points of contact, facilitating interactions with key external players, translation assignments, and some negotiations. It is important to point out that a minority of these professionals now play a role that is primarily focused on supporting senior international staff who are also responsible for implementing the security management of project teams. Whilst they are frequently consulted, however, locally hired staff are rarely involved in making security-related decisions.

The Changing Role of Locally Hired Staff: Specific Aspects

With regard to security management in humanitarian organisations, the role of locally hired staff is evolving against a backdrop of changing perceptions of risk, influenced by the complex security challenges now emerging in many environments. In 2009, access to the population of Sudan's Darfur region was limited due to both humanitarian agencies' measures to address the uncertain security situation and government restrictions on international presence. Thirteen major international NGOs were expelled, which reduced aid delivery capacity by around 40%, and some organisations lost contact with their locally

DOI: 10.4324/9781003542247-7

hired colleagues.[2] Such restrictions mean that humanitarian actors have to adapt and, therefore, rely entirely on their national staff to maintain operations. In 2011, during the famine that affected several regions of Somalia, an international NGO working in the country managed to gain secure access by deploying expatriate Somalis to supervise and administer its projects. Thanks to their local networks and in-depth knowledge of the context, they were able to visit difficult-to-access areas regularly and increase the organisation's operational presence.[3]

Today's humanitarian response strategies focus on the management of risk rather than its systematic avoidance. Consequently, various intervention models have been used in recent years to facilitate access to affected populations and simultaneously safeguard staff security. MSF has introduced a so-called profiling policy, which involves selecting international mobile staff based on non-professional criteria such as nationality or skin colour. Although this practice reduces the risk of Western personnel being kidnapped, it does not appear to have an impact on other dangers, such as arrests, attacks on convoys, bombings, or suicide attacks.[4]

Regarding remotely managed projects,[5] locally hired staff frequently come under intense pressure from local and national actors, especially if they are deemed to have an influence on resource management or are perceived as having a higher economic status.[6] The deployment of international staff on-site is, therefore, crucial to the continuity of operations. It allows regular contact with the authorities and other stakeholders to be established, thus ensuring transparency and answering any questions about the nature of the project. The constant deterioration of humanitarian space,[7] exacerbated by domestic and inter-state conflicts, as well as the proliferation of non-state armed actors, who are often hostile to the presence and activities of humanitarian organisations in many parts of the world, particularly in the Sahel and the Middle East, have only added to the list of strategic security options required to enable humanitarian staff to operate with greater reassurance in these complex environments.

The matter of programmes being managed by national teams has given rise to doubts and sometimes heated debate within international organisations, but the changing nature of conflicts has made this partial delegation to locally hired staff necessary. The role of these professionals has, therefore, developed considerably, thanks in particular to their proximity to the realities of the context and their knowledge of sociopolitical issues. In many cases, this has facilitated the acceptance of humanitarian activities and negotiations with stakeholders.

During the 1999 conflict in Chechnya, where access for humanitarian actors was limited due to the constant threat of kidnapping or murder, security became the top priority, affecting the feasibility of operations and prompting many NGOs to reduce the number of international staff while gradually shifting responsibility to Chechen staff, who were then tasked with distributing the majority of assistance. In an emblematic way, this example illustrates the need for humanitarian organisations to adapt, taking not just local resources into account, but also the resilience of their teams on the ground, to the extent of profoundly changing the traditional relationships between international and locally hired staff, with the former relying on the latter to implement operations and security protocols.[8]

Professionals on the Front Line

In some cases, locally hired staff have to contend with the dangers associated with working for an international NGO whose reputation may suffer from accusations that are often spurious. Such hostility indirectly affects this category of professionals, especially when the international managers of these organisations are not visible in the areas of intervention. Teams operating in their own countries are frequently caught in a vice-like grip between their ties with their employer and their proximity to the local population, and are particularly at risk when they are mobile or involved in negotiations.[9] Furthermore, working for an international organisation gives locally hired staff a professional and symbolic advantage that carries social prestige but also brings risks, as they are often the first to fall victim to crimes committed against humanitarian workers.[10] The violence suffered by this category of staff in connection with their employment can spill over into their personal lives, taking the form of threats, blackmail, or attempts at extortion.[11] Whether they are involved in gathering information about ongoing violence or acting as mediators with state or non-state armed actors, locally hired professionals contribute to the regular analysis of the context and general security conditions. They reconcile the roles of "*'fixers', intermediaries and humanitarians*", thus allowing NGOs to act and evolve cautiously in increasingly fragmented and constantly changing environments.[12]

Caught Between Domestic Laws and Political and Social Pressures

As interventions are marked by complex security challenges and respect for humanitarian actors and health structures is fragile, questions can be raised about the relevance of conventional humanitarian norms supposed to protect aid providers.[13] This is even more problematic for locally hired staff, who are subject to the laws of their country and to pressure from the authorities in states, which sometimes introduce new legislation criminalising certain forms of aid. Other threats include arbitrary arrest and detention with no respect for the relevant legal procedures. The same trend is also common among non-state armed actors who commit acts of violence against humanitarian staff, for reasons that are not always clear. In response to Sudan's "nationalisation" policy, one NGO in Darfur drew up a set of principles to guide its activities. It recruited international staff only if the skills and experience sought were not available locally, and was prepared to justify its decision if necessary.[14]

Embodying the Principles of the Organisation: A Complex Exercise?

The sociocultural affiliations of locally hired staff can sometimes lead to friction, and in some cases local actors can find it difficult to accept their neutrality, especially in areas where intercommunal tension is running high and where practising professionals belong to one of the parties involved in the conflict. In such situations, these individuals are perceived as both humanitarian actors and stakeholders in the crisis in which they are working, and mitigation strategies that are supposed to protect them prove ineffective.[15] It is also vitally important to understand the specific challenges and risks associated with their involvement in crisis situations and to listen to their analyses of the dangers they face. While the principles of neutrality and impartiality are sometimes difficult for locally hired staff to uphold, many succeed in maintaining a distance from the sociopolitical nature of the events they operate in, as do their international colleagues.[16]

A Few Concluding Thoughts

The issue of transferring risk from international mobile staff to locally hired professionals has been discussed at length by MSF.[17] It implies that the dangers faced by some staff – mainly Western – are being shifted to their national or international counterparts from the Global South. If this tendency does exist, and if it can sometimes be justified by previous instances of explicit threats or even violence against the presence of international actors, it could undermine the autonomy of decisions made by professionals who are all too aware of the risks. In theory, the same security measures should apply to all employees; but, in practice, this fairness is proving fragile, especially for locally hired staff, whose protection becomes difficult to ensure outside the workplace. Given their increased exposure to major risks,[18] the organisation should carry out a specific analysis of security policies for locally hired staff.[19]

While job profiles or titles may vary from context to context, the need for locally hired staff acting as intermediaries in NGO security management has grown considerably, becoming a standard model for humanitarian programme implementation in most organisations operating in unsafe environments. This is a relatively new phenomenon, driven by MSF's current consideration for this category of staff, and whose primary role has long been overlooked by their international counterparts.[20]

Notes

* Translated from French by Derek Scoins.
1 MSF, 2024.
2 Stoddard, Harmer, and Renouf, 2010.
3 Egeland, Harmer, and Stoddard, 2011.
4 Duroch and Neuman, 2021.
5 DG-ECHO (The Directorate-General for European Civil Protection and Humanitarian Aid Operations) defines remote management as *"an operational approach used to provide relief in situations where humanitarian access to disaster-affected populations is limited by security concerns and/or formal or informal decisions imposed by de jure or de facto authorities"*.

6 *"In South Sudan, for instance, armed men entered hospitals at night demanding food. In CAR and in the Nairobi slum of Kibera, thieves stole cash from MSF staff, knowing they earn a salary."*: MSF, 2016, p. 21.
7 Groupe URD defines humanitarian space as *"a symbolic space in which there is freedom to conduct operations, and where working methods and respect for principles preserve the flexibility, independence, and impartiality that are necessary in humanitarian action. It exists to provide people affected by crises with security and protection, and to provide them with access to the aid that is essential to their survival."*
8 Arki, 2010.
9 Duroch and Neuman, 2021.
10 UN News, 2025.
11 MSF, 2016, chapter 8.
12 Atlani-Duault, et al. (eds), 2021.
13 As discussed in Chapter 3. See also the articles on international humanitarian law in 'International humanitarian law: the great step… backwards?', 2023.
14 Egeland, Harmer, and Stoddard, 2011.
15 See Chedorge and Neuman, 2016, p. 170.
16 *"Neutrality can be adopted by anyone. There are many examples where, for instance, medics in a country have tried to stand outside a conflict, make their clinics a zone of safety and provide care to all. Such service is not only in the gift of international humanitarian agencies."*: Healy, 2021.
17 The Global Interagency Security Forum defines risk transfer as *"the intentional or unintentional creation, transformation, or shifting of risks (either increasing or decreasing in severity) for one actor due to the presence or action of another"*.
18 Internal MSF data between 2010 and 2024 show that locally hired staff account for two-thirds of the victims of kidnapping and arrests, as well as for a large majority of work-related deaths.
19 *"In none of the projects studied did the MSF security policies or risk analysis contain a specific section on national staff, nor had they identified staff who were more likely to be at risk of incidents because of issues surrounding ethnicity, religion or job profile."*: MSF, 2016, p. 56.
20 *"In 2006, an internal study of the position of 'national staff' (to use the language of the time) in MSF found that, with two modest exceptions, issues concerning them had 'not been systematically addressed in any international platform'. There were significant gaps in knowledge about and provisions for national staff – no reliable numbers for how many people MSF employed on such contracts, for example; limited efforts to inform national staff about complaint mechanisms; few policies to support their security and no data about incidents affecting them. […] Since that period, significant inroads have been made and meaningful – albeit uneven – improvements across a range of internal inequalities."* Davey, 2024.

References

Arki, Annabelle (2010), 'Quatorze ans de mission Médecins du Monde en Tchétchénie'. *Humanitaire. Enjeux, pratiques, débats*, n° 25. [https://journals.openedition.org/humanitaire/764].

Atlani-Duault, Laëtitia, Jean-Hervé Bradol, Marc Le Pape, and Claudine Vidal (eds) (2021), *Violences extrêmes. Enquêter, secourir, juger: Syrie, Rwanda, République démocratique du Congo*, Paris: Éditions de la Maison des sciences de l'homme.

Chedorge, Delphine, and Michaël Neuman (2016), 'The Duty of a Head of Mission', in Neuman, Michaël and Fabrice Weissman (eds), *Saving Lives and Staying Alive: Humanitarian Security in the Age of Risk Management*, London: Hurst & Co.

Davey, Eleanor (2024), 'The Road from La Mancha: Narratives of Failure and Institutional Reform', *Centre de réflexion sur l'action et les savoirs humanitaires*. [https://msf-crash.org/en/humanitarian-actors-and-practices/road-la-mancha-narratives-failure-and-institutional-reform].

Duroch, Françoise, and Michaël Neuman (2021), 'Should We Discriminate in Order to Act? Profiling: A Necessary but Debated Practice', *Humanitarian Practice Network*. [https://odihpn.org/publication/should-we-discriminate-in-order-to-act-profiling-a-necessary-but-debated-practice/].

Egeland, Jan, Adele Harmer, and Abby Stoddard (2011), 'To Stay and Deliver - Good Practice for Humanitarians in Complex Security Environments', OCHA.

Healy, Sean (2021), 'Neutrality: Principle or Tool?' *Humanitarian Practice Network*. [https://odihpn.org/publication/neutrality-principle-or-tool/].

'International humanitarian law: the great step… backwards?' (2023), *Humanitarian Alternatives*, n° 23. [https://www.alternatives-humanitaires.org/en/category/focus-en/international-humanitarian-law-the-great-step-backwards/].

MSF (2016), 'Medical Care Under Fire: An Analysis of MSF's Experience of Violence and Insecurity in the Field', MSF internal report.

MSF (2024), '2023 Staff Data and Trends Report', MSF internal report.

Stoddard, Abby, Adele Harmer, and Jean S.Renouf (2010), 'Once Removed: Lessons and Challenges in Remote Management of Humanitarian Operations for Insecure Areas', Humanitarian Outcomes.

UN News (2025), '"Attacks on Aid Workers Must End," Security Council Told', 2 April. [https://news.un.org/en/story/2025/04/1161786].

Part II

Navigating Expectations

4 From Technique to Technicity

Evolving Aims in MSF's Medical Practice

Jacob Burns and Natalie Roberts

Given that MSF has grown into a 2 billion-euros-a-year behemoth with interventions in more than 70 countries around the world, we would like to start this chapter with a surprising statement: the medical humanitarian gesture, as it was first conceived by MSF practitioners, was a humble one. It was a gesture that aimed to use what was available to the doctor in a difficult or low-resource setting to address a specific problem, often one that posed an immediate and grave threat to the patient's health.

Considering the stakes of that intervention, it may seem odd to say that it was humble. Yet what set it apart from the prevailing humanitarian-development ethos at the time was that the humanitarian medic was not attempting to change everything; there was no pretension that an entire health system would be built or that an entire population would view their well-being differently after the presence of the doctor. What was proposed, instead, was an intervention that might not make a difference to the population as a whole, but which would make a world of difference for those who were treated.[1]

Inherent in that humility was an acceptance of limitations: at the end of the 1970s, doctors coming from France acknowledged that resources available to them at home would not be available in the camps of Thailand; some problems, they would not be able to address at all. In order to try and tackle those that could be dealt with, humanitarian medicine developed as a *technique*: the adaptation of Western medical practices and tools for application in the sites where humanitarianism was being practised, particularly refugee camps.[2] The technique was a creative application of medical tools to situations where they had not been designed to function rather than a complete transposition of Western medical practices to humanitarian settings. Gradually, humanitarian medics began to trial the use of simplified tools and protocols, conceived with the aim of being better adapted to the environment in which they were working and the pathologies they were treating.[3] These tools were most successful when they gained political traction with the local practitioners or authorities tasked with tackling those pathologies, and, most importantly, with the patients suffering from them.

Two obvious routes from humility to hubris emerge in this history. The first is the hubris of the doctor who puts themselves forward to do the work of the

DOI: 10.4324/9781003542247-9

humanitarian. There is inevitably a little conceit in all of us who leave home to go to difficult places – or who stay in their home when their home becomes too difficult for many to stay in – because we think we can make a difference. For some of us, that hubris has been more pronounced than others, leading, in some cases, to the creation of "hero" narratives[4] around certain persons and interventions that quickly belie any notion of humility, and which do not accurately reflect the importance of social and political engagement between the humanitarian and the individual or individuals that they aim to assist.

The second route is more structural. The history of MSF is one of professionalisation: of giving our medical personnel better chances to make their encounter with the patient a successful one by standardising the tools available to them and broadening the support – in logistics, human resources, and other fields – necessary to ensure efficient medical interventions at scale. As our financial resources increase and our material capacities improve, it is tempting for us to lose sight of the idea of humanitarian medicine as a technique and let hubris enter into the practice through an obsession with *technicity*: that is, the replication (or even bettering) of Western medical standards in humanitarian settings. Technicity is where the technique becomes divorced from politics: it forgets the political and cultural site in which it was designed to operate. And, as pointed out by Jean-Hervé Bradol, innovation can only really take place when sociopolitical conditions permit and encourage it.

Of course, aiming to do things well is not a problem. What becomes problematic with technicity is when it becomes an obsession to the point of leading us to forget to ask what is right for the patient or for the setting of our intervention.

The last decade has been marked by the posing of important questions about inequality and inequity in humanitarian practices, as well as a reappraisal of whether humanitarians should engage with the roots of the issues that they are trying to treat. They mirror longer-running debates on, amongst other things, the value of high-cost individual treatment versus public health interventions. These questions are important and valid, and what we write here is not intended to invalidate them. Nor do we suggest that there is only one right answer. What we seek to argue, however, through our four case studies, is that the technique of humanitarian medicine is at its most powerful when it marries a deep understanding of contextual realities to a drive to do better for our patients. It is not only *what* we do, but where we do it, how, who for, and who with.

This is not simply a rehashing of the humanitarian vs. development debate, but rather an exploration of what humanitarian medicine can (and perhaps should) look like, and which technical objectives it should set for itself. As the humanitarian project expands and evolves, and the contexts in which humanitarians intervene change, it is important to review our own expectations, the expectations of the authorities in the countries where we operate, and, most importantly, the expectations of the people we treat, regarding the quality and form of humanitarian interventions. What tools are useful in the places where we work? How do we develop new tools and techniques? And how do we judge what creatively disrupts the practice of medicine in a particular place, bringing benefits to patients, and that which needlessly destabilises practices that deploy techniques adapted to their context, just for the sake of technicity?

I Syria: Finding Relevance

In March 2011, large numbers of people began demonstrating in the streets of Daraa, demanding the fall of the Syrian government led by President Bashar al-Assad. The protests quickly spread to all of Syria's major cities. They were met by police and military violence: mass arrests, detention and torture of protesters; a brutal crackdown on what had started as peaceful demonstrations. By the end of April, the Syrian government had deployed warplanes and ground troops. By July, a diffuse collection of newly formed opposition militia groups had coalesced into the Free Syrian Army. The armed insurgency rapidly descended into a savage civil war. In the ten years that followed, an estimated 306,887 civilians would be killed, many of them by relentless Syrian government air strikes against its own population.[5]

As the violence escalated, MSF attempted to negotiate access into the country to provide direct medical assistance to the Syrian people. Denied permission to even meet with the Syrian regime, MSF began donating supplies to networks of Syrian medics working in clandestine health structures that were springing up across the country. Eventually abandoning efforts to obtain official access, an MSF team took the decision to cross the border into Idlib Governorate, from Turkey, in May 2012, opening the first MSF-run hospital in Syria in a converted house a couple of weeks later.[6] Over the following months, further teams were sent cross-border by multiple MSF sections into Syria's north-western governorates of Idlib, Aleppo, and Latakia.

After months of powerlessly watching videos and images of bombs falling on hospitals and civilians, and of hearing the stories of exhausted medics dealing with mass casualty events in urban centres and on the front lines, MSF's initial priority was to offer emergency care to war-wounded patients, primarily via the provision of acute trauma surgery. The Middle East was *"not like Africa"*, where in conflict zones MSF would usually focus on supporting displaced people, preventing outbreaks, and delivering essential maternal and paediatric care. The Syrian population would expect a *"higher level of care"* in response to the relentless shelling they were subject to, and that meant trauma surgery.[7] Emulating the Syrian doctors that they had been supporting, MSF teams set up a series of "field hospitals": trauma units located outside existing medical structures, in converted houses and warehouses, disused chicken farms, and even a cave. The ambition was to receive the wounded as quickly as possible after their injury and stabilise them via damage-control surgery, before referring any who needed more complex secondary interventions across the border to Turkey. However, given the extreme level of risk, most MSF facilities were positioned at a certain distance from the front lines, often in small villages close to the Turkish border.

Despite the huge numbers of wounded generated by the conflict, including from a massive escalation in violence in the nearby city of Aleppo, MSF initially struggled to find relevance. After a preliminary surge of acute injuries, the relatively few wounded patients who came to MSF facilities consisted mainly of "cold cases": individuals seeking the removal of sutures or superficial remnants of bullets and shrapnel that remained after receiving first aid at a field hospital on the front lines several weeks earlier. MSF also received people suffering from severe brain, spine, or nerve injuries that – if repairable at all – were well beyond the capabilities of a makeshift facility. By September, the majority of patients arriving at MSF's trauma centre in Atmeh were suffering from minor ailments or were looking for medicines for their chronic disease. Finding that MSF did not have the drugs that they were seeking, many requested a referral to Turkey to allow them to visit a pharmacy or clinic there before returning to Syria the next day.

Newly recruited Syrian MSF staff explained the underlying issue. Before the war, Syrians considered their health system to be highly sophisticated; at the forefront of advances in technicity and technology. However, the system was essentially run as a private enterprise. Injectable broad-spectrum antibiotics, of the type that in European hospitals would be reserved only for the most severe antibiotic-resistant infections, were freely available at every pharmacy, for those that could afford to pay. Elective Caesarean sections and other non-essential surgical procedures were routinely provided, at a price. Corruption and profiteering inevitably resulted in poor outcomes and massive inequality, but to the Syrian public, that level of technology-on-demand and highly interventional approach was a marker of quality, and that expectation was still maintained now the country had descended into civil war. Even as hospitals were being destroyed, as CT and MRI scanners gathered dust due to the lack of electricity, as laboratories ran out of reagents, and as huge numbers of Syrian medics and surgeons had fled the country, the care that MSF was offering – prescriptions of oral antibiotics, conducting surgery in a converted kitchen – was considered less than acceptable.[8] Operating in such poor conditions could be justified in a field hospital on the front lines (such as the cave hospital, which was so dangerous that the MSF team evacuated after a short time), but even the armed groups preferred their wounded to then be referred to private Syrian facilities or across the border to Turkey. People that could afford to pay for their care were suspicious that MSF provided everything for free and assumed that MSF hospitals were mainly providing basic medical treatment for the poor and the displaced.

In addition, MSF had inadvertently entered into competition with the Syrian private system. Although many had fled, the remaining Syrian medics continued to operate from private clinics and hospitals away from the front lines, in the same pro-opposition areas where MSF was now setting up its centres. They received huge support from Arab states, sympathetic to the opposition cause, and from Syrian diaspora groups. Newly appointed "civil councils" were tasked with distributing a steady flow of medical supplies, equipment, and cash, which in the initial years of the war could still relatively easily cross the porous

Turkish border. MSF could not – and did not want to – compete with a support system that provided shipments of thousands of blood bags when there was no capacity for screening the blood for viruses and no electricity to refrigerate it after collection, nor with a system which encouraged the over-prescription of intravenous antibiotics, and which supplied surgical equipment for Caesarean sections and routine surgeries without any reassurance regarding the competence of the surgical team, and without the necessary means of sterilising the equipment between patients. In one newly installed field hospital, the MSF team was instructed to leave by the local militia within weeks of opening, after consistently refusing access to the local surgeon to conduct private non-urgent surgeries using MSF drugs and equipment.

MSF had entered Syria with the logical ambition to offer trauma surgery, which from the outside seemed to be the most pressing need, but had ended up trying to provide that care in the wrong places. Newly arriving international staff, expecting to be managing mass casualties day and night, quickly became frustrated. After accepting an extremely high level of risk by crossing the border without the authorisation of the Syrian government, they did not feel that their work was adequately useful to justify that risk.

At the end of 2012, having established a foothold in northern Syria, MSF decided to move closer to the epicentre of the violence: the city of Aleppo. They hoped there to find more operational relevance for MSF, thereby justifying the risks taken. After a couple of assessment visits made by two separate teams, a two-person international team was sent to Al-Bab, a city just to the east of Aleppo where it was reported that the majority of the wounded were being treated after initial first aid. Preliminary instructions were to establish a base location where MSF could offer trauma surgery in Al-Bab, to support the Syrian field hospitals in the eastern half of Aleppo city, and to implement a referral system of ambulances between the two cities.

The Al-Bab team initially faced much the same welcome to MSF's medical intentions as elsewhere, but at much higher risk. Al-Bab, seen as a heartland of the resistance, was bombed nightly. Cars travelling towards East Aleppo were shot at by Syrian Air Force planes and helicopters, and the clandestine field hospitals that MSF was aiming to support were regularly hit by air strikes, or forced to move when informants leaked their locations to Damascus. Huge suspicion was directed towards the two foreigners who had arrived at the front lines of a brutal war claiming to want to provide medical care to the wounded, but who offered only dressings and sterilisation equipment rather than the CT scanners and neurosurgeons that the Syrian medics felt were lacking. Despite intense negotiations, the MSF team was persistently refused permission to set up a trauma surgery service in Al-Bab.

Making a tactical switch, MSF followed the advice of the public health leader of the newly created local civil council to move away from trying to provide MSF-led trauma surgery and focus on supporting the medical system to adapt to the new wartime reality: massive population displacement, an economy in crisis, and the collapse of public services. He recommended starting with the blood bank: East Aleppo's main blood bank had been destroyed in an air strike in the early days of the war, and now there was no access to safe transfusion. MSF set up a clandestine blood bank in an Al-Bab apartment, calling for donations at the local mosques, then screening and manually cross-matching the blood using simple rapid diagnostic tests, before storing it in a fridge powered by a generator and an improvised power bank made from car batteries. Medical structures across the city were provided with blood sample tubes and request forms: anyone arriving at the apartment with both a blood sample and the correct form was issued a unit of safe blood of the appropriate blood type. MSF blood bags were soon being used by all the same hospitals in the city that had refused MSF access to offer trauma care.

MSF began looking for other ways to be useful, introducing tools and protocols to the region that were unfamiliar to Syrian medics but better adapted to the now-collapsed health system. The MSF team worked alongside the volunteers in the field hospitals in Aleppo City, demonstrating the basic principles of triage and trauma resuscitation and the organisation of a response to a mass casualty event. Faced with a shortage of oxygen production facilities, hospitals and ambulances were equipped with oxygen concentrators that could be run by small generators or batteries. Simple protocols were written and rapidly translated into Arabic to guide nurses and pharmacists in how to manage chronic diseases using the limited range of medicines available locally or across the border in Turkey. When MSF was finally allowed to open a new hospital to the east of Al-Bab, the surgical unit was set up to provide Caesarean sections as well as trauma surgery, and the care on offer ranged the full spectrum of emergency medicine, including safe abortion care and the management of acute complications of chronic disease.

Initially, MSF's ambitions in Syria were shaped by the same hubris held by the Syrian medics: that war in Syria was somehow different from war elsewhere; that quality of care was demonstrated through cutting-edge technology and high prices; and that trauma surgery was the pinnacle of sophistication, requiring high-tech equipment and specialists. The gradual recognition by MSF teams and local medics of the value of simple humanitarian medical practices and tools, developed over decades of working in health systems collapsed by conflict, was key to creating the political traction necessary for MSF to negotiate access to act, and to ensure that MSF teams were offered protection by the local authorities. It took moving past the shared hubris to come to a shared understanding of quality for MSF to begin contributing to better patient outcomes, or at least to limiting the harm caused by well-intentioned gestures of support for a system ill-adapted to war.

II Gaza: Between Ambition and Expectation

30 March 2018 marked the beginning of a series of protests in Gaza that would come to be called "The Great March of Return". Demonstrators approached the fence that separated the blockaded territory from Israel, and in some cases

tried to enter it. Israeli forces responded with a hail of bullets, killing 15 people and injuring 773 with live ammunition on that first day alone.[9] Over the next year and a half, some 214 Palestinians were killed during the demonstrations and more than 8,000 were injured by live fire.[10] The vast majority of those people were shot in the lower limbs, causing catastrophic injuries: huge areas of missing bone, large volumes of muscle destroyed, nerves and blood vessels pulverised and severed.

The Gazan health authorities were quickly overwhelmed by the number and severity of the injuries, despite their experience in dealing with mass casualty incidents during the repeated wars that have marked Gaza's recent history. On the bloodiest day of the protests, 14 May 2018, 1,359 people were shot and injured by Israeli forces.[11] Waves of the seriously wounded flooded the emergency rooms of Gaza, causing chaos. While the wounded generally received lifesaving surgery from Ministry of Health (MoH) teams to stop the bleeding, debridement of the wounds was often rushed due to the volume of patients waiting for surgery, and follow-up care was less than optimal. Many patients were discharged from hospital to make room for new wounded before having the further debridement and wound closure that they would require. The risk of infection of the wounds and of the shattered bones within was huge.

The Gazan health authorities were not generally willing to let MSF teams be involved in first-line surgeries. As MSF was already running outpatient clinics for the post-operative follow-up of trauma and burns patients, it initially saw its contribution as being to increase capacity there, performing *"specialised nursing care and wound dressings"*.[12] This quickly expanded to adding surgical resources to *"operate – or re-operate – on the more severe cases"*, as the teams noticed the exceptional severity of the wounds that were being caused:[13]

> *Our patients can be divided into three groups of roughly equal sizes: those who will eventually heal, those who will need extra surgeries to heal, and those who will need specialist reconstructive surgery over the course of years if they are to have any chance of healing.*[14]

The phrasing of the diagnosis of one of the surgeons working in the summer of 2018 in Gaza is telling: the only outcome mentioned is healing, even if the possibility of not healing is implied. No category exists for hopeless cases: those for whom no healing is realistic. And there is no category of people for whom the ordeal of such a long duration of intensely painful treatment, punctuated by recurrent life-threatening infections, might outweigh any potential benefit of keeping a poorly functioning limb.

Our ambition took form over the first few months of the crisis: to quickly implement the specialist reconstructive surgery that we felt was lacking in Gaza in order to save the limbs of our patients, and to eventually return them to a functionality that was as close to their pre-injury state as possible. This was partially influenced by the views of many local medical colleagues, who said that amputation would never be "culturally accepted".[15] The plan for such an advanced programme was built around three poles: introducing new reconstructive surgery techniques, which would rely, at least in part, on outside expertise and the importation of surgical material; the creation of inpatient antibiotic treatment programmes to combat the high prevalence of osteomyelitis, much of it antibiotic resistant;[16] and a pain management plan to care for patients during their long course of treatment, much of which would be extremely arduous.

The implementation of such ambitious medical activities in a context like Gaza was obviously complicated: it needed many different components to work and faced many delays. Often the impression was that the introduction of a long-awaited element of the programme, once up and running, exposed more gaps and issues with the organisation of the project than the gaps and issues that it had been designed to solve.

One challenge was that MSF was not acting alone: teams from two MSF operational centres were present, which resulted in competition and problems in collaboration; the MoH was a strong actor; the World Health Organization (WHO) was supporting the MoH while also trying to guide it in the direction of their own trauma protocols; and other NGOs, like Medical Aid for Palestinians, were also present. Each actor was pushing for the implementation of technically advanced reconstructive surgery, but in ways that differed from one another, with different expectations, different quality standards, and different working methods. This led to occasions where communication was lacking and continuity between surgeries was inadequate: a problem exacerbated by the habit of patients "shopping" around various NGOs when the doctor at one gave them an answer that they did not like.

Fundamentally, however, MSF was locked in a cycle of ambition and expectation: we wanted to help, and we evidently came to consider the primary indicator of success of that help as being limb salvage and complete restoration of limb functionality. That ambition came partially from what we saw as our expertise in reconstruction, given our long-running reconstructive surgery project in Amman,[17] but was also influenced by the expectations of the MoH, who were unwilling to countenance programmes that they viewed as "degraded" medicine. Their expectations expressed themselves in the sophistication of surgical expertise that they wanted to see developed in Gaza, an ambition that went above and beyond the immediate treatment of the wounded. Our vertical programme only partially responded to their lofty institutional ambitions, which led to further demands for support from MSF: support that we did not necessarily want to give. The "quality" and ambition of our proposals, therefore, became a way in which we could justify our added value to the authorities as well as to ourselves.

Another way in which our objectives were shaped by the expectations of the authorities was in their refusal to authorise amputations. All amputations had to be approved by a committee of three MoH surgeons, who, for a mix of personal and political reasons, were very hesitant to do so, even when all medical NGO actors agreed that further treatment would only prolong the patient's suffering, for no gain in functionality.

These ambitions led to sharp debates amongst MSF teams: some surgeons were convinced that with the introduction of new techniques and better antimicrobial stewardship, the limbs could eventually be saved. Others held that the likelihood of a return to the kind of functionality we were aiming for – and that the patient was expecting – was slim in many cases, and that meanwhile the psychological and social costs of the treatment were greater than its benefit. It was necessary to try and arbitrate between metrics of different orders to decide whether we had succeeded in our objectives. Which was more important: freedom from infection, limb functionality, or mental and social well-being? How far should we place the onus on patients to make an "informed choice" about their own future when we could not agree amongst ourselves on what outcomes were technically possible?

Often, we seemed to be motivated by the idea that the lack of access to treatment in Gaza reflected the fundamental injustice of a population locked up in a blockaded, occupied territory. Yet non-MSF surgeons we spoke with said that even in the best-equipped hospitals in the West, the objective of attempting to restore function to potentially unsalvageable limbs would be considered overly ambitious.[18] They pointed to studies from a British military complex trauma rehabilitation centre that demonstrated superior functional gains amongst amputees compared to patients that underwent limb salvage.[19] We can wonder if technicity had come to serve as a sign of solidarity with Palestinians in Gaza – they *should* have access to the same level of care as other people, and therefore we *would* do that, whether it truly reflected their needs and desires and the realities of their situation or not.

For many patients, however, our interventions did permit useful outcomes: around half of all the wounded from the Great March of Return passed through MSF programmes. An osteomyelitis unit run by MSF in collaboration with the MoH finally opened towards the end of 2019, just as the protests were winding down, providing a level of advanced treatment for some of the most complicated cases until it closed in 2022. In parallel, the attitude of the MoH softened towards amputations after it became clear that some cases would require it, no matter what, and the decision-making process was changed, with the abolition of the amputation committee.

We had wanted to do something noble: to provide a level of care that was unavailable in a place suffering the double violence of a blockade and repression. Yet we had come up against both the practical difficulty of instituting that care in a form that was effective for the people we were trying to help, and the medico-ethical dilemma of whether it was really the best option for some of those same people.[20] In both cases, we were simultaneously negotiating and renegotiating our own expectations and those of the MoH about what MSF should and could do – and in both cases, we can ask where and if the voice of the patient was truly heard.

III Aden: Missing the Essentials

In the early part of 2020, the news of, and rumours about, COVID-19 swept Aden, in southern Yemen, just like the rest of the world. There was, for a time, a hope that Yemen could somehow be different; a belief that it would avoid the virus. Perhaps that was born from the fear of what consequences the pandemic might have for a country that had been at war for years, whose authorities were divided, and whose health system was already on its knees.[21]

The first case of COVID-19 was confirmed in Hadhramout on 10 April. In Aden, it became clear through the CT scans being shared in doctors' WhatsApp groups that the disease was also circulating there, and the first cases in the city were confirmed by polymerase chain reaction (PCR) tests on 29 April.

Deciding how to try to respond to the spread of the virus was complicated for the authorities by a strong fear of the disease within the general population and amongst healthcare workers. Some inhabitants of the area around MSF's trauma hospital threatened to kill the director of a neighbouring hospital if she let the MoH place an isolation centre there. Staff fled from emergency departments and intensive care units when suspected COVID-19 cases presented, complaining of a lack of protective material.

Finally, the southern separatists, who had taken control of the city in 2019 – but allowed certain government institutions, including the health authorities, to continue working – grew impatient with the MoH's faltering efforts to lead a response, and identified a disused cancer hospital ten kilometres from the centre of the city as the structure where suspected cases would be isolated and care provided to those infected.

Very quickly, however, it became clear that the health authorities could not cope with even the few cases a day that managed to make it out to the centre. The MSF coordinator at the time said that they knew that they were going to be asked by the authorities to take over the centre, and that there was an expectation from MSF headquarters to do something about COVID-19, even though the necessary staff, equipment, and medications were not available. Despite the lack of resources, the coordinator proposed to the authorities to do more at the hospital, and was glad when it was suggested that MSF take over running the structure entirely at the beginning of May, because – he said – it was easier to manage something 100% MSF than to try working in a mixed set-up.[22]

"We were immediately overwhelmed: we built the project around the patients" was the conclusion of a logistician who went on to be one of the project coordinators.[23] The challenges were huge: the patients were initially split between two buildings, some hundreds of metres apart, which had none of the essential oxygen supply infrastructure; given the need to be up and running immediately, recruiting skilled staff proved impossible, and the staff that were seconded by the MoH lacked the intensive care skills necessary to care for the patients; protective equipment and the basic drugs needed to safely sedate and paralyse ventilated patients remained absent; and MSF was working in an instable security situation where fear and anger surrounding COVID-19 exposed the staff to serious risk.

By the time the project closed in July, the monumental efforts of the team had overcome many of these issues. Yet some problems had been insurmountable, particularly the late arrival and serious conditions of the patients. Of the 365 patients admitted to the structure, 59% died. The peak of admissions, in

May, coincided with the time when much of what was needed for the project to provide even basic care at an acceptable level was still under construction.

When the project began, the general medical consensus worldwide was still that early intubation and invasive ventilation was the best course of action for serious COVID-19 patients.[24] MSF medics also initially adopted this approach. Even though it was known to be a challenging and technically demanding medical intervention, requiring extensive training and clinical expertise, it accorded with what was thought to be best practice, and it aligned with the expectations of healthcare staff and the relatives of patients in Aden. The cultural norm there tended to lead to a desire to see all possible tools used in the effort to save a life, and palliation did not form part of usual medical practice. It remained difficult to convince Yemeni staff and relatives that early intubation was not the right decision. Even when later evidence demonstrated that better results emerged with non-invasive ventilation, we were expected to "do everything" although it was clear that a patient was dying, despite intubation and invasive ventilation sometimes prolonging life for people for whom the chance of survival was almost nil and whose suffering we could not rule out, due to the low quality of the sedatives available.

In light of the poor outcomes, the decision to continue to intubate and ventilate patients was later called into question by other intensivists and operational staff:

> *I think if our outcomes were different I'd be all in favour of doing everything we possibly can but at the moment, we don't have all the steps in that chain that you need for someone to survive ICU and so what we're doing at the moment is not even a half-measure, it's a quarter-measure for what they need, it's enough for people to feel like they've made a start but it's not enough for people to finish, and I guess there's a moral quandary in that, which I don't know the answer to.*[25]

In the end, only one patient who was intubated would live to be extubated, following a transfer to another facility. The death rate in the intensive care unit (ICU) was 84%; the 16% of patients that survived were those who were treated with non-invasive ventilation.

Again, as in Gaza, there is a conjunction between a desire, internal to MSF, to do as much as possible to help – including by opening an ICU in conditions where we knew that we would not have all the necessary resources – and an external expectation around the type of care to be offered, which led us to an attempt to implement technically advanced solutions in a setting where it was difficult to do so.

The logistician-turned-project coordinator who closed the project noted in his report that, while it was technically feasible to intubate patients, we were missing all the other essential components to produce good outcomes for those patients: nursing skills, physiotherapy, drugs to maintain and control sedation, and dialysis. Had we let the technicity of intubation come to be the symbol of our dedication in the face of insurmountable odds, even when other techniques emerged as possibilities? There were further debates in the team about the wisdom of having chosen to be so intensively involved in case management when there was also potential to participate in community activities.

Again, the desire to save lives, combined with the expectations of the authorities and a preference for doing things "our" way, led us to set up a programme whose ambitions were difficult, if not impossible, to realise. Our push for technicity had made sense at the time, but in the end put staff in positions that exposed them to intense stress and trauma and meant that some patients had less than ideal end-of-life care.

IV Niger: Missing the Mark

Sometimes MSF's political or medical ambitions are represented through technology – even a product – rather than a technique. From early 2020, as the COVID-19 pandemic spread rapidly across the globe, it did not affect all countries and all populations equally. During the initial months of the outbreak, scientists, public health physicians, and epidemiologists worldwide struggled to understand this novel disease: how it was transmitted, the clinical consequences of infection, and, most crucially, how best to respond, with no techniques or products proven to effectively treat or prevent infection. Most countries initially adopted the same approach as China, swiftly setting up COVID-19 centres to isolate en masse not only the sick but also their immediate contacts, in an attempt to stop the spread of the virus. The futility of this strategy was reinforced in later months and years, when it was demonstrated that infected people could remain asymptomatic yet still pass on the disease to others, and that the virus could spread via airborne transmission.[26]

In high-income countries of the Global North, the worst-affected categories of patients became immediately clear: people of older ages, particularly those over 80 years old or confined to nursing homes, and people with certain comorbidities.[27] The world watched in horror as military vehicles carried coffins out of Bergamo, Italy, where more than 600 nursing home residents died between 7 and 27 March 2020.[28] However, the same pattern of disease was not necessarily seen elsewhere. In the Middle East and North Africa, South Asia, and Latin America, the cohorts developing critical illnesses and dying appeared to be younger. Early predictions suggested that when the pandemic finally "hit" sub-Saharan African countries, with their fragile health systems and limited capacity for hospitalisation and provision of intensive care, the consequences would be catastrophic.[29]

MSF, as detailed above in relation to Yemen, initially focused on the care of COVID-19 patients. In MSF projects across the world, teams concentrated their efforts on setting up treatment centres, trying to obtain or generate oxygen supplies, and acquiring ventilators. In some locations, MSF suspended routine activities entirely. In others, MSF teams developed innovative ways of continuing to deliver care to existing patients, despite being hampered by global supply chain issues, local curfews and lockdowns, and fear.[30] In many countries, MSF had to tackle new medical crises that were created or exacerbated by the restrictive measures imposed by authorities in an attempt to contain the spread of the pandemic.[31]

In the meantime, new vaccines against COVID-19 were developed, trialled, manufactured, and rolled out in record time.[32] The different vaccine technologies all produced the same result: they could not prevent infection or eradicate the virus, but they did make infection significantly more trivial. The UK was the first country to launch its national COVID-19 vaccination programme; perhaps justified, given that England and Wales had some of the highest excess mortality rates by the time the first vaccine was administered on 8 December 2020.[33] Other high-income countries soon followed suit. Actors from the Access to Medicines movement, including MSF's Access Campaign,[34] quickly called foul. For them, the fact that vaccines were initially being rolled out in high-income countries, mainly in the Global North, was just another example of systemic global injustice and the perpetuation of inequalities for countries in the Global South, rooted in legacies of colonialism, globalisation, and capitalism. The new vaccine became a symbol to support a global political campaign that ran wider than MSF's medical operations.

MSF was also not satisfied with the efforts of COVAX, a multilateral collaboration between the Global Alliance for Vaccines and Immunization (GAVI), the Coalition for Epidemic Preparedness Innovations (CEPI), the United Nations Children's Fund (UNICEF), and WHO, which aimed at delivering *"a truly global solution to this pandemic"*, where *"people in all corners of the world will get access to COVID-19 vaccines once they are available, regardless of their wealth"*.[35] In late 2021, MSF's Access Campaign condemned COVAX as *"a broken promise to the world"*, and recommended immediate adjustments to secure increased and more equitable distribution of COVID vaccines to low-income countries.[36] Lively internal debates ensued within MSF about how far – and how – to try to influence COVAX, including by pushing for the creation of a humanitarian buffer mechanism that would ensure vaccine access for excluded populations.

Meanwhile in Niger, as in most other sub-Saharan African countries, the predicted COVID-19 catastrophe never transpired. After adapting to the initial disruption caused by travel bans and closed borders, MSF project teams in Niger continued their usual activities, which for 20 years have mainly aimed at limiting child mortality linked to high rates of malnutrition, malaria, and other infectious diseases.[37] During 2021, the second year of the COVID-19 pandemic, MSF teams supported the response to multiple infectious disease epidemics, namely a larger-than-usual measles outbreak, and a cholera outbreak that spread across seven regions of the country, including the capital, Niamey.[38] However, throughout the country, the dedicated COVID isolation units, generally tents that had rapidly been erected in the compounds of district hospitals, remained empty.

In November 2021, the West African experience of the COVID-19 pandemic was the theme at the annual scientific conference of CERMES, Niger's national centre for medical and public health research.[39] This was an opportunity for the region's leading scientists and public health authorities to recap the situation and consider what lessons West African countries could learn for the future, including regarding the COVID-19 vaccination programme.

Data presented at the conference determined that, in contrast to the experience of countries like the UK and Italy, COVID-19 in Niger appeared to be a relatively benign disease. Despite performing nearly 200,000 COVID-19 PCR tests, and detecting 6,589 confirmed cases, only 227 deaths of people infected with COVID-19 had occurred across the whole country since March 2020. Seroprevalence surveys amongst healthcare workers demonstrated that the vast majority had antibodies, and so had contracted the virus, yet only a small proportion could remember having had any symptoms consistent with COVID-19 infection, and those were invariably mild.

By the time the conference was held, Niger had received 2.2 million doses of COVID-19 vaccine, mainly via the COVAX mechanism. Vaccination teams were struggling to convince people who did not fully trust the vaccine to accept the doses that were offered to them. Almost half the population did not believe that the disease was real; the rest just assumed that COVID-19 was unlikely to cause them a serious problem.[40] Despite only managing to administer just under half of the vaccines they had, the country was due to receive a further 3 million doses over the coming months. Given logistical and human resource limitations, routine vaccination programmes – including for childhood diseases such as measles, meningitis, and diphtheria – had been suspended to divert capacity towards the COVID-19 campaign.

During a lively debate about the situation, attendees at the conference expressed concern at Niger receiving far more COVID-19 vaccines than it could deliver, and at the pressure the country was under to use them. They questioned the need to continue such huge efforts towards the mass administration of a vaccine which only results in an infection being more trivial, given that the disease was anyway so benign in Niger. One participant noted an apparent hypocrisy: while Niger faced ten times more deaths from rabies than COVID-19 annually, it had never been supported to obtain and administer rabies vaccines on anywhere near the necessary scale, by WHO, MSF, or any other actor. Another pointed out that Niger, due to multiple obstacles, had also never achieved adequate measles vaccine coverage; now that routine measles vaccination had been suspended, the country was likely to face an imminent catastrophic outbreak.

The conclusion of the discussion was that this was just yet another example of the lack of power that resource-limited countries like Niger have against the dominant discourse of wealthy states, and of "Western" global health actors, such as WHO and GAVI. Not without precedent, the West was offering poor countries a solution to a problem they did not have, and ignoring the problems they did have. Yet, if Niger was to challenge the necessity to vaccinate the majority of its population against COVID-19, it would be labelled as "ignorant".

We acknowledge that not every country in the Global South was spared the direct consequences of the COVID-19 pandemic: India experienced a massive outbreak; Peru had one of the highest mortality rates linked to COVID-19 infection globally. However, we can question if, by not adequately challenging COVAX's ambition to vaccinate the whole world, whatever the epidemiological situation, and publicly pushing for increased distribution of vaccines across every country in the Global South in order to support a long-standing global political campaign, MSF inadvertently contributed to the disruption of health systems and the reduced provision of vital prevention of other infectious diseases in countries like Niger.

This illustration may seem slightly different from the others in this chapter, but what it reveals is the process by which a technique or a technology can become mere technicity when it is divorced from political and social realities. MSF's ambition to bring about systemic global change, using the example of the COVID-19 vaccine, ultimately contributed to – or at least did not adequately argue against – the imposition of a new technology that Niger did not need, and reduced access to the existing technologies that they did: technologies that were already in critically short supply.

V Conclusion

At the beginning of this chapter, we said that the humanitarian medical gesture was a humble one, but one whose aspirations could easily grow. Through these four case studies, we have seen how a combination of good intentions and poorly defined or unrealistic expectations prompted MSF to try to implement ambitious actions that caused logistical, operational, and ethical problems and led us to question aspects of our response, in one way or another.

Frequently, what MSF teams attempted was previously untested or untried: implementing a level 3 ICU in a wedding hall in Yemen; creating the capacity for high-level reconstructive surgery in a blockaded Gaza. This might seem to align with the same daring innovative spirit that marks MSF's contributions to the development of the technique of humanitarian medicine: trying something new in order to give people access to care that they did not have before.

Yet, as our examples have shown, these efforts to implement technicity differ subtly but importantly from the development and innovation of humanitarian medicine as a technique. While medical humanitarian technique aims to adapt the tool or the practice to the context in which it is being applied, ambitions towards the global implementation of technicity attempt to bypass or ignore the contextual difficulties: they assume a neutral field on which technicity can be brought to bear.

This can lead to an ironic outcome, in which efforts to erase differences in access to healthcare can result in proposing solutions that ignore the specificities of the people that we are trying to treat, as well as the characteristics of their societies. In wanting to see everyone as the same, we eventually pay less attention to what each individual wants or needs. In deciding not to negotiate or adapt our response to fit the specific environment or ecosystem in which we are working, we end up imposing a top-down "solution" on those whose needs and demands could have produced another form of response.

For humanitarianism to remain fit for purpose when operating at the expansive global scale of today, medical humanitarians will have to continue to reflect on their level of ambition, to ensure that we do not prioritise technicity over technique and that we do not succumb to an egalitarian ideal where everyone in the whole world has access to the "standards" set by Western medicine. That does not mean that some people deserve less good care than others; rather, what counts as good care will differ from place to place and situation to situation. This cuts both ways, of course: local authorities are often just as invested in proposing technically advanced solutions, sometimes for "good" reasons – wanting to develop the level of the local health system – and sometimes for "bad" ones – continuing their own private gains.

Finally, if medical humanitarian organisations do manage to maintain the momentum towards "person-centred" innovation,[41] then it is possible to refrain from continuing the binary debates of the past about humanitarianism vs. development. By introducing, improving, and ensuring access to tools and techniques that are adapted to the problems faced by the people they aim to assist, humanitarian medics contribute to providing better care in the short-term – and when they marry medical innovation with political savvy, the techniques they develop can even make a lasting difference.

Notes

1 See Melissa McRae's contribution on the "greater good" in humanitarian medicine (Chapter 5).
2 Brauman, 2009.
3 Bradol and Vidal (eds), 2011.
4 See Neuman, 2017.
5 OHCHR, 2023.
6 Khaldi, 2020, pp. 48–57.
7 2012 briefing to one of the authors, in MSF Paris HQ.
8 2012 conversations between one of the authors and Syrian MSF staff in Idlib and Aleppo.
9 Balousha and Holmes, 2018.
10 OCHA, 2020.
11 OCHA, 2018.
12 MSF, 2018a.
13 MSF, 2018b.
14 MSF, 2018c.
15 It remains a matter of some debate as to how true this is – is it that amputation is not culturally accepted, or is any amputation that is not adequately explained often instinctively rejected by many people around the world? Who gets to be the "local expert", and what legitimacy they have to speak on behalf of those they claim to represent, is always a fraught question in humanitarian operations. Most

importantly, what those wounded individuals truly would have wanted remains unknown, and this chapter can get no closer to really answering that question.

16 Kanapathipillai et al., 2018.
17 MSF, 2017.
18 Advice to one of the authors from a selection of British civilian and military trauma and orthopaedic surgeons.
19 Ladlow et al., 2016, pp. 1996–2005.
20 The medical ethical dilemma can be summed up as, should you continue doing painful surgeries on people for whom you know that they are essentially useless? Some medical personnel felt that we drifted into doing harm in a limited number of cases, despite – or perhaps because of – our good intentions.
21 See MSF, 2020b and Koum Besson et al., 2021.
22 Details taken from interview with Thierry Durand, project coordinator, May 2020.
23 Taken from the person concerned's end-of-mission report.
24 Grotberg and Kraft, 2023.
25 Interview with Dr Rachel Lister, intensive care doctor for the project, 29 June 2020.
26 The WHO did not describe COVID-19 transmission as "airborne" until December 2021, two years after the emergence of the virus. Studies demonstrating that asymptomatic carriers were able to transmit COVID-19 were initially published in early 2021.
27 Jalil, 2020.
28 Trabucchi and Leo, 2020, pp. 387–8.
29 Paintsil, 2020, pp. 2741–4.
30 MSF, 2020a.
31 MSF, 2020c.
32 Glassman, Kenny, and Yang, 2022.
33 Islam et al., 2021.
34 The Access Campaign is an international project within MSF, launched in 1999 to support MSF's work by advocating for improved access to treatment and the development of better medicines. See https://msfaccess.org/.
35 Berkley, 2020.
36 MSF Access Campaign, 2021.
37 See https://www.msf.org/niger.
38 IFRC, 2022.
39 Ibrahim and Yahaya, 2021.
40 Anecdotal evidence reported at the 2022 CERMES Scientific Conference.
41 Person-centred care considers the individual needs of patients and respects their autonomy to manage their own healthcare choices, based on advice from healthcare professionals.

References

Balousha, Hazem, and Oliver Holmes (2018), 'Palestinians Hold Day of Mourning after 773 "Shot with Live Ammunition"', *The Guardian*, 31 March. [https://www.theguardian.com/world/2018/mar/31/palestinians-hold-day-of-mourning-after-773-shot-with-live-ammunition].

Berkley, Seth (2020), 'COVAX Explained', *VaccinesWork*. [https://www.gavi.org/vaccineswork/covax-explained].

Bradol, Jean-Hervé, and Claudine Vidal (eds), *Medical Innovations in Humanitarian Situations: The Work of Médecins Sans Frontières*, CreateSpace Independent Publishing Platform, 2011.

Brauman, Rony (2009), *Humanitarian Medicine*, Paris: Presses Universitaires de France. [https://msf-crash.org/en/medicine-and-public-health/humanitarian-medicine].

Glassman, Amanda, Charles Kenny, and George Yang (2022), 'COVID-19 Vaccine Development and Rollout in Historical Perspective', Center for Global Development (Working Paper 607). [https://www.cgdev.org/publication/covid-19-vaccine-development-and-rollout-historical-perspective].

Grotberg, John C., and Bryan D.Kraft (2023), 'Timing of Intubation in COVID-19: When It Is Too Early and When It Is Too Late', *Critical Care Explorations*, vol. 5, n° 2, p. e0863. doi:10.1097/CCE.0000000000000863.

Ibrahim, Abdoul-Aziz, and Nafissa Yahaya (2021), '3èmes Journées Scientifiques du CERMES: Echanges et réflexions sur la situation de la COVID-19 en Afrique de l'Ouest', *Le Sahel*, 11 November. [https://www.lesahel.org/3emes-journees-scientifiques-du-cermes-echanges-et-reflexions-sur-la-situation-de-la-covid-19-en-afrique-de-louest/].

IFRC (2022), 'Niger: Cholera Outbreak Final Report'. 2 September. [https://reliefweb.int/report/niger/niger-cholera-outbreak-2021-final-report-dref-operation-mdrne025].

Islam, Nazrul, Vladimir M. Shkolnikov, Rolando J. Acosta, Ilya Klimkin, Ichiro Kawachi, Rafael A. Irizarry, Gianfranco Alicandro, et al. (2021), 'Excess Deaths Associated with Covid-19 Pandemic in 2020: Age and Sex Disaggregated Time Series Analysis in 29 High Income Countries', *BMJ*, vol. 373, p. n1137. doi:10.1136/bmj.n1137.

Jalil, Abduladheem Turki (2020), 'COVID-19 Most Affected Age Groups and Lethality in Europe', *Global Journal of Public Health Medicine*, vol. 2, n° SP1, pp. 179–184. doi:10.37557/gjphm.v2iSP1.51.

Kanapathipillai, Rupa, Nada Malou, Kate Baldwin, Pascale Marty, Camille Rodaix, Clair Mills, Patrick Herard, and Malika Saim (2018), 'Antibiotic Resistance in Palestine: An Emerging Part of a Larger Crisis', *BMJ*, vol. 363, p. k4273. doi:10.1136/bmj.k4273.

Khaldi, Hakim (2020), 'Humanitarian Field Practices in the Context of the Syrian Conflict from 2011 to 2018', *Journal of Humanitarian Affairs*, vol. 2, n° 2, pp. 48–57. doi:10.7227/JHA.043.

Koum Besson, Emilie S., Andy Norris, Abdulla S. Bin Ghouth, Terri Freemantle, Mervat Alhaffar, Yolanda Vazquez, Chris Reeve, Patrick J. Curran, and Francesco Checchi (2021), 'Excess Mortality during the COVID-19 Pandemic: A Geospatial and Statistical Analysis in Aden Governorate, Yemen', *BMJ Global Health*, vol. 6, n° 3, p. e004564. doi:10.1136/bmjgh-2020–004564.

Ladlow, Peter, Rhodri Phillip, Russell Coppack, John Etherington, James Bilzon, M. Polly McGuigan, and Alexander N. Bennett (2016), 'Influence of Immediate and Delayed Lower-Limb Amputation Compared with Lower-Limb Salvage on Functional and Mental Health Outcomes Post-Rehabilitation in the U.K. Military', *JBJS*, vol. 98, n° 23, pp. 1996–2005. doi:10.2106/JBJS.15.01210.

MSF, 'Niger | MSF Medical and Humanitarian Aid'. [https://www.msf.org/niger].

MSF (2017), 'Jordan: A Decade of Healing at MSF's Reconstructive Surgery Hospital', 20 December. [https://www.msf.org/jordan-decade-healing-msf%E2%80%99s-reconstructive-surgery-hospital].

MSF (2018a), 'Palestine: MSF Increases Medical Efforts for Wounded in Gaza Strip', 5 April. [https://www.msf.org/palestine-msf-increases-medical-efforts-wounded-gaza-strip].

MSF (2018b), 'Palestine: MSF Teams in Gaza Observe Unusually Severe and Devastating Gunshot Injuries', 19 April. [https://www.msf.org/palestine-msf-teams-gaza-observe-unusually-severe-and-devastating-gunshot-injuries].

MSF (2018c), 'Gaza: A Long Ordeal Awaits Hundreds of Wounded from the March of Return', 8 August. [https://www.msf.org/gaza-long-ordeal-awaits-hundreds-wounded-march-return].

MSF (2020a), 'COVID-19: "It Was Never an Option for Us to Drop Our Regular Medical Services"', 3 June. [https://msf.org.uk/article/covid-19-it-was-never-option-us-drop-our-regular-medical-services].

MSF (2020b), 'Coronavirus COVID-19 has made Yemen's health system collapse complete', 10 June. [https://www.msf.org/covid-19-has-made-yemen-health-system-collapse-complete].

MSF (2020c), 'Women Face Greater Danger during COVID-19 Pandemic', 2 July. [https://www.msf.org/women-and-girls-face-greater-dangers-during-covid-19-pandemic].

MSF Access Campaign (2021), 'COVAX: A Broken Promise to the World', 21 December. [https://msfaccess.org/covax-broken-promise-world].

Neuman, Michaël (2017), 'Dying for humanitarian ideas: Using images and statistics to manufacture humanitarian martyrdom', *Centre de réflexion sur l'action et les savoirs humanitaires*. [https://msf-crash.org/en/humanitarian-actors-and-practices/dying-humanitarian-ideas-using-images-and-statistics-manufacture].

OCHA (2018), 'Fifty-Five Palestinians killed and thousands injured in Gaza', 14 May. [https://www.ochaopt.org/content/fifty-five-palestinians-killed-and-thousands-injured-gaza].

OCHA (2020), 'Two years on: people injured and traumatized during the "Great March of Return" are still struggling', 6 April. [https://www.ochaopt.org/content/two-years-people-injured-and-traumatized-during-great-march-return-are-still-struggling].

OHCHR (2023), 'Behind the data: Recording civilian casualties in Syria', 11 May. [https://www.ohchr.org/en/stories/2023/05/behind-data-recording-civilian-casualties-syria].

Paintsil, Elijah (2020), 'COVID-19 Threatens Health Systems in Sub-Saharan Africa: The Eye of the Crocodile', *The Journal of Clinical Investigation*, vol. 130, n° 6, pp. 2741–2744. doi:10.1172/JCI138493.

Trabucchi, Marco, and Diego De Leo (2020), 'Nursing Homes or Besieged Castles: COVID-19 in Northern Italy', *The Lancet Psychiatry*, vol. 7, n° 5, pp. 387–388. doi:10.1016/S2215–0366(20)30149–30148.

5 Global Health Security in Humanitarian Medicine

What Is the Greater Good?

Melissa McRae

Over the past four decades, health issues, in particular emerging infectious diseases, have been increasingly framed as security threats, legitimising the use of restrictive public health emergency measures and, at times, portraying less wealthy states as vectors of disease threats.[1] Conflating health with security was originally conceptualised to reduce the degree of health inequity faced by vulnerable individuals and minorities. However, in practice, it is now a state-led public health approach that prioritises the needs of the population majority as they align with state strategic interests.[2] Wealthy countries are accused of dominating this space to prioritise emerging diseases from afar which pose the greatest threat to their military, political, and economic interests. Consequently, global health funds are diverted away from non-emerging infectious diseases which continue to cause preventable morbidity and mortality in conflict zones and less wealthy states.[3] The role of humanitarian assistance within global health security is not well-defined, despite calls for Médecins Sans Frontières (MSF) to increase its "health security actorness".[4] This raises an ethical dilemma: what is the greater good? Supporting state-led health services will reach more people and help promptly end an outbreak. On the other hand, the humanitarian imperative guides MSF to assist those most in need, often disadvantaged or oppressed by state-led structural barriers – reaching fewer people, but likely addressing health equity gaps within state populations and perhaps delivering a more morally impactful humanitarian greater good.

Global health security (hereinafter referred to as "health security") is a popular but fluid concept, constantly adapted to overcome the disconnect between theory and practice. Alongside the World Health Organization (WHO), the United States (US) remains at the forefront of defining it: *"the existence of strong and resilient public health systems that can prevent, detect, and respond to emerging infectious disease threats, wherever they occur in the world"*.[5] However, other health security frameworks now extend well beyond outbreak preparedness and response, to address weak health systems, health financing, and universal health coverage (UHC). WHO includes infectious diseases, biological or chemical agents, and ionising radiation among threats leading to a public health emergency of international concern (PHEIC), whether accidental, natural, or deliberate.[6] The International Health Regulations (IHR) of 2005

DOI: 10.4324/9781003542247-10

outline states' minimum legal obligations in such events, both to their citizens and to other states.[7] As far as guiding ethical frameworks, health security leans heavily on public health ethics, in particular consequentialist utilitarianism: the right moral action is what brings the greatest good to the greatest number of people, often knowingly accepting a smaller calculated harm.[8] Interestingly, utilitarianism also guides humanitarian medical action, although, as explored in this chapter, determining the greater good is limited to a narrowed humanitarian target population rather than the entire state population. MSF is self-mandated to act according to the humanitarian imperative, helping those most in need, which does not necessarily mean the largest number.[9]

A handful of outbreaks have been instrumental in shaping the current health security narrative: avian flu (H5N1), swine flu (H1N1), Ebola, COVID-19, and, most recently, mpox. Despite the COVID-19 pandemic making existing global and national health inequities glaringly obvious, health security "in practice" did not emerge stronger. Many states enacted nationalistic and protectionist health policies, with little uniformity in how governments adapted their containment and response measures (quarantine and lockdown). In different corners of the globe, individuals' lived COVID-19 experiences were contingent on how *their* state's pandemic response secured *their* health. For lower-income states, the pandemic reinforced their status quo; preventable but persistent diseases linked to hunger and poverty remained the highest threat to their population's health, especially those under five years of age.[10] As all resources pivoted towards the fight against COVID-19, the wealthiest 1% of the globe took nearly two-thirds of new wealth generated.[11] Both during the COVID-19 pandemic and other outbreaks, socially disadvantaged groups were the worst off within state populations.[12] These world realities remain implementation barriers, reinforcing sceptics' views that health security demands an unrealistic level of global governance reform led by altruistic leaders concerned about the plight of those beyond their borders.[13] Conceptually, health security is a borderless solution to complex global health inequities which refer to different health outcomes for different groups of people. Health inequities are not biological but structurally created by macro-level social forces (such as poverty, racism, gender inequality, political violence, and conflict), which are underpinned by state policies, global governance, and cultural norms. They expand with unfair wealth and power distribution, poor governance, corruption, and political indifference to the highest health needs, both within state populations and between states. Inequities can also be forced upon one state by a more powerful state through trade agreements, financial loans, foreign policy agendas, and health security frameworks.[14]

Much has already been written on health security, predominantly by those who believe it to be the solution to creating a better world in a postcolonial era: United Nations organisations, wealthy states, and public health academics. This chapter adds to the discourse by unpacking the ethical dilemma faced by MSF in terms of the greater good: should the organisation assist as many people as possible or fewer people who are disproportionally suffering? The briefest of accounts of health security's evolution follows, acknowledging that more in-depth accounts can be found elsewhere, then an overview of two different health security approaches: one that puts state needs and the population majority first, while the other prioritises vulnerable minorities. Both can be framed as a greater good; hence the ethical dilemma. Finally, MSF's approach within what is argued as an increasingly state-dominated health security space is reflected upon. Two important limitations exist: firstly, health security is far broader than this chapter's deliberate focus on emerging infectious diseases, but any complete analysis would fill a book, not a chapter; secondly, while the author portrays MSF's positioning from their own experience, MSF does not represent all that is humanitarian, but is one among many who collaboratively deliver humanitarian assistance.

I From Human Security in 1994 to Health Security in 2024

> *Pandemics, health emergencies and weak health systems not only cost lives but pose some of the greatest risks to the global economy and security faced today.*[15]
>
> (WHO)

The Briefest of Histories

The motivation to converge human health with the security domain is not hard to conceptually grasp: diseases do not respect borders; conflict and other forms of violence cause preventable mortality and morbidity; and morally problematic health inequities exist between and within states. Like security, health is a state obligation, and investing in citizens' health not only improves well-being but ensures an economically viable and military-ready population.[16] However, national security is limited to protecting the people and interests of one sovereign state, whilst global health is borderless, working to improve the health of all people within and across states.[17] This raises questions of how the humanitarian objectives, public health, and national security interests can really intersect to address health inequities faced by populations, minorities, and disadvantaged groups.

The HIV/AIDS epidemic (1980s–1990s) is cited as the origin of both the terms "emerging infectious diseases" and "health security".[18] HIV/AIDS' high transmissibility and fatality coincided with increasing political willingness to extend security thinking beyond the nationalistic military models of the Cold War era.[19] In its *Human Development Report*, the UN Development Programme (UNDP) introduced the concept of "human security", including health, economic, food, political, and environmental security.[20] UNDP outlined states' responsibilities towards individual human rights: foremost, upholding human rights and ensuring individual and societal welfare rather than strengthening state interests. The report claimed that, for most people, it is not military threats abroad, the traditional focus on national security, that bring a sense of insecurity, but threats closer to home that disrupt daily life: insufficient food, no access to healthcare, gender-based violence, or living in an oppressive state.[21] This framing linked "structural violence"[22] as the driving force behind inequities: systemic inequitable social forces or arrangements, perpetuated by state institutions and formal social structures that prevent individuals or populations from meeting their basic needs.[23] Framing threats of torture by a state and violence directed against women (rape, domestic violence) as security challenges was considered pioneering at the time, within UN circles.[24]

Ultimately, human security's acceptance and policy impact were marginal.[25] Two subsequent events helped frame the state-led health security narrative we have today. In 2000, the UN Security Council (UNSC) urged the security community to reprioritise resources to mitigate the impact of high HIV/AIDS prevalence among strategically important populations: soldiers and peacekeepers. Acknowledging the complexity of this analysis, concerns included peacekeepers spreading HIV/AIDS while on mission, loss of military staffing capacity, and high HIV treatment costs, leading militaries to seek higher proportions of public expenditure whilst less able to protect national interests. To many, health security had become a vehicle to prioritise the health of military troops above vulnerable civilians – a perspective that took decades to shift. Then, the leading authority in global public health joined the discussion, rebranding health security as a responsibility of states towards other states and their own populations at large. WHO's 2007 World Health Report, titled *A Safer Future: Global Public Health Security in the 21st Century*, supported the "*highest level of global health security possible*".[26] The report did not mention individual security or humanitarian medicine, nor did it acknowledge that state actions may be a threat to individual health.[27] WHO advocated to reduce global health inequities, measured by comparing the health status of one state population with that of another (e.g. Germany and Sierra Leone), putting the emphasis on helping the greatest number of people. Without being sidetracked by the IHR, WHO's report coincided with the implementation of the IHR revision (2005), promoting strengthened detection, reporting, and cooperation between states. This rebranding was not warmly received by all UN member states: in 2008, Brazil argued that health security "*had no clear meaning and enjoyed no consensus among members of the World Health Assembly*",[28] and Indonesia controversially halted the sharing of human avian flu viral samples with WHO until assured of an equal benefit from intellectual property rights and profits.[29] In 2007, Indonesia had the highest number of human cases, and health minister Siti Fadilah Supari claimed samples provided freely were leveraged by companies in wealthy countries for profit, producing biotechnologies that Indonesia would not be able to afford: "*If the world continues to operate in this way [...] The poor will become poorer, and the rich become richer. It is the responsibility of all nations to change this situation.*"[30]

Jumping forward to 2014, and two-thirds of WHO member states were not IHR-compliant. In the midst of the West African Ebola epidemic (2014–16), the US launched the Global Health Security Agenda (GHSA) network[31] to accelerate IHR implementation.[32] The immense scale of the outbreak, but also the fear of haemorrhagic fever entering Western countries, enticed GHSA membership.[33] Nevertheless, forthcoming support was criticised for being hyper-focused on Ebola symptomatic detection and containment in "war" time (during an outbreak), whilst ignoring health system strengthening in peacetime.[34] Therefore, WHO incorporated health system strengthening and UHC under the expanding umbrella of health security frameworks, as well as non-communicable chronic diseases, which account for two-thirds of global morbidity and mortality.[35] Finally, post-COVID-19, WHO is coordinating a new pandemic agreement in which states' obligations towards global equity and access to health products are explicitly stated for the first time, via a new IHR amendment. With a dose of cynicism, health security has become a convenient buzzword used to justify many agendas.

An Academic Analysis of Health Security in Theory and in Practice

Is health security a government apparatus to protect state interests and their chosen population majority, or a mechanism to prioritise vulnerable minorities most disadvantaged by health events?

Davies[36] and Lakoff[37] have unpacked health security's historical evolution into two comparable approaches: (i) state-centric health security, a mechanism that widens national security agendas and prioritises the needs of the state population at large; and (ii) individual-centric health security, which protects the needs of vulnerable individuals regardless of their statehood. Relying on international relations and state security theories, Davies presents the two approaches as overlapping on a spectrum, using the terms "statist" and "globalist". With practical examples, such as the comparison of Indonesia and WHO's interactions in the H5N1 outbreak (2006–08) with MSF's advocacy towards equitable access to global pharmaceutical supplies for neglected tropical diseases (NTDs), Lakoff frames "global health security" and "humanitarian biomedicine" as two opposing regimes with competing ethical principles and incompatible visions of social order. Davies' and Lakoff's complementary analyses explore the persistent tension resulting from the fact that health security can protect the health of states, populations, and vulnerable individuals, but not at the same time and not to equal degrees. Choices must be made regarding whose interests to protect.

Positioning 1: State-centric

A state-centric health security approach aims to protect and maintain state order at any cost. International cooperation is secondary, with no guilt wasted on the reality that states are not on an equal footing. A disease – usually a single one – is reimagined as a threat of "*proportional menace to war, nuclear proliferation, or terrorism*"[38] to be securitised[39] and the source identified, eliminated, or contained via emergency response, executed with military assistance, if required. Psychologically influential tactics, such as vague but ominous language, are employed to create fear among the population: "*a threat to one is a threat to all*".[40] Reinforcing loyalty to the nation above membership of other groups helps protect the state by establishing an internal/external dynamic that "something over there" endangers "our safe space".[41] Border closures during the HIV/AIDS epidemic, to prevent "*massive influxes of disease infected refugees*", were justified in this way.[42] More recently, this tactic is superbly exploited by right and centrist liberal politicians who claim that inhumane immigration policies are nationally protective.[43]

Cultivating fear also helps legitimise swiftly imposed emergency public health measures, potentially extraordinarily restrictive to individuals and minority communities, with little time for ethical considerations;[44] measures enacted to achieve a greater good, simultaneously safeguarding state interests by protecting the largest number of the most "useful" citizens. When analysed within a humanitarian context, it is easy to think inequity is driven by a lack of resources, and yet structural barriers to health equity also exist in wealthy nations. Essentially, state-centric health security is one way of optimising the public health of a large population and reducing inequities between countries, yet it is also, ultimately, undesirable for individuals' health when security measures are used to discriminate further against minorities and other structurally underserved groups.[45]

Positioning 2: Individual-centric

At the other end of the health security spectrum, closer to UNDP's initial framing, are actors who support individual security in order to uphold human rights, alleviate suffering, and promote human well-being, regardless of individual statehood or social standing.[46] Akin to critical human security studies, individual-centric health security "*exposes and challenges structural conditions*" that foster insecurity.[47] Security threats are social constructs shaped by value-based choices from those in power to protect their needs whilst risking deprioritising or excluding population minorities. As such, health security approaches must be community-driven and tailored to meet individual vulnerabilities.[48] In this case, the greater good is achieved by reducing the health inequity faced by the most disadvantaged, whilst accepting some cost to the state, the population at large, and those privileged by power. Lakoff claims that individual-centric health security must remain external to state sovereignty, relying on diverse healthcare actors (NGOs, civil, and intergovernmental) to drive bottom-up solutions that can rebalance state power.[49]

The following section reviews how these two positions have been enacted during major recent outbreaks: Ebola and COVID-19.

II Health Security in Action: Whose Interests Are Actually Prioritised?

Ebola Outbreaks: State-centred Responses

The UNSC declared the massive Ebola outbreak in West Africa (2013–15) a "*threat to international peace and stability*".[50] An analysis of the health security positioning, performed by Harman and Wenham, found a state-centric approach between states and from the state towards the population majority, whilst local and international NGOs focused on individuals' and vulnerable minorities' needs. The latter delivered technical expertise, flexible financing, and an emergency response mindset that the authors felt many states could not, or would not, have provided. A lack of investment in health systems and insufficient, inconsistent engagement of communities and local actors was an early critique of all actors.[51] An insight into IFRC's community-driven approach during an Ebola outbreak in the Democratic Republic of the Congo (DRC, 2017–18) is provided in a dedicated section at the end of this chapter.

This state-centric approach included a Western protectionist agenda and the generation of fear, via internal and external threat tactics, to justify border closures.[52] Wealthy states blamed the outbreak's immense scale and slow response on chronically underfunded local health systems, attributed in part to government corruption. There were concerns that funding funnelled via the state was not reaching the most affected population, especially in remote areas. Corruption and a lack of accountability on the part of affected governments seemingly contributed to wealthy states feeling morally absolved of any obligation to assist beyond their own borders, a mechanism that penalised individuals more than states.[53] Seven months into the outbreak, global collaboration, including military support, finally arrived. However, this coincided with a significant risk of transmission in Western countries, leading to suspicions that the actions were more about self-protection than genuine international solidarity.[54] Three years later, during a smaller Ebola outbreak in the DRC (2017–19), Canada, the United Kingdom, the US,[55] Germany, Italy, and Norway gave timely pledges, and again economic motivation was surmised, given that DRC mines half of the global cobalt resources.[56]

COVID-19 Pandemic: The Pitfalls of Standardised Strategies

Reflecting on the COVID-19 pandemic (2020–23), many people will recall the widespread fear and the swift, restrictive public health measures implemented by states. Guided by utilitarian frameworks, these measures frequently overshadowed individual needs to protect the interests of the population at large. A one-size-fits-all approach was critiqued as being Western-orientated: for example, using social distancing and mask-wearing to facilitate economic activity increased welfare values by 30–40% in the US and UK, but only 9–10% in India and Bangladesh.[57] A consequence of rediverting global funding towards COVID-19 was 23 million children in the DRC missing routine vaccinations in 2020, the highest number in more than a decade.[58] Furthermore, reliably curable diseases like malaria, pneumonia, diarrhoea, and tuberculosis became harder to detect and treat due to diagnostic and medication shortages, as pharmaceutical and biotechnology companies shifted production in favour of more profitable COVID-19 products that not all states could equitably access.[59]

At the extreme end of state-centric approaches, vulnerable individuals were targeted by states in the name of health security. Amnesty International documented how state leaders instrumentalised public health restrictions to order or condone abuses of state power towards civilians, citing India, the Philippines, and Nigeria as examples.[60] In Mexico, authorities suspended the legally mandated processing of asylum claims despite a 33% rise in forced migration, and when the DRC–Uganda border closed, 10,000 people were stranded, with no exceptions made for refugees and asylum seekers.[61] Finally, when international solidarity was offered to support populations in Afghanistan, the Taliban refused a donation of COVID-19 vaccines.

In academic literature, Kennedy retrospectively applied Davies' and Lakoff's two approaches to the COVID-19 responses of three organisations: WHO, the US Centers for Disease Control and Prevention (CDC), and MSF.[62] Based on public communications between 13 January 2020 and 11 March 2022, the conclusion that MSF was individual-centric, focused on marginalised and vulnerable individuals, condemning nationalistic measures that reduced healthcare access, is reassuring. The US CDC coming out as state-centric and protective of the US population – a stance defended by contemporary liberals as successful governance – is also not a surprise.[63] Interestingly, despite its reputation as a securitising actor, WHO shifting its approach as the pandemic evolved was unexpected, but supports Davies' theory that state- and individual-centric approaches exist on a spectrum. During the first COVID-19 wave, WHO concentrated on fulfilling the surveillance demands of wealthy states and driving biotechnology innovations that would likely disproportionately benefit them. This catered to the needs of state population majorities, as minorities are frequently under-reported or absent from surveillance mechanisms unless specifically sought out. However, in subsequent waves, WHO's communication urged states to provide equitable healthcare access, promoted the COVAX mechanism[64] for global vaccine distribution, and advocated for marginalised communities to be at the centre of decision-making.[65] WHO's shift highlights a practical challenge in health security conceptualisation: supporting the state population majority can effectively reduce global health inequities between states, but risks perpetuating health equity gaps for minorities within a state.

III MSF Cannot Do It All and Do It Well

The portrayal of MSF as an individual-centric health security actor likely resonates for many readers because it is accurate, especially in conflict zones, emergency responses, and humanitarian crises impacted by the intentional or unintentional oppressive actions of state and non-state actors. However, MSF's ethical dilemma regarding health security does not emerge in these contexts, and also is not linked to MSF advocacy examined by Lakoff; MSF can always be relied upon to speak out, particularly regarding multinational global health funding reductions which necessitate MSF to cover critical gaps in NTDs, HIV, tuberculosis, and malaria care.[66] The dilemma arises in protracted, complex humanitarian crises in low-income states where MSF remains year after year. Staff begin to ask if the greater good is to prop up the failing state healthcare system to have a wider impact, such that MSF's target humanitarian population becomes the local state population. The benefits of reaching more people are weighed against the cost of compromise, if aligning MSF service delivery with the state healthcare system approach means diverting energy away from tailored humanitarian assistance for disadvantaged groups. This raises the ethical question of what morally matters: the number of people assisted or that the most disadvantaged are helped?

Rising to the Needs

> *The problem is that organisations have a spontaneous tendency to grow... and to justify their growth by incessant new needs. And in terms of humanitarian aid there is always something more to do.*[67]
>
> (Rony Brauman)

In countries like South Sudan, DRC, and the Central African Republic, among others, large sub-populations are disadvantaged by structural social forces that contribute to humanitarian needs; forces influenced by state corruption, the health priorities of wealthy states, and other global governance issues that health security cannot adequately address, but that keep populations in poverty. MSF staff witness widespread poor access to basic healthcare and extreme levels of structural violence that have become normalised and tolerated by states. MSF's moral and operational limits are tested, and staff experience moral distress, as selecting a humanitarian target population from within this sub-population feels wrong, given the scale of the needs, especially when large proportions of the demographic are women and children. An impartial needs-based logic no longer serves its purpose, and MSF is pulled towards a more state-centric health security approach.

For some years now, the majority of MSF operations in these states have been delivered in partnership with Ministry of Health facilities, helpfully assisting them to fulfil their health obligations to the local population. This choice is also influenced by reflections within the humanitarian sector regarding improved local ownership and coordination. For instance, MSF invested more money in DRC (139 million euros) than any other country in 2023, employing 2,576 locally hired and 313 international staff across projects in 16 of 25 provinces, plus paying incentives to state health workers.[68] MSF supports state inpatient, outpatient, and community care, including public health interventions, supplies, and training. However, the direct care provided to patients by MSF staff is limited, questioning the degree to which MSF values humanity and proximity – core principles that contributed to its success. While MSF selects locations with the highest needs, working from a state hospital means the target population is determined by the hospital's official catchment area. Also, MSF's support attracts patients from afar, widening the demand–supply gap but improving health access for many.

These operations begin with targeted assistance for vulnerable groups but experience "mission creep", expanding the range and target demographics of MSF activities over the years due to the unwavering determination of MSF staff to address the needs of the people they encounter. There is, however, an overly optimistic internal view that partnering with the state increases the systemic value of these operations or is morally superior, assuming that MSF's contribution renders state services more sustainable in the long run – assumptions to be tested in each context. While present, MSF's support does make that state facility functional and addresses the outcomes of locally driven health inequities, but not political systemic failures, structural societal transformation, or financing issues that sustain health inequities. In fact, MSF's expanding presence can deter longer-term investors, and even the state, from supporting that sub-population. Even when MSF specifically targets a health policy change via a multi-year advocacy campaign or operational research, MSF's expertise is primarily technical, not social justice reform.

Too Big Not to Act?

> *MSF will undoubtedly have more means on the ground after a certain time, but will arrive later, or the wrong place or the wrong time.*[69]
>
> (Rony Brauman)

Whilst MSF teams feel compelled to act when witnessing rising unmet humanitarian needs, there is a more pressing internal factor influencing where the limits of moral responsibility lie: the growth of MSF itself.[70] Recent massive organisational growth lulls MSF teams into a false impression, especially in rural areas, that MSF's budget is higher than, or comparable to, the state health budget, hence imposing a sense of responsibility towards the population. On a global scale, MSF now succumbs to "brand" name considerations, knowing that the MSF brand is influential at the highest levels of global health governance (UNSC, WHO Executive Board), where state partnerships are positively received. The trade-off is an aversion for being "politically incorrect" and taking risks with smaller, local civil society alliances or independent MSF operations, even if these might be the optimal way to meet minority needs. MSF's inherently rebellious activist spirit feels harder to locate at the centre of this expanding organisation.

With larger budgets comes higher accountability for MSF "deliverables", most objectively met by reporting the number of people reached. MSF is not alone in this well-accepted practice, yet it drives the organisation to measure success by patient volumes rather than the humanitarian imperative of whom is helped. While counting people who benefit or lives saved is a public health interpretation of utilitarianism, particularly justified in outbreak response or vaccination campaigns, it is not the only way to determine the greater good. Utilitarianism ultimately determines the net benefit by the quality of happiness or another metric measure of utility, not merely quantity.[71] Under consequentialism, the action that achieves the right end result is what ethically matters, which, according to the MSF Charter, is to provide assistance to *"populations in distress, to victims of natural or man-made disasters and to victims of armed conflict"*[72] – accepting the trade-off that not everyone can be helped. For a growing MSF, the challenge is that smaller, more targeted operations require a non-volumetric accountability logic, and measuring the degree of vulnerability and/or suffering is difficult to objectively achieve.

IV Ensuring "Fairness for All" Remains Insufficient

> *Corrupt and inefficient governments around the world should no longer be able to escape their moral duty to respond to humanitarian need in their own countries by passing them on to the system of Western-funded aid.*[73]
>
> (Hugo Slim)

With good intentions, MSF teams often ask why the organisation cannot be state-centric and individual-centric at the same time. They further argue that supporting the state will also serve minorities. However, a consequential analysis of who benefits most is needed, in the eyes of MSF and the state, acknowledging that both hold defensible claims to a greater good. COVID-19, yet again, proved what other outbreak responses have demonstrated: that a utilitarian public health approach is not tailored to benefit minorities and at-risk groups. These groups are less able to protect themselves via generic preventative strategies and disproportionately burdened by public health interventions imposed to protect the population majority. Too often, pandemic frameworks are focused on ensuring fairness for all and removing biases that drive inequities, yet this remains insufficient. At-risk groups need bias in their favour via individual-centric approaches to address their specific barriers to care; specific support either not required by the population at large or not feasible to deliver on a wider scale.[74] Where national outbreak frameworks do single out exceptional categories of people, the logic is based on the group's utility to society, such as healthcare professionals, rather than their disadvantage within society.[75] Beyond the moral question of whether MSF should invest their donations into inequitable state structures, pragmatically trying to simultaneously cater to state- and individual-centric health security approaches will likely create tension for front-line staff, as they will be faced with explaining why MSF is treating people from the same population differently within the same facility. Organisational transparency and community acceptance can be jeopardised, misunderstood as favouritism, and not accepted by local leaders who have their own interpretation of the greater good within their community. Furthermore, at-risk groups often have a mistrust of state entities, and linking MSF support to the state may create another barrier to care.

As MSF grows, there seems to be constant pressure, both internally and externally, for the organisation to evolve into something more. At present, MSF risks trying to do it all but doing it badly, with minority groups potentially becoming the accepted trade-off. By deviating from the humanitarian imperative, MSF may unwittingly take focus off the most vulnerable individuals to deliver operations at scale that meet the demands of states and large populations. Despite significant financial growth and a healthy ego, MSF is not a state, nor is it an implementing partner of the UN system to support member states. MSF has no moral obligation to step in for states that perpetuate disadvantage, especially if driven by inefficient governance or corruption. MSF remains a private medical humanitarian organisation, trusted by generous donors to deliver the humanitarian imperative, and a "middle-of-the-road" health security positioning might divert our focus or diminish our ability to achieve just that.

V Conclusion

Whilst health security remains alive as a concept, its ethics and implementation face considerable challenges. Many popular global health security approaches do warrant scrutiny, as they are as much about politics and global power between states as they are about health. Despite states demonstrating their capability to produce multiple COVID-19 vaccines in under a year, it took 35 years to develop a single malaria vaccine, requiring the Gates Foundation's funds to reach the last mile.[76] Many wealthy states are unwilling to make the necessary sacrifices to assist less wealthy states to battle the health challenges they face.[77] Originally rooted in addressing individual insecurity, today health security operates as a state-centric mechanism to promote the greater good of states and the population at large; efforts which nobly reduce health inequities between states but are insufficient to tackle health inequities within states. This state-centric approach prevails not because of its superior means of achieving health security, but because humanitarian-orientated, individual-centric approaches are too easily dismissed by public health utilitarian accountability mechanisms that measure success by the number of people benefitting.

In some states, the scale of humanitarian needs makes it challenging for MSF project teams to focus on the humanitarian imperative without being sidetracked by systemic state failures to deliver basic healthcare. Whilst MSF's sense of its own moral responsibility is expanding, believing that MSF partnering with the state will address the structural health inequity faced by minorities is, in most cases, mere well-intentioned optimism. An organisation whose moral responsibility becomes overstretched risks spreading itself thin and failing to support individuals most in need of its help. As MSF grapples with the temptation of further growth, this ethical dilemma will continue to arise for project teams. Maintaining a disciplined focus on the most urgent humanitarian needs while simultaneously supporting states to achieve their greater good is not without compromises. MSF maintaining an individual-centric approach will likely lead us to areas where other health security actors are present, but more importantly, also where they are not, and where assisting those most in need regardless of their statehood or volume is the greater good.

Notes

1 Malik, Barlow, and Johnson, 2021.
2 McCoy et al., 2023.
3 Rushton, 2011; Lakoff, 2010, pp. 59–79; Abraham, 2011, pp. 797–812; Global Health Council, 2023.
4 Nunes, 2017, pp. 3–21.
5 See https://www.usaid.gov/global-health/health-areas/global-health-security.
6 See https://www.who.int/health-topics/health-security.
7 The International Health Regulations are a legally binding instrument for 196 countries, including 194 WHO member states, that address the inherent threats of globalisation on disease control. See https://www.who.int/health-topics/international-health-regulations.
8 Goodin, 1985; Nunes, 2017, pp. 3–21.
9 Glasman, 2020.
10 See https://www.unicef.org/health/childhood-diseases.
11 Oxfam International, 2023.
12 McGowan and Bambra, 2022, pp. e966-e975; Antipova, 2022.
13 Weir, 2014, cited by Harman and Wenham, 2018, pp. 362–76.
14 National Academies of Sciences, Engineering, and Medicine, 2017.
15 See https://www.who.int/health-topics/health-security.
16 Brown, 2015, pp. 340–55.
17 Feldbaum, Lee, and Patel, 2006.
18 Snowden, 2020, pp. 457–8, cited by Kennedy, 2023.
19 In the Cold War era, health was valued for its utility/benefit to the state, then secondarily the individual, as the state required a healthy workforce population to achieve state economic and political modernisation: Newman, 2022, pp. 431–54.
20 UN, 1994, p. 23.
21 UN, 1994, p. 22; Feldbaum, Lee, and Patel, 2006.
22 Paul Farmer later reframed structural violence within public health thinking as the social arrangements that put individuals and populations in harm's way: *"The arrangements are structural because they are embedded in the political and economic organisation of our social world; they are violent because they cause injury to people. Structural violence remains a high-ranking cause of premature death and disability."* (Farmer et al., 2006).
23 See Galtung, 1969, pp. 167–91.
24 Newman, 2022, pp. 431–54.
25 Newman, 2022; Rushton, 2011, pp. 779–96.
26 WHO, 2007.
27 Newman, 2022; Ferhani and Rushton, 2020, pp. 458–77.
28 Fidler, 2024; Aldis, 2008, pp. 369–75.
29 Lakoff, 2010, pp. 59–79; Sedyaningsih et al., 2008, pp. 482–8; Holbrooke and Garrett, 2008.
30 Sedyaningsih et al., 2008.
31 By 2023, GHSA had grown to include 71 countries and 12 organisations, including international organisations, intergovernmental organisations, and coalitions, that respectively represented more than 30 non-governmental organisations and private sector actors. Another key initiative is the Global Health Security Initiative (GHSI), launched in November 2001 by Canada and the European Commission, France, Italy, Japan, Mexico, the United Kingdom, and the United States, with WHO as observer. Its aim is to strengthen public health preparedness and response to the threat of international biological, chemical, and radio-nuclear terrorism. See https://globalhealthsecurityagenda.org/about/.
32 Tappero et al., 2017.
33 Johnson, Walsh, and Olonisakin, 2022, pp. 11–6.

34 El-Jardali and Fadlallah, 2022; Lal et al., 2022, pp. e1675-e1683.
35 See https://www.who.int/news-room/fact-sheets/detail/noncommunicable-diseases.
36 Davies, 2010, pp. 1167–90.
37 Lakoff, 2010 and 2017.
38 Davies, 2010.
39 Securitisation is a political process whereby an actor securitising an issue is able to persuade an audience to accept the claim. Its success requires trust in leadership as, according to securitisation theory, a threat is a social construct put forward as an existential danger that justifies exceptional mitigation mechanisms: Buzan, Wæver, and de Wilde, 1998, cited by Nunes, 2017. Whether health security's aim is to securitise medicine or medicalise security remains unclear; the former frames disease as a threat (akin to terrorism), whilst the latter optimises political control of health to protect state stability (military outbreak response readiness or reconceptualising pharmaceuticals as security-related technologies).
40 UN, 2004.
41 Bell and Aronoff-Spencer, 2020, pp. 1175–7.
42 Davies, 2010, p. 1173.
43 Su, 2024.
44 Fehross, Pahlman, and Silva, 2024, pp. 131–50; Malik, Barlow, and Johnson, 2021.
45 Goodin, 1985.
46 Some iterations of globalist thinking encompass all threats to individual well-being, beyond direct healthcare implications: Davies, 2010.
47 Newman, 2022, pp. 431–54.
48 Lakoff, 2010.
49 Lakoff, 2010.
50 UN, 2014; UN News, 2018.
51 Piot, Muyembe, and Edmunds, 2014, pp. 1034–5; Piot, 2014; Harman and Wenham, 2018, pp. 362–76.
52 Harman and Wenham, 2018.
53 Davies, 2010, pp. 1167–90.
54 Johnson, Walsh, and Olonisakin, 2022, pp. 11–6.
55 The Trump administration made a small pledge but, in parallel, they ceased funding a health security advisor position and wanted to cancel USD 252 million the government had previously set aside for future epidemics.
56 Armstrong, 2018.
57 Barnett-Howell, Watson, and Mobarak, 2021, pp. 807–19.
58 UNICEF, 2021.
59 Aborode et al., 2021, pp. 26–9. Also see https://www.unicef.org/health/childhood-diseases.
60 Amnesty International, 2021.
61 UNHCR, 2020; Amnesty International, 2021.
62 Kennedy, 2023.
63 Davies, 2010.
64 Specifically, the ACT-Accelerator focused on accelerating development in four pillars: diagnostics, therapeutics, vaccines (called COVAX), and health systems strengthening. See https://www.acted.org/en/covid-19-what-are-we-doing-what-can-you-do/.
65 Alakija, 2023, pp. e310–e317.
66 MSF, 2022.
67 Quoted by Elzas, 2021.
68 These figures exclude Ministry of Health staff working in the MSF supported facility, who are employed by the state but paid a per diem equivalent to a salary by MSF: MSF, 2024.
69 Quoted by Elzas, 2021.
70 World Bank, 2024.

71 Driver, 2022.
72 See https://www.msf.org/msf-charter.
73 Slim, 2024.
74 DeBruin, Liaschenko, and Marshall, 2012, pp. 586–91.
75 McGowan and Bambra, 2022.
76 Pawar, 2022.
77 Rushton, 2011.

References

Aborode, Abdullahi Tunde, Kenneth Bitrus David, Olivier Uwishema, Agbendeh Lubem Nathaniel, Jegede Oluwatoyin Imisioluwa, Sherifdeen Bamidele Onigbinde, and Fozia Farooq (2021), 'Fighting COVID-19 at the Expense of Malaria in Africa: The Consequences and Policy Options', *The American Journal of Tropical Medicine and Hygiene*, vol. 104, n° 1, pp. 26–29. doi:10.4269/ajtmh.20–1181.

Abraham, Thomas (2011), 'The Chronicle of a Disease Foretold: Pandemic H1N1 and the Construction of a Global Health Security Threat', *Political Studies*, vol. 59, n° 4, pp. 797–812.

Acted, 'Covid-19: What Are We Doing? What Can You Do?'. [https://www.acted.org/en/covid-19-what-are-we-doing-what-can-you-do/].

Alakija, Ayoade (2023), 'Leveraging Lessons from the COVID-19 Pandemic to Strengthen Low-Income and Middle-Income Country Preparedness for Future Global Health Threats', *The Lancet Infectious Diseases*, vol. 23, n° 8, pp. e310–317. doi:10.1016/S1473–3099(23)00279–00277.

Aldis, William (2008), 'Health Security as a Public Health Concept: A Critical Analysis', *Health Policy and Planning*, vol. 23, n° 6, pp. 369–375. doi:10.1093/heapol/czn030.

Amnesty International (2021), '"Virulent Strain of Leaders" Weaponizing Pandemic', 7 April. [https://www.amnesty.org/en/latest/press-release/2021/04/annual-report-covid19-decades-of-oppression-inequality-abuse/].

Antipova, Anzhelika (2022), 'Analysis of Disease Burden in Socially Disadvantaged Areas: Mapping of Geographical Inequalities in COVID-19 Morbidity and Mortality Using a Social Disadvantage Index in Tennessee', *Frontiers in Sustainable Cities*, vol. 4. doi:10.3389/frsc.2022.876945.

Armstrong, Michael J. (2018), 'Stopping Ebola before the Virus Goes Viral', *The Conversation*. [http://theconversation.com/stopping-ebola-before-the-virus-goes-viral-97234].

Barnett-Howell, Zachary, Oliver John Watson, and Ahmed Mushfiq Mobarak (2021), 'The Benefits and Costs of Social Distancing in High- and Low-Income Countries', *Transactions of The Royal Society of Tropical Medicine and Hygiene*, vol. 115, n° 7, pp. 807–819. doi:10.1093/trstmh/traa140.

Bell, David, and Eliah Aronoff-Spencer (2020), '"Global Health": Time to Refocus While We Still Have Time', *The American Journal of Tropical Medicine and Hygiene*, vol. 102, n° 6, pp. 1175–1177. doi:10.4269/ajtmh.20–0081.

Brown, Hannah (2015), 'Global Health Partnerships, Governance, and Sovereign Responsibility in Western Kenya', *American Ethnologist*, vol. 42, n° 2, pp. 340–355. doi:10.1111/amet.12134.

Buzan, Barry, Ole Wæver, and Jaap de Wilde (1998), *Security: A New Framework for Analysis*, Boulder, CO: Lynne Rienner Publishers.

Davies, Sara E. (2010), 'What Contribution Can International Relations Make to the Evolving Global Health Agenda?', *International Affairs (Royal Institute of International Affairs 1944–)*, vol. 86, n° 5, pp. 1167–1190.

DeBruin, Debra, Joan Liaschenko, and Mary Faith Marshall (2012), 'Social Justice in Pandemic Preparedness', *American Journal of Public Health*, vol. 102, n° 4, pp. 586–591. doi:10.2105/AJPH.2011.300483.

Driver, Julia (2022), 'The History of Utilitarianism', in Edward N. Zalta, and Uri Nodelman (eds), *The Stanford Encyclopedia of Philosophy*, Metaphysics Research Lab, Stanford University. [https://plato.stanford.edu/archives/win2022/entries/utilitarianism-history/].

El-Jardali, Fadi, and Racha Fadlallah (2022), 'No Global Health Security without Strong and Resilient Health Systems in the Mediterranean', *FOCUS*, n° 9. [https://www.iemed.org/publication/no-global-health-security-without-strong-and-resilient-health-systems-in-the-mediterranean/].

Elzas, Sarah (2021), 'From a Scrappy Group of Doctors to a Massive Global Aid NGO, MSF Marks 50 Years', *RFI*, 21 December. [https://www.rfi.fr/en/france/20211221-from-a-scrappy-group-of-doctors-to-a-massive-global-aid-ngo-msf-marks-50-years].

Farmer, Paul E., Bruce Nizeye, Sara Stulac, and Salmaan Keshavjee (2006), 'Structural Violence and Clinical Medicine', *PLOS Medicine*, vol. 3, n° 10. doi:10.1371/journal.pmed.0030449.

Fehross, Anson, Kari Pahlman, and Diego S. Silva (2024), 'Ethics and Health Security in the Australian COVID-19 Context: A Critical Interpretive Literature Review', *Journal of Bioethical Inquiry*, vol. 21, n° 1, pp. 131–150. doi:10.1007/s11673–11023–10255–10256.

Feldbaum, Harley, Kelley Lee, and Preeti Patel (2006), 'The National Security Implications of HIV/AIDS', *PLoS Medicine*, vol. 3, n° 6. doi:10.1371/journal.pmed.0030171.

Ferhani, Adam, and Simon Rushton (2020), 'The International Health Regulations, COVID-19, and Bordering Practices: Who Gets in, What Gets out, and Who Gets Rescued?', *Contemporary Security Policy*, vol. 41, n° 3, pp. 458–477. doi:10.1080/13523260.2020.1771955.

Fidler, David P. (2024), 'The Amendments to the International Health Regulations Are Not a Breakthrough', *Think Global Health*. [https://www.thinkglobalhealth.org/article/amendments-international-health-regulations-are-not-breakthrough].

Galtung, Johan (1969), 'Violence, Peace, and Peace Research', *Journal of Peace Research*, vol. 6, n° 3, pp. 167–191.

GHSA, 'What Is the Global Health Security Agenda?' [https://globalhealthsecurityagenda.org/about/].

Glasman, Joël (2020), 'The Invention of Impartiality: The History of a Humanitarian Principle, from a Legal, Strategic and Algorithmic Perspective'. [https://msf-crash.org/en/publications/invention-impartiality-history-humanitarian-principle-legal-strategic-and-algorithmic].

Global Health Council (2023), 'Shaping a New Narrative on Global Health Security'. [https://globalhealth.org/shaping-a-new-narrative-on-global-health-security/].

Goodin, Robert E. (1985), 'Protecting the Vulnerable: A Reanalysis of Our Social Responsibilities', Conference Paper.

Harman, Sophie, and Clare Wenham (2018), 'Governing Ebola: Between Global Health and Medical Humanitarianism', *Globalizations*, vol. 15, n° 3, pp. 362–376. doi:10.1080/14747731.2017.1414410.

Holbrooke, Richard, and Laurie Garrett (2008), 'When "Sovereignty" Risks Global Health', *Project Syndicate*. [https://www.project-syndicate.org/commentary/when–sovereignty–risks-global-health].

Johnson, Oliver, Sinead Walsh, and Funmi Olonisakin (2022), 'The Role of the UN Security Council in Health Emergencies: Lessons from the Ebola Response in Sierra Leone', *Australian Journal of International Affairs*, vol. 76, n° 1, pp. 11–16. doi:10.1080/10357718.2021.2017841.

Kennedy, Denis (2023), 'Global Health Governance Responds to COVID-19: Does the Security/Access Divide Persist?', *Global Public Health*, vol. 18, n° 1. doi:10.1080/17441692.2023.2200296.

Lakoff, Andrew (2010), 'Two Regimes of Global Health', *Humanity: An International Journal of Human Rights, Humanitarianism, and Development*, vol. 1, pp. 59–79.

Lakoff, Andrew (2017), *Unprepared: Global Health in a Time of Emergency*, Oakland, CA: University of California Press.

Lal, Arush, Salma M. Abdalla, Vijay Kumar Chattu, Ngozi Adaeze Erondu, Tsung-Ling Lee, Sudhvir Singh, Hala Abou-Taleb, Jeanette Vega Morales, and Alexandra Phelan (2022), 'Pandemic Preparedness and Response: Exploring the Role of Universal Health Coverage within the Global Health Security Architecture', *The Lancet Global Health*, vol. 10, n° 11, pp. e1675–1683. doi:10.1016/S2214–2109X(22)00341–00342.

McCoy, David, Stephen Roberts, Salma Daoudi, and Jonathan Kennedy (2023), 'Global Health Security and the Health-Security Nexus: Principles, Politics and Praxis', *BMJ Global Health*, vol. 8, n° 9. doi:10.1136/bmjgh-2023–013067.

McGowan, Victoria J, and Clare Bambra (2022), 'COVID-19 Mortality and Deprivation: Pandemic, Syndemic, and Endemic Health Inequalities', *The Lancet Public Health*, vol. 7, n° 11, pp. e966–975. doi:10.1016/S2468–2667(22)00223–00227.

Malik, Sadia Mariam, Amy Barlow, and Benjamin Johnson (2021), 'Reconceptualising Health Security in Post-COVID-19 World', *BMJ Global Health*, vol. 6, n° 7. doi:10.1136/bmjgh-2021–006520.

MSF, 'MSF Charter'. [https://www.msf.org/msf-charter].

MSF (2022), 'Countries Must Re-Engage on HIV, TB and Malaria', 7 September. [https://www.msf.org/countries-must-re-engage-hiv-tb-and-malaria].

MSF (2024), 'International Financial Report 2023', MSF Internal Report.

National Academies of Sciences, Engineering, and Medicine (2017), *Communities in Action: Pathways to Health Equity*, Washington, DC: The National Academies Press. doi:10.17226/24624.

Newman, Edward (2022), 'Covid-19: A Human Security Analysis', *Global Society*, vol. 36, n° 4, pp. 431–454. doi:10.1080/13600826.2021.2010034.

Nunes, João (2017), 'Doctors Against Borders: Médecins Sans Frontières and Global Health Security', in Michiel Hofman and Sokhieng Au (eds), *The Politics of Fear: Médecins Sans Frontières and the West African Ebola Epidemic*, New York, NY: Oxford University Press, pp. 3–21. doi:10.1093/acprof:oso/9780190624477.001.0001.

Oxfam International (2023), 'Survival of the Richest'. [https://www.oxfam.org/en/research/survival-richest].

Pawar, Pratik (2022), 'It Took 35 Years to Get a Malaria Vaccine. Why?', *Undark Magazine*. [https://undark.org/2022/05/25/it-took-35-years-to-get-a-malaria-vaccine-why/].

Piot, Peter (2014), 'Ebola's Perfect Storm', *Science (New York, N.Y.)*, vol. 345, n° 6202. doi:10.1126/science.1260695.

Piot, Peter, Jean-Jacques Muyembe, and W. John Edmunds (2014), 'Ebola in West Africa: From Disease Outbreak to Humanitarian Crisis', *The Lancet Infectious Diseases*, vol. 14, n° 11, pp. 1034–1035. doi:10.1016/S1473–3099(14)70956–70959.

Rushton, Simon (2011), 'Global Health Security: Security for Whom? Security from What?', *Political Studies*, vol. 59, n° 4, pp. 779–796. doi:10.1111/j.1467–9248.2011.00919.x.

Sedyaningsih, Endang R., Siti Isfandari, Triono Soendoro, and Siti Fadilah Supari (2008), 'Towards Mutual Trust, Transparency and Equity in Virus Sharing Mechanism: The Avian Influenza Case of Indonesia', *Annals of the Academy of Medicine, Singapore*, vol. 37, n° 6, pp. 482–488.

Slim, Hugo (2024), 'Painful Choices: How Humanitarians Can Prioritize in a World of Rising Need', *Global Public Policy Institute*. [https://gppi.net/2024/01/11/how-humanitarians-can-prioritize].

Snowden, Frank M. (2020), *Epidemics and Society: From the Black Death to the Present*, New Haven, CT/London: Yale University Press.

Su, Yvonne (2024), 'Beyond the Harris-Trump Debate: How Politicians Use Anti-Immigrant Rhetoric to Mask Systemic Failures', *The Conversation*, 12 September. [http://theconversation.com/beyond-the-harris-trump-debate-how-politicians-use-anti-immigrant-rhetoric-to-mask-systemic-failures-238851].

Tappero, Jordan W., Cynthia H. Cassell, Rebecca E. Bunnell, Frederick J. Angulo, Allen Craig, Nicki Pesik, Benjamin A. Dahl, et al. (2017), 'US Centers for Disease Control and Prevention and Its Partners' Contributions to Global Health Security', *Emerging Infectious Diseases*, vol. 23, n° 10. doi:10.3201/eid23S1.170946.

UN (1994), *Human Development Report 1994*, Oxford/New York, NY: Oxford University Press.

UN (2004), 'Report of the High-Level Panel on Threats, Challenges and Change'. [https://www.securitycouncilreport.org/atf/cf/%7B65BFCF9B-6D27-4E9C-8CD3-CF6E4FF96FF9%7D/CPR%20A%2059%20565.pdf].

UN (2014), 'With Spread of Ebola Outpacing Response, Security Council Adopts Resolution 2177 (2014) Urging Immediate Action, End to Isolation of Affected States', 18 September. [https://press.un.org/en/2014/sc11566.doc.htm].

UN News (2018), 'Security Council Urges Responder-Safety Focus, as DR Congo Ebola Outbreak Worsens', 30 October. [https://news.un.org/en/story/2018/10/1024442].

UNHCR (2020), 'Despite Pandemic Restrictions, People Fleeing Violence and Persecution Continue to Seek Asylum in Mexico', 28 April. [https://www.unhcr.org/news/briefing-notes/despite-pandemic-restrictions-people-fleeing-violence-and-persecution-continue].

UNICEF, 'Childhood Diseases'. [https://www.unicef.org/health/childhood-diseases].

UNICEF (2021), 'COVID-19 Pandemic Leads to Major Backsliding on Childhood Vaccinations, New WHO, UNICEF Data Shows', 15 July. [https://www.unicef.org/press-releases/covid-19-pandemic-leads-major-backsliding-childhood-vaccinations-new-who-unicef-data].

USAID, 'Global Health Security: Protecting the World from Health Emergencies'. [https://www.usaid.gov/global-health/health-areas/global-health-security], original web page accessed October 2024, now only available at [https://web.archive.org/web/20250131211100/https:/www.usaid.gov/global-health/health-areas/global-health-security].

Weir, Lorna (2014), 'Inventing Global Health Security, 1994–2005', in Simon Rushton and Jeremy Youde (eds), *Routledge Handbook of Global Health Security*, London: Routledge.

WHO, 'Health Security'. [https://www.who.int/health-topics/health-security].

WHO, 'International Health Regulations'. [https://www.who.int/health-topics/international-health-regulations].

WHO (2007), 'The World Health Report 2007: A Safer Future: Global Public Health Security in the 21st Century'. [https://iris.who.int/handle/10665/43713].

WHO (2024), 'Noncommunicable Diseases'. [https://www.who.int/news-room/fact-sheets/detail/noncommunicable-diseases].

World Bank (2024), 'Aid Architecture: A Changing Landscape'. [https://www.worldbank.org/en/publication/a-changing-landscape-aid-architecture].

Zoom-in: The IFRC's Community-driven Approach in DRC's Ebola Outbreak

Ombretta Baggio

Despite extensive evidence that community-led approaches and accountability systems are key to effective epidemic response, systematically and deliberately seeking affected communities' perspectives and engagement in the design of health interventions remains scattered and reactive. In recent times, particularly during the Ebola outbreaks and the COVID-19 pandemic, we have observed a persistent lack of sustained investments in community systems that amplify the voices and perspectives of people, especially those who are often voiceless and marginalised.

Ebola epidemics create fear due to the severity of the symptoms, misunderstanding of the causes, the high number of deaths, and the control measures, which are *"generally perceived as intrusive and as such often interfere with local social, cultural, and religious practices"*.[1] Ebola myths and rumours spring from entrenched belief systems and can cause denial and spark sometimes fatal community violence towards healthcare workers and local staff and volunteers, as we witnessed in the Democratic Republic of the Congo.

During the Ebola outbreak in North Kivu (2017–18), the Red Cross invested in feedback systems that enabled communities to voice their understanding of Ebola-related issues and provide timely and regular input regarding response mechanisms.[2] With this near-real-time perception data, the Red Cross were able to appreciate the reasons why safe and dignified burial teams were denied access and jointly define some alternative traditional rituals and prayers designed to help a deceased person's spirit make its journey to the ancestors.

Since then, the IFRC has focused on systematically collecting and using community feedback to adapt response strategies, enhancing engagement with vulnerable populations and building trust. Here are three key insights from the IFRC on why investing in community-inclusive and community-led strategies is essential for effectively reaching the most vulnerable:

- Localised approaches are crucial to ensure we listen often and act locally and in a timely manner to course-correct our health interventions. Understanding local beliefs, practices, and community insights helps responders to effectively involve communities locally, especially the most vulnerable, in ways that specifically and promptly address their anxieties and fears.[3]

DOI: 10.4324/9781003542247-11

- Investing in stronger community systems fosters trust and engagement between healthcare providers and the local population.[4] When local actors and communities participate in the planning and implementation of health interventions, they are more likely to accept and adhere to the recommended practices.
- Community-led strategies are inherently more relevant to the specific needs and cultural contexts of the populations they serve.[5]

Excluding community-led approaches from health frameworks limits funding and attention to proactive investments needed for their effective integration in preparedness and readiness plans and health systems strengthening approaches overall.

Community-inclusive and community-led strategies may be more time-consuming, difficult, and require more widespread resources, but there is not one "silver bullet" to solving the complex challenges of health insecurity today.

Notes

1 Dickmann et al., 2015.
2 McKay et al., 2022; Earle-Richardson et al., 2021, pp. 332–3.
3 Earle-Richardson et al., 2021.
4 Erlach et al., 2021, pp. 13–20.
5 IFRC, 2023.

References

Dickmann, Petra, Andrew Kitua, Paul Kaczmarek, Julius Lutwama, Justin Masumu, Esron Karimuribo, Yunus Karsan, Nigel Lightfoot, and Mark Rweyemamu (2015), 'Using Lessons Learned from Previous Ebola Outbreaks to Inform Current Risk Management', *Emerging Infectious Diseases*, vol. 21, n° 5. doi:10.3201/eid2105.142016.

Earle-Richardson, Giulia, Eva Erlach, Vivienne Walz, Ombretta Baggio, Molly Kurnit, Cheick Abdoulaye Camara, Christina Craig, et al. (2021), 'New Mixed Methods Approach for Monitoring Community Perceptions of Ebola and Response Efforts in the Democratic Republic of the Congo', *Global Health: Science and Practice*, vol. 9, n° 2, pp. 332–343. doi:10.9745/GHSP-D-21–00144.

Erlach, Eva, Bronwyn Nichol, Sharon Reader, and Ombretta Baggio (2021), 'Using Community Feedback to Guide the COVID-19 Response in Sub-Saharan Africa: Red Cross and Red Crescent Approach and Lessons Learned from Ebola', *Health Security*, vol. 19, n° 1, pp. 13–20. doi:10.1089/hs.2020.0195.

IFRC (2023), 'Community Engagement and Accountability (CEA) Strategy 2023–2025'. [https://www.ifrc.org/document/community-engagement-and-accountability-cea-strategy-2023-2025].

McKay, Gillian, Ombretta Baggio, Cheick Abdoulaye Camara, Eva Erlach, Lucia Robles Dios, Francesco Checchi, and Hana Rohan (2022), 'The Response Is like a Big Ship: Community Feedback as a Case Study of Evidence Uptake and Use in the 2018–2020 Ebola Epidemic in the Democratic Republic of the Congo', *BMJ Global Health*, vol. 7, n° 2. doi:10.1136/bmjgh-2021–005971.

6 Caught in the Crossfire?

International NGOs and Contemporary Forms of Protest and Resistance

*Maelle L'Homme**

In today's globalised societies, the notion that international non-governmental organisations (INGOs) – and human rights non-governmental organisations (NGOs) in particular – help bring about structural and political change beyond the borders of their home countries is relatively uncontroversial. The extent to which this actually applies to humanitarian INGOs, however, is much more open to debate. The role of foreign humanitarian agencies in a given country is, in fact, ambivalent insofar as they have to negotiate a space for intervention and sometimes overcome government-imposed restrictions on their activities without necessarily being a force for progress in the public debate or a forum for political protest for the societies in which they operate. Furthermore, their relations with the authorities are usually less strained than those enjoyed by other players in civil society – an old catch-all concept in Western political philosophy understood here as a *"place for contestation or opposition, or even social innovation"; "an arena where individual interests fight for recognition"*; a crossroads of *"sources of power outside the State and, more often than not, acting against the State"*.[1]

When faced with the repression of popular uprisings, the relations between humanitarian organisations and regimes whose practices are illiberal, if not authoritarian, can easily put them at odds with the people they are trying to help. It is not uncommon for opposition forces within local civil society to exert a kind of collective pressure on humanitarian INGOs to adopt a clear stance in support of their demands, and to refrain from cooperating with governments perceived as violent and illegitimate. For aid organisations working in such contexts of high political expectations, however, it is a particularly delicate matter to become associated with protest or resistance movements whose objectives might provoke sympathy but are outside the scope of humanitarian assistance, and whose methods they do not share. The question, then, is how separate, detached, or even aloof these organisations must remain from opposition groups fighting for their emancipation.

How do international humanitarian organisations deal with the effects of violence when it takes the form of political repression? How do they delineate a humanitarian response in situations of civil unrest, and how do they see the potential for convergence with the protest movements that permeate the

DOI: 10.4324/9781003542247-12

societies in which they operate? Drawing on the experience of Médecins Sans Frontières (MSF), this chapter examines the interplay – and the interference – between humanitarian action and contemporary forms of protest and resistance. Without wishing to deny the profoundly diverse nature of these movements and the contexts in which they arise, the analysis focuses on the way in which their protagonists interact with aid actors (MSF in particular). It explores the bonds of solidarity they seek to forge, the leverage methods they deploy, and the dilemmas this poses for the organisation. Many examples will serve to illustrate the point, two of which will be examined in greater detail: the Sudanese revolution in 2019, and the civil disobedience movement in Myanmar following the *coup d'état* in 2021. The analysis of these two situations is largely based on the points of view of humanitarian staff and activists alike, interviewed by the author between March and June 2024.

I Contemporary Protests and Humanitarian Response

Many countries in which MSF teams work regularly experience popular uprisings that are violently suppressed, particularly during election periods. These phenomena are, therefore, not unprecedented in the history of the organisation, but they have taken on a new dimension over the last 15 years with the Arab Spring revolts in Tunisia, Egypt, Bahrain, and Yemen in 2011, followed by Morocco, Jordan, Sudan, Algeria, Iraq, and Lebanon in 2018–19. Other parts of the world have also seen similar protests, including Europe, with the anti-austerity movements in Greece (2010–12) and Spain (2011–15).

Between 2008 and 2020, MSF addressed the needs that arose during "moments of protest" in 14 countries.[2] The aid provided consisted of donations of equipment and medicines; training courses; support for ambulance networks; and the deployment of mobile teams and/or support for displaced people. The difficulty of mounting a humanitarian response against a backdrop of insurrection always lies in the fact that, even though repression generates its share of victims and hinders access to basic services (including healthcare), these crises do not generally result in a humanitarian emergency in the traditional sense of the term, as the medical needs are not necessarily immense and the capacity of the local healthcare system to address them is sometimes sufficient. MSF's experience, however, shows that the intervention of an independent medical organisation can be relevant – especially if that organisation is already present in the country at the start of the protest – particularly to facilitate access to care for demonstrators afraid of being treated and arrested in public hospitals.

During the protests against the ruling monarchy in Bahrain in 2011, MSF teams supported the doctors' networks established to treat the injured away from Ministry of Health hospitals. Even though few patients were treated, several members of staff were detained, and the organisation was eventually expelled from the country, MSF's medical work nonetheless allowed it to witness the use of torture by the security forces. That same year, in Egypt, MSF provided medical equipment on Tahrir Square in central Cairo, sent a surgeon to support a local team, and trained mental-health volunteers working with survivors of sexual violence. In South Africa in 2015, during student demonstrations suppressed by the police, MSF donated first aid kits and joined forces with other civil society organisations to lobby for safe access to healthcare facilities for ill and injured demonstrators.[3]

MSF has also been criticised more than once for not supporting protest movements that were harshly suppressed (or not supporting them enough). In 2022, for example, the organisation came under pressure from the Iranian diaspora to help demonstrators injured during the "Women, Life, Freedom" uprising, which set the country ablaze following the death of Mahsa Amini.[4] A few years earlier, in Hong Kong in 2019, when a massive public protest met with a heavy-handed police response, disagreements within MSF about the appropriateness of doing something and/or speaking out developed into an internal crisis. On the one hand, the management team believed that needs were being covered, and that the situation could not be classed as a humanitarian or medical crisis, and therefore did not meet MSF's criteria for intervening. On the other, locally recruited staff and some members of the Board thought that the level of violence of the clashes and the fact that some demonstrators were afraid of seeking treatment in hospital justified an intervention. Even today, opposing views persist about the extent of the medical needs and the role and responsibilities of MSF during the protest:[5]

> *It was extremely frustrating that we could not intervene. We thought of lots of things, but it would only have been cosmetic. Needs were clearly covered by numerous first-aid teams, 40 very modern hospitals, mental health services ... Furthermore, it would have been complicated for MSF to offer quality care discreetly, as only Hong Kong doctors could practise, and finding these volunteers would have been difficult.*[6]

Sometimes, for a foreign organisation, having a local foothold can be "*a means of gaining the space it need[s] to develop its activity*".[7] The Hong Kong context is unique, however, in that MSF does not have an operational presence there, although it has always been very active in terms of recruitment and raising funds. The population's expectations are, therefore, based on a kind of "moral contract" whereby MSF is part of the local social fabric. As a result, not becoming involved in the country's politics (unlike Amnesty International, for example, which issues regular statements about police violence) poses a reputational risk and a potential loss of revenue for the organisation. In fact, in 2019, when MSF tried to justify itself by publishing a clumsy declaration to the effect that this was not a humanitarian crisis, a torrent of insults poured in online and thousands of donations were cancelled, resulting in an estimated loss of revenue of 12 million euros for 2020.[8]

II New Forms of Mobilisation

The debates, if not the tension, surrounding the decision by a medical humanitarian actor such as MSF to join forces with an overtly militant organisation with very strong political methods and leanings are nothing new.[9] The experience of Hong Kong, however, demonstrates the extent to which the actions and public stances of humanitarian INGOs are scrutinised in times of political and emotional turmoil. It also shows how the increasing use of digital technology and the emergence of new forms of activism online, particularly on social media, have transformed the way that people mobilise, and generated a greater risk of misinformation.[10] The presence of national and international NGOs on these platforms, and their exposure to the social movements that use them, makes it necessary for them to account for the consistency of their positions and the relevance of their operations.

In Greece, social media has allowed people organised in collectives, independent volunteers, and "solidarity activists" to mobilise outside conventional aid frameworks.[11] During the mass influx of migrants in 2015, relations between these various actors and humanitarian organisations were at times openly antagonistic, illustrating the former's distrust of well-financed institutional INGOs, with their paid workforces.[12]

With the changing humanitarian landscape reflected in these new forms of mutual aid – even though there is long-standing tension between a supposedly militant volunteer humanitarianism and a professional, almost technical, humanitarianism deemed to be dehumanising – the operating principles and methods, and the declarations or silence emanating from traditional humanitarian organisations are coming under increasing public scrutiny. The greater the attention generated in the media, the more the debate becomes polarised, and the more organisations such as MSF are likely to be subjected to pressure, criticism, and sometimes intimidation and threats, which, for example, take the form of campaigns on social media or waves of more or less targeted emails.[13]

Note that this pressure can also be internal. Over the past few years, many people within the aid community have been calling for humanitarian action to be more concerned with issues of solidarity, and for the advent of a *"humanitarian resistance"*.[14] If the issue of the interaction between aid actors and political militants is a pressing one, it is no doubt because the expectations of the latter have simply kept pace with the expansion of the sector in terms of means and mandate. But it is also because, in many situations, the individuals and groups that oppose a regime, or that are committed to defending the rights of those whom it oppresses, play a major role in providing relief; even more so when widespread insecurity limits international aid organisations' access to the most-affected areas, as was the case in Sudan, for example, following the 2018 revolution.

III The Sudanese Revolution

In the wake of the various popular protest movements that affected the Arab world from December 2010 onwards, the people of Sudan staged several uprisings between 2013 and 2016, and again in 2018, to demonstrate against austerity measures introduced by President Omar al-Bashir. Anger over a deteriorating economic situation was gradually joined by demands for individual freedoms, as evidenced by the increasingly anti-regime slogans.[15] The protest was led by various civil society actors, including professional associations and student unions, grouped together in two urban movements which appeared in the late 2010s: Girifna ("We are fed up"/"We've had enough") and Sudan Change Now. These movements operate underground, and made and continue to make massive use of social media to reclaim the public space under authoritarian rule.[16]

Alongside these two organisations, "resistance committees" were at the forefront of demanding the fall of the regime. Organised in the form of neighbourhood committees, these groups, which have little or no hierarchical structure, are particularly active at the local level. They gained the trust of the local population by carrying out specific actions, such as repairing water pipes, cleaning and monitoring streets, denouncing (on social media) acts of violence committed by forces loyal to the regime, rebuilding schools, and organising solidarity markets where products were sold at cost price. It is these committees which, in November 2016, following on from the events of 2013, called for strike action and civil disobedience. Although there was little support for it, the strike showed how important professional associations had become in Sudan's political life, on the fringes of the official unions controlled by the regime and the political parties deemed ineffective and obsolete by some of the country's urban youth.[17]

When the revolution broke out in December 2018, resistance committees played a vital role in raising awareness and mobilising the people. They acted as field relays for the Sudanese Professionals Association (SPA), a network of independent unions relaunched on this occasion to join forces with other opposition groups within the Forces of Freedom and Change (FFC), in January 2019. On 11 April 2019, Omar al-Bashir was deposed, but the demonstrations continued, demanding the end of the Transitional Military Council and the return of power to civilian hands. The population gathered in front of army headquarters. The al-Qiyadah sit-in became the heart of the Sudanese revolution for nearly two months. On 3 June 2019, the sit-in was dispersed at the cost of 150 dead, dozens missing, and hundreds injured.[18] Even though the *coup d'état* of 25 October 2021 dashed hopes of a democratic transition, the resistance committees are organising massive demonstrations in the regions spared by the fighting, to express their rejection of the two warring parties: the Sudanese Army and the Rapid Support Forces (RSF).

Reckoning with the Expectations of Sudanese Activists

It is difficult to understand Sudanese civil society's expectations of MSF without a brief review of the organisation's history in the country. MSF has been present in Sudan since 1979, and continuously so since 2004. In March 2005, at a time when the international community was debating how to classify the violence perpetrated by the Sudanese Army and pro-government militias against civilians in Darfur, and when Western diplomatic circles were mentioning the risk of genocide, the Dutch section of MSF published a report entitled *The crushing burden of rape: sexual violence in Darfur.*[19] A few weeks later, the head of mission and field coordinator were arrested for *"crimes against the State, publishing false reports, spying, and undermining Sudanese society"*.[20] Deeply rooted in people's memories, this story has helped forge MSF's identity and reputation in the country, both in the eyes of the authorities and of the local population. It has also influenced the profile of those who applied to work at MSF after 2005: *"At that time, the [Sudanese] doctors who worked with MSF in Khartoum and Darfur had a similar political background. They were known to have engaged against [Omar al-Bashir's] government during their university years."*[21] Incidentally, regarded by the authorities as a disruptive influence and an organisation that was out of control, MSF earned the support of Darfur's civilian population and the diaspora by establishing itself as *"the organisation capable of putting into words the suffering of the population in Darfur"*.[22]

In March 2009, after President Omar al-Bashir was charged with genocide by the International Criminal Court (ICC), the Dutch and French sections – both operating in the Darfur region – were expelled from the country. Along with 12 other NGOs, they were accused of having *"violated [their] mission as humanitarian organisations"* by cooperating with the ICC.[23]

This reputation as a potential "troublemaker" led to specific expectations of MSF. For Sudanese civil society movements, and particularly the professional associations which opposed the regime, MSF was a prospective ally from which they could hope to obtain material support and recognition, if not protection, insofar as its statements are a means of exerting pressure. During the 2019 revolution, resistance committees were especially keen to use MSF's voice to attract attention and establish themselves as legitimate players. It is not because they would have had a direct or immediate impact on people's suffering that MSF's statements were solicited, but because they represented *"a step towards the recognition of this suffering"*.[24] On the one hand, *"[it] was necessary for someone to bear witness to the fact that the demonstrators, including the doctors who had come to treat the wounded, were being killed"*; and, on the other, *"resistance committees used MSF's name in interviews and on public channels because for them, being supported by a recognised international organisation was a guarantee of political credibility"*.[25]

Incidentally, this quest for legitimacy is not the prerogative of popular movements. In many instances it even sits at the very heart of opposition groups' engagement strategies with humanitarian organisations. Sometimes it is akin to searching for symbolic – even discreet – support. At the start of the Sudanese revolution, MSF's response, therefore, remained clandestine: (limited) donations of equipment and medicine to a network of doctors running safe spaces to treat injured demonstrators. When two Sudanese members of MSF were arrested because of these activities, *"the very fact that we were arrested was appreciated more than the medical aid we were actually able to provide. Because it showed that MSF was on their side."*[26]

This snapshot of MSF's experiences in Sudan is a clear illustration of the ambiguity, if not the inscrutability – at least in the eyes of an outside observer – of the bonds of solidarity some humanitarian organisations forge with protest movements. The trade-off between making these bonds public or remaining discreet in order to preserve an operational response capability is a complex matter, especially as it does not depend solely on an objective assessment of the associated risks or other factors external to the organisation. In some countries, the close links between local civil societies and aid agencies are largely due to the fact that locally recruited staff are very politically active and committed. For certain positions, this closeness is even sought out by INGOs, which gain a clear advantage from the partisan loyalties of their employees. It should, therefore, come as no surprise to learn that the political culture of employees has a bearing on the manner in which an organisation takes up certain issues. In this respect, Myanmar is an interesting case study, in that activists themselves perceive the influence of an INGO such as MSF on the local political landscape as very limited.

IV The Civil Disobedience Movement in Myanmar

In Myanmar, resistance to the military coup of 1 February 2021 against Aung San Suu Kyi's government very quickly found tangible form in the Civil Disobedience Movement (CDM). The CDM was formed the day after the coup, following a call for a general strike launched by a group of doctors in Mandalay. Over the following days, peaceful demonstrations grew in scale, coinciding with a rise in the severity of the repressive measures. The highest proportion of CDM participants came from the health and education sectors. At its peak in February–March 2021, as many as 420,000 employees joined the strike,[27] and civil servants were under immense pressure to join it. "Social punishment" campaigns were organised on social media to publicise the fact that an individual belonged to one camp or the other, in an attempt to shame members of military families or business communities with close links to the Myanmar military authorities. Boycott campaigns were launched, thanks to tools such as the *Way Way Nay* ("Stay away") app, which allows anti-coup militants to make informed decisions about what they buy.[28]

Over the following months, the peaceful demonstrations gave way to violent clashes between the military forces (the *Tatmadaw*) and the pro-democracy forces organised into a rebel army consisting of resistance groups.[29] In April 2021, the opposition formed a National Unity Government (NUG), a shadow authority based partly in rebel-held areas, and partly abroad. Finally, in May 2021, it created an armed wing, the People's Defence Force (PDF), and in September 2021 the NUG declared a "defensive war". Under the command of the NUG, the PDF has between 60,000 and 80,000 soldiers, plus troops from dozens of armed ethnic groups which hold the country's border regions and have been intermittently fighting the *Tatmadaw* since independence in 1948.[30]

Whilst the CDM is an unprecedented popular uprising in Myanmar, in terms of its scale and lifespan, *"its organisers acknowledge that the movement has not reached its primary goal of pushing a crippled junta to cede power"*.[31] In October 2023, the military authorities admittedly experienced some serious setbacks during Operation 1027, in which an alliance of armed ethnic groups, the Three Brotherhood Alliance (TBA), simultaneously attacked several army, police, and other security force positions in the states of Shan, Kayah, and Rakhine. The NUG, however, still faces the challenge of obtaining genuine recognition and tangible support from the international community. Fighting aside, the repression has generated its own share of victims: since the coup, over 2,600 civilians are thought to have been killed, and 16,500 arrested during demonstrations. Activists and journalists have been imprisoned, tortured, raped, and murdered, forcing thousands of others to go into hiding or flee the country.[32]

Reckoning with the Expectations of Burmese Activists

In the immediate aftermath of the popular uprising which followed the coup in February 2021, thousands of healthcare workers joined the CDM, leaving the public health system, which represents around 80% of the country's hospitals and clinics, virtually unstaffed. Secret clinics were established by the strikers. Though they were not present at the demonstrations, because of the violence of the repression, some humanitarian organisations donated a small number of emergency kits – a strong symbolic gesture, but one with limited medical impact.

In one specific project run jointly between an INGO and the Ministry of Health, all the civil servants resigned following the coup. The subsequent decision by the INGO to take over the management of the entire hospital was controversial, as it undermined the CDM's strategy of trying to ensure that the system collapsed. The main request of locally hired humanitarian staff was that their organisation stop negotiating and cooperating with the government and refuse all contact.

Since Operation 1027 and the reversal of the balance of power between the *Tatmadaw* – which is facing a massive number of desertions – and the revolutionary forces, some aid actors are reporting increasing pressure for the humanitarian system to stop operating in government-controlled parts of the country and step up their activities in the rebel-occupied areas instead. Some activists think that the humanitarian response in government-controlled areas should be the prerogative of United Nations agencies, whilst the primary responsibility of an independent organisation such as MSF should be to circumvent access restrictions by operating more from neighbouring countries.

Two weeks after the movement began, MSF issued a press release expressing concern for the welfare of people in Myanmar, particularly healthcare workers, and deploring the restrictions imposed on its activities following the declaration of a state of emergency.[33] Those citizens who expected INGOs to stop collaborating with the military authorities were soon disappointed, however, even though many of them now understand the impact such a decision would have had:

> *Citizens did not feel supported in their political struggle. They lost confidence. At the same time, they know the limits of an organisation like MSF. They are quite realistic. While they'd prefer it if INGOs didn't pay incentives to Ministry of Health staff, they think [they] have hardly any political influence.*[34]

Time has also dampened hopes and led to a sense of fatalism for those who wanted MSF to continue its activities: "*People are tired of it. They've become pragmatic.*"[35] Beyond the passage of time and the specific characteristics of the operational environment in which MSF works in Myanmar, however, perhaps also a cultural dimension underlies this pragmatism: "*Burmese people are reserved in nature. We tend not to challenge or question others. Including MSF, I would say. We rely on ourselves and our close circle and continue working or doing what we are supposed to do.*"[36] It is, therefore, clear how the diversity of contexts prevents us from thinking in general terms about the relationships between humanitarian actors and local civil societies, as the expectations – and the constraints – are not the same everywhere. MSF's experience in Sudan, Myanmar, and elsewhere, however, would suggest that, beyond the strictly humanitarian impact, an identity issue underlies the interplay between aid actors and protest movements: when does an INGO start to be perceived as, or consider itself to be, part of the civil society of the country in which it operates? Who defines its role and limits? In the service of which agenda and according to which criteria?

V Navigating a Workable Distance

Far from limiting itself to discussions about the localisation of aid and a better sharing of the decision-making power in the humanitarian sector, the issue of how aid organisations become rooted in the communities with, and for which, they work helps shed light on the gap that may exist between the way they perceive themselves and the way they are perceived. In this respect, ambiguity can be beneficial. As a Sudanese colleague said, "*there's nothing to be gained by labelling ourselves [MSF] as part of Sudanese civil society. If they think we're their allies, so much the better, but there's no point in presenting ourselves as such.*"[37]

This ambiguity, however, can also generate a feeling of frustration: even when they consider the possibilities of aligning objectives with the social movements in the societies in which they work, humanitarian organisations adopt – consciously or not – strategies of distancing and differentiation. The reasons for this are known and repeated everywhere: fear of not having the legitimacy to lead internal political struggles and being accused of interfering; fear of being manipulated by an insurrection movement busy building its local and international credibility; fear of a backlash from authorities being challenged; fear that an outwardly peaceful and legitimate protest movement will be taken over by forces that are neither more legitimate nor more reputable than the government in place.

Are some of these fears exaggerated? While MSF's decision to speak out about massacres, or what it deems to be violations of the dignity of entire populations, has at times prevented it from working in part or all of the country concerned,[38] the fear of reprisals from disputed governments can also lead to a kind of self-censorship.[39] With regard to the risk of manipulation, it works both ways, as shown by MSF's experience in Pakistan, where international aid played the role of auxiliary to the government's counter-insurgency strategy.[40]

Apart from the real risks which may explain the initial reticence of humanitarian INGOs to intervene in times of protest, MSF may well be reluctant to get involved in political dynamics which are beyond its control and which it struggles to understand. Additionally, the organisation still has difficulty formulating interventions whose value is more symbolic than medical. Perhaps this stems, in part, from insufficient contact with civil society prior to moments of protest, weak links with the diasporas, and no real roots in the societies in which MSF works, thus creating excessive dependence on locally recruited staff. The ability of the latter to convince – even to put pressure on – the organisation to adopt a position, therefore, logically has a significant influence on the decision-making process.

In other words, the possibility for closer links between humanitarian INGOs and protest movements is shaped by the political affiliations and partisan loyalties of locally recruited employees. Subject to external influences, MSF is also a very diverse organisation. Its size, mode of governance, and complex structure reflect the divisions that run through the societies in which it operates. In that regard, the support that a cause can elicit as a result of the sense of closeness that it generates contributes to the inscrutability of certain operational choices or certain statements. For humanitarian organisations, striking a balance between a workable distance and some degree of proximity to opposition groups is not primarily a matter of preventing manipulation. From the point of view of some activists who observe what MSF does or says elsewhere, it is, rather, a question of consistency and fairness. It is only a matter of time before the new forms of online activism, which rely on public questioning as a method of civic expression and mobilisation, force humanitarian INGOs to rise to the challenge.

Notes

* Translated from French by Derek Scoins.

1 Pirotte, 2007, p. 4; Sibony, 2016, p. 3; Dahrendorf, 1990, cited by Ghils, 1994, p. 131. Translated from French by Derek Scoins.

2 MSF, 2020.

3 Whittall, 2019.

4 Jina Mahsa Amini, a 22-year-old Iranian Kurdish student, died on 16 September 2022 after being detained by the morality police in Tehran. Her death heralded the start of a series of demonstrations, during which many women removed their veils as a sign of protest.

5 Martin et al., 2020.
6 Former MSF senior executive in Hong Kong, correspondence with the author, November 2024.
7 Neuman, 2011, p. 166.
8 Martin et al., 2020.
9 See Neuman, 2011, on the history of the alliances between MSF and South African civil society.
10 See Sandrine Tiller's contribution in the zoom-in at the end of this chapter.
11 The Greek word *allilegyos* means "one who shows solidarity". It was largely used in the 2000s by refugee and migrant support groups. See Rozakou, 2017a and Papataxiarchis, 2016.
12 Rozakou, 2017b; Cabot, 2018.
13 These methods have, for example, been used by Ukrainian activists since the Russian invasion in 2022, and Israeli activists since the attacks of 7 October 2023.
14 Slim, 2022.
15 Deshayes, 2019.
16 Deshayes, 2016.
17 Deshayes and Vezzadini, 2019.
18 Bach et al., 2020.
19 MSF, 2005.
20 Binet, 2024.
21 MSF employee and Sudanese activist, interviewed by the author on 4 April 2024.
22 *Ibid.*
23 Weissman, 2011, p. 196.
24 MSF Sudanese employee, interviewed by the author on 24 April 2024.
25 Former MSF employee and Sudanese activist, interviewed by the author on 26 March 2024.
26 MSF employee and Sudanese activist, interviewed by the author on 4 April 2024.
27 Fishbein, 2023.
28 Witteking, 2021.
29 Paddock, 2022.
30 RTS, 2023.
31 Htet, 2023.
32 Aakash and Ellis-Petersen, 2023.
33 MSF, 2021.
34 Former MSF senior executive, interviewed by the author on 2 May 2024.
35 Locally hired MSF employee, interviewed by the author on 16 April 2024.
36 *Ibid.*
37 MSF employee and Sudanese activist, interviewed by the author on 4 April 2024.
38 In addition to Bahrain and Sudan, as discussed above, other examples include Ethiopia in 2007 and Panama in 2024.
39 It must also be said that, "*[i]n a growing number of countries such as Ethiopia, Russia, Zimbabwe and Sri Lanka, national laws and government framework agreements oblige MSF to strict confidentiality.*" (Weissman, 2011, p. 177).
40 Whittall, 2011.

References

Aakash, Hassan, and Hannah Ellis-Petersen (2023), 'On the frontline with the rebel army fighting Myanmar's brutal junta', *The Guardian*, 8 January. [https://www.theguardian.com/world/2023/jan/08/on-the-frontline-with-the-rebel-army-fighting-myanmars-brutal-junta].

Bach, Jean-Nicolas, Raphaëlle Chevrillon-Guibert, and Alice Franck (2020), 'Introduction to the topic: An end to authoritarian rule in Sudan?', *Politique africaine*, vol. 158, n° 2, pp. 5–31.

Binet, Laurence (2024), 'MSF and Darfur 2003–2009', Speaking Out Case Studies, Médecins Sans Frontières. [https://www.msf.org/speakingout/msf-and-darfur-2003-2009].

Cabot, Heath (2018), 'The European Refugee Crisis and Humanitarian Citizenship in Greece', *Ethnos, Journal of Anthropology*, vol. 84, n° 5, pp. 747–771. [https://www.tandfonline.com/doi/full/10.1080/00141844.2018.1529693].

Dahrendorf, Ralf (1990), *Reflections on the Revolution in Europe*, London: Chatto & Windus.

Deshayes, Clément (2016), 'Emergence de nouveaux groupes contestataires urbains et dynamiques de la semi-clandestinité au Soudan', *Confluences Méditerranée*, vol. 98, n° 3, pp. 61–73.

Deshayes, Clément (2019), 'The Sudanese Revolution: the Climax of a Decade of challenging the Political Order', *Noria*, 7 May. [https://noria-research.com/mena/the-sudanese-revolution-or-the-climax-of-a-decade-of-challenging-the-political-order/].

Deshayes, Clément, and Elena Vezzadini (2019), 'Quand le consensus se fissure. Processus révolutionnaire et spatialisation du soulèvement soudanais', *Politique africaine*, vol. 154, n° 2, pp. 149–178.

Fishbein, Emily (2023), 'Myanmar's striking civil servants: Displaced, forgotten, but holding on', *Al Jazeera*, 29 August. [https://www.aljazeera.com/news/2023/8/29/myanmars-striking-civil-servants-displaced-forgotten-but-holding-on].

Ghils, Paul (1994), 'Le concept et les notions de société civile', *Equivalences*, 24e année-n°2; 25e année-n°1–2, pp. 119–152.

Htet, Ye (2023), 'It's time to re-think the CDM', *Frontier*, 28 August. [https://www.frontiermyanmar.net/en/its-time-to-re-think-the-cdm/].

Martin, Cédric, Sandrine Tiller, and Carmen Lee (2020), 'The Hong Kong Protests of 2019 and MSF Hong Kong's Response', MSF Internal Review Paper.

MSF (2005), 'The Crushing Burden of Rape: Sexual Violence in Darfur', 8 March. [https://www.msf.org/crushing-burden-rape-sexual-violence-darfur].

MSF (2020), *Pocket Guide for Popular Uprisings*, Brussels Operational Centre.

MSF (2021), 'Myanmar: Our Statement of Solidarity', 17 February. [https://msf.org.au/article/statements-opinion/myanmar-our-statement-solidarity].

Neuman, Michaël (2011), 'South Africa: MSF, an African NGO?', in Claire Magone, Michaël Neuman, and Fabrice Weissman (eds), *Humanitarian Negotiations Revealed, The MSF Experience*, London: Hurst & Co, pp. 163–169.

Paddock, Richard (2022), 'Myanmar's Coup and Its Aftermath Explained', *The New York Times*, 9 December. [https://www.nytimes.com/article/myanmar-news-protests-coup.html].

Papataxiarchis, Evthymios (2016), 'Being "there": At the front line of the 'European refugee crisis' – part 1', *Anthropology Today*, vol. 32, n° 3, pp. 3–7.

Pirotte, Gautier (2007), *La notion de société civile*, Paris: Collection Repères, Editions La Découverte.

Rozakou, Katerina (2017a), 'Solidarians in the land of Xenios Zeus: Migrant deportability and the radicalisation of solidarity', in Dimitris Dalakoglou and Georgios Agelopoulos (eds), *Critical Times in Greece*, Abingdon: Routledge, pp. 188–201.

Rozakou, Katerina (2017b), 'Solidarity Humanitarianism: The blurred boundaries of humanitarianism in Greece', *Allegra Lab*. [https://allegralaboratory.net/solidarity-humanitarianism/].

RTS (2023), 'L'armée au pouvoir en Birmanie ébranlée par l'offensive rebelle', 1 December. [https://www.rts.ch/info/monde/14519420-larmee-au-pouvoir-en-birmanie-ebranlee-par-loffensive-des-rebelles.html#:~:text=L%27arm%C3%A9e%2C%20connue%20sous%20le,par%20divers%20groupes%20ethniques%20minoritaires].

Sibony, Denis (2016), 'La société civile: deux perspectives d'analyse', *Sciences & Actions Sociales*, vol. 2, n° 4, pp. 10–30.

Slim, Hugo (2022), 'Humanitarian resistance: Its ethical and operational importance', Humanitarian Practice Network, Network Paper n° 87.

Weissman, Fabrice (2011), 'Silence Heals… From the Cold War to the War on Terror, MSF Speaks Out: A Brief History', in Claire Magone, Michaël Neuman, and Fabrice Weissman (eds), *Humanitarian Negotiations Revealed, The MSF Experience*, London: Hurst & Co, pp. 177–197.

Whittall, Jonathan (2011), 'Pakistan: The Other Side of the Coin', in Claire Magone, Michaël Neuman, and Fabrice Weissman (eds), *Humanitarian Negotiations Revealed, The MSF Experience*, London: Hurst & Co, pp. 69–74.

Whittall, Jonathan (2019), 'Popular uprisings and humanitarian action', MSF Internal Document.

Witteking, Courtney T. (2021), 'Learning from 'Social Punishment': Neutrality in Myanmar is no longer tenable', *ISEAS Fulcrum*, 16 April. [https://fulcrum.sg/learning-from-social-punishment-neutrality-in-myanmar-is-no-longer-tenable/].

Zoom-in: Protecting Humanitarian Action in an Age of Disinformation

Sandrine Tiller

Transformative advances in digital technology in the last two decades and the creation of an "online environment" have generated a new type of risk for humanitarian practitioners. The rise of online disinformation campaigns is a direct threat to the relation of trust between humanitarians and the communities with whom they work. Trust is vital for humanitarian agencies; if the people they assist lose confidence in them, their work will be untenable. This was clearly illustrated during the COVID-19 pandemic, when the rapid spread of medical misinformation – false information shared without intent to harm – and disinformation – false or out of context information shared with harmful intent – provoked a rise in vaccine hesitancy and fuelled doubt and distrust towards medical providers.[1] In the Democratic Republic of the Congo, medical mistrust went even further, with the incitement of violence online, which led to the burning of Ebola clinics.[2]

Targeted disinformation campaigns maligning the work of humanitarians by sowing doubt on the motives of Non-governmental Organisations (NGOs) or the safety of medicines can jeopardise the provision of assistance by humanitarian actors and become a direct risk for aid-worker safety. Political actors understand the usefulness of online disinformation campaigns to push their narratives. Independent organisations providing humanitarian aid are vulnerable to these campaigns, particularly when they are seen as treating or assisting people considered "undesirable" or "enemies of the state" (e.g. migrants or certain population groups in conflict zones). The campaign waged by Israel against the United Nations Relief and Works Agency for Palestine Refugees (UNRWA) is an egregious example, with paid Google Ads being used to associate the term "terrorist" with UNRWA and effectively discredit the agency.[3]

The online environment has radically magnified the scale and spread of rumours and harmful information on social media. With the line between hostility online and real-life threats more porous than ever, how do humanitarian organisations confront damaging and false narratives?[4] This text reflects on the experience of Médecins Sans Frontières (MSF) to look at the challenges humanitarians face to retain access and protect their operations, teams, and reputation.

DOI: 10.4324/9781003542247-13

What Does the Information Landscape Look Like in Humanitarian Contexts?

Over the past 15 or so years, the world has become increasingly interconnected, with the advancement of mobile technology and the introduction of social media platforms. This has dramatically changed the information landscape. Whilst many countries where MSF works are still lagging behind in terms of access to the internet and uptake of social media, internet penetration is increasing steadily.[5]

Crisis or conflict contexts are particularly prone to toxic, fragmented, and chaotic information environments, as there are few reliable local media outlets. Online disinformation is pervasive. It is part of the propaganda toolbox:[6] an ancient, tried and tested method to promote a political point of view, influence public opinion, denigrate enemies, and set the narrative. What is different now is that social media allows it to spread incredibly fast and incredibly far.

The use of artificial intelligence (AI) to create content has allowed low-grade or irrelevant "slop" to fill social media spaces, leading to reliable information being crowded out. AI-powered automated bots are being used by states to create fake accounts to push narratives, but also to silence activists. AI can also create convincing false images and text that seem to come from real sources.[7] The rising prevalence and sophistication of AI-generated deepfake images, voice recordings, and videos thus allow the promotion of biased content, as seen in recent conflicts, such as Ukraine and in the Gaza Strip.[8]

Globally, there is little legislation to regulate content moderation and control harmful or misleading content. The recent decisions by major platforms to rescind and reduce fact-checking and content moderation policies in the United States will likely further contribute to online hate speech, harassment, and disinformation.[9] In other states, disinformation laws have been enacted, but with the aim to censor or harass opposition voices. In countries with minority languages, such as Myanmar and Ethiopia (which have unique alphabets and dialects), social media companies do not find it profitable to invest in local-language content moderation. This has allowed hate speech and disinformation to flourish.

New laws and mechanisms are being used to curtail freedom of expression and to control the media. In 2020, Sudan enacted a cybercrime law targeting the spreading of fake news, which includes penalties against anyone insulting or defaming the military online. Serious and sustained internet shutdowns have been used in Myanmar, Iraq, Sudan, Pakistan, and Ethiopia. Refugee communities in Bangladesh have additionally been banned from accessing mobile services.[10] In Ukraine, people were subjected to micro-targeted disinformation, where Russian campaigns promoted false information about the location of shelters or aid distribution to provoke population movements and create panic.[11]

Humanitarian agencies, both local and international, struggle to have their messages heard in these environments, and often end up in the crossfire: accused of portraying a country in a negative light, or of exaggerating humanitarian needs, and even of being foreign agents, of siding with armed groups, or of having ulterior motives.

What Kind of Disinformation Campaigns Has MSF Been Confronted with and How Did It Affect the Organisation?

In Hong Kong in 2019, MSF and other NGOs were targeted in an online campaign by pro-democracy protesters which aimed to garner the support of international organisations to their cause. The campaign quickly evolved into a flood of "shaming" posts, denouncing those organisations that did not seem to be standing up for democracy. In this highly political crisis, MSF's low-profile communication strategy and non-intervention led to a torrent of abuse online, as well as in person at the Hong Kong office. Thousands of donations were cancelled. Conflicting views about MSF's role in that context, as well as its identity as a civil society actor, led to an internal crisis.

Similarly to the online scrutiny observed in Hong Kong, "social punishment" was used by protesters in Myanmar after the coup in 2021, to chastise those deemed to be supportive of the military authorities. Although the doxxing campaign primarily focused on those connected to the military elite, some civil servants perceived to be collaborating with the government were also targeted and publicly shamed. MSF staff were working very closely with the Ministry of Health, and this had the effect of creating an atmosphere of anxiety amongst them. However, MSF's reputation of independence and neutrality provided a degree of protection for locally hired teams in that they could present themselves as working with an international NGO rather than with the government. Nevertheless, in order to mitigate the exposure of staff, the frequency and visibility of interactions with the authorities was diminished and, wherever possible, international staff took the lead.[12]

The Tigray war produced a very toxic online information environment in Ethiopia. Disinformation and hate speech were rampant, with frequent attacks on journalists and organisations that were seen to be helping "the enemy". The World Food Programme (WFP) in particular was subjected to an online campaign that falsified its logo (to make it look like the sheaves of wheat were guns). Meanwhile, diaspora groups used fake profiles to sow doubt on an MSF report about attacks on health facilities in Tigray.[13]

In Lebanon, anti-NGO narratives have developed online, accusing humanitarian agencies of exacerbating humanitarian crises for financial gain and being part of foreign countries' agendas. International NGOs are accused of being culturally insensitive and of creating parallel structures, thus undermining local organisations.[14] More general "anti-NGO" narratives mentioning MSF sometimes mix legitimate criticism (cultural insensitivity, for example) with unfair claims (that NGOs are enriching themselves). Responding to those would require a more in-depth, self-reflective approach, which itself could then be manipulated or misunderstood.

In the Sahel, online campaigns funded by state actors and their proxies have claimed that NGOs have ulterior motives or are deliberately causing crises.[15] There have been online stories accusing MSF of being in collusion with non-state armed groups (providing military or communications materials to them) or of being undercover for the French intelligence services. These have not had large viewing figures, but there are a variety of channels used, from videos on YouTube to WhatsApp messages and Facebook posts. Sometimes these narratives have spilled out into the real world, contributing to anti-Western sentiment in the region.[16]

In the Central African Republic, a similar campaign has echoed false accusations of MSF having links to terrorist groups, or of being a front for Western intelligence services. These claims have been published in official media outlets, with these narratives elaborated and embellished by local YouTubers.

How Did MSF Respond to Disinformation Campaigns and How Could the Organisation Be Better Prepared in the Future?

Overall, teams on the ground often struggle to assess the level of threat posed by disinformation campaigns and to anticipate tangible consequences on the organisation's activities, in order to decide on the best means of mitigation.

MSF monitors and reports any direct attacks or clear falsehoods about its operations. Debunking (countering disinformation directly online) can be done by MSF itself or through local fact-checking organisations. Pre-bunking (providing reliable information in anticipation of the escalation of a wave of disinformation) is a method that MSF and other humanitarian agencies are trialling, but it has been difficult to assess the effectiveness of this approach to date.

However, the insidiousness of "slow-burning" disinformation campaigns is much harder to counter. Firstly, there is the challenge of mapping the spread of disinformation narratives over fragmented social media "ecosystems" in different countries. Connecting the dots between online and traditional media is also difficult. Developing monitoring systems that cover multiple countries and sources over time is an essential task, but it requires trained staff who can understand the local information culture.

Project teams need an extensive analysis of the specific information environment of each context, understanding which accounts may be false, which may be "proxies" of state or non-state actors, and which of these are most influential. Anticipating the risk of online attacks targeting humanitarian staff and assessing to what extent they might translate into direct physical or psychological threats must be incorporated more clearly into MSF's security approach.

Understanding and responding to online influence campaigns which undermine the credibility of the humanitarian enterprise requires a more in-depth and long-term engagement. A multidisciplinary approach that brings together the digital communications teams with advocacy, legal, security, IT, and operations teams is needed, because what happens online goes beyond being a "comms" issue.

The current online environment that humanitarians are navigating calls for investment in context-specific analysis and communication to protect their reputation, secure their operations, and ensure that they are seen as trustworthy by the communities with whom they work.

Notes

1 Kisa and Kisa, 2024.
2 Ratcliffe, 2019.
3 Dave, 2024.
4 Global Interagency Security Forum, and Humanitarian Outcomes, 2024.
5 In places where MSF has large-scale, long-running operations, internet penetration varies between 44.5% in Bangladesh and 27.2% in the Democratic Republic of the Congo. South Sudan and the Central African Republic still have low internet penetration, at 12.1% and 10.6%, respectively. Data available at https://datareportal.com/reports.
6 Wardle and Derakhshan, 2017.
7 Jones, 2024.
8 Iacucci, 2024.
9 Newton, 2025.
10 See https://www.accessnow.org/campaign/keepiton/.
11 Center for Civilians in Conflict, 2023.
12 MSF, 2021.
13 Mwai, 2021.
14 MSF, 2024.
15 Insecurity Insight, 2024.
16 Guiffard, 2023.

References

Access Now, '#KeepItOn: Fighting Internet Shutdowns around the World'. [https://www.accessnow.org/campaign/keepiton/].

Center for Civilians in Conflict (2023), 'When Words Become Weapons: The Unprecedented Risks to Civilians from the Spread of Disinformation in Ukraine'. [https://civiliansinconflict.org/publications/research/when-words-become-weapons-the-unprecedented-risks-to-civilians-from-the-spread-of-disinformation-in-ukraine/].

DataReportal (2024), 'Reports', DataReportal – Global Digital Insights. [https://datareportal.com/reports].

Dave, Paresh (2024), 'Israel Is Buying Google Ads to Discredit the UN's Top Gaza Aid Agency', *Wired*, 26 August. [https://www.wired.com/story/israel-unrwa-usa-hamas-google-search-ads/].

Global Interagency Security Forum, and Humanitarian Outcomes (2024), 'State of Practice: The Evolution of Security Risk Management in the Humanitarian Space'. [https://humanitarianoutcomes.org/security_risk_mgmt_humanitarian_space_2024].

Guiffard, Jonathan (2023), 'Le sentiment anti-français en Afrique de l'Ouest, reflet de la confrontation autoritaire contre "l'Occident collectif"', *Institut Montaigne*. [https://www.institutmontaigne.org/expressions/le-sentiment-anti-francais-en-afrique-de-louest-reflet-de-la-confrontation-autoritaire-contre].

Iacucci, Anahi Ayala (2024), 'Misinformation, Disinformation and Hate Speech in Conflict', Grand Challenges Canada.

Insecurity Insight (2024), 'Social Media Watch: Protecting the Humanitarian Space in Mali'. [https://insecurityinsight.org/wp-content/uploads/2024/12/13.-Protecting-the-Humanitarian-Space-in-Mali-Dec-2024.pdf].

Jones, Marc Owen (2024), 'How Do States and Non-State Actors Use Social Media for Deception and Disinformation?', in Anna Reuss, and Stephan Stetter (eds), *Social*

Media and Peacebuilding, Cham: Springer Nature Switzerland (Rethinking Peace and Conflict Studies), pp. 25–48. doi:10.1007/978-3-031-73917-0_2.

Kisa, Sezer, and Adnan Kisa (2024), 'A Comprehensive Analysis of COVID-19 Misinformation, Public Health Impacts, and Communication Strategies: Scoping Review', *Journal of Medical Internet Research*, vol. 26. doi:10.2196/56931.

MSF (2021), 'Mis/Disinformation Project Report', MSF Internal Report.

MSF (2024), 'Anti-NGO Rhetoric in Lebanon', MSF Internal Report.

Mwai, Peter (2021), 'Tigray Conflict: The Fake UN Diplomat and Other Misleading Stories', *BBC*, 25 March. [https://www.bbc.com/news/56456535].

Newton, Casey (2025), 'Meta Just Flipped the Switch That Prevents Misinformation from Spreading in the United States', *Platformer*, 14 January. [https://www.platformer.news/meta-ends-misinformation-enforcement-zuckerberg/].

Ratcliffe, Rebecca (2019), 'Arsonists Attack Ebola Clinics in DRC as Climate of Distrust Grows', *The Guardian*, 28 February. [https://www.theguardian.com/global-development/2019/feb/28/arsonists-attack-ebola-clinics-in-drc-as-climate-of-distrust-grows].

Wardle, Claire, and Hossein Derakhshan (2017), 'Information Disorder: Toward an Interdisciplinary Framework for Research and Policy Making', Council of Europe.

7 Speaking Out With, Not For

Rethinking Humanitarian Narratives

*Sophie Désoulières and Juliette Garms**

> *[I]t is clear that all sections of MSF have a common understanding of the basis for our action as both medical and humanitarian, and inextricably linked with the expression of public positions and describing our experiences ("temoignage") to the point that the separation of the concept of "temoignage" from operations has disappeared.*[1]

Denouncing the situations of widespread human suffering that teams from Médecins Sans Frontières (MSF) have periodically witnessed is an integral part of the organisation's identity. Indeed, speaking out is the cornerstone of the MSF foundation story: doctors who, in reaction to the silence imposed by the International Committee of the Red Cross during the Biafra War in Nigeria, created MSF with journalists, in 1971. *"Speaking out, denouncing, standing up for victims against their murderers, such was to be the thrust of the new humanitarian commitment embodied by MSF."*[2] While this interpretation is often criticised and questioned, it remains deeply embedded in the organisation's culture.[3]

On 10 December 1999, when MSF was awarded the Nobel Peace Prize, the president of the MSF International Council gave a speech that began by calling on Russian authorities to halt the bombing of civilians in Chechnya, highlighting the fact that staying silent in the face of mass crimes undoubtedly helps to prolong them.[4] Although MSF does not labour under the illusion that it can improve crisis situations simply by speaking out, its current strategic vision for public communications, "Telling It As It Is", demonstrates a continuing determination to provide accounts of events that reflect reality as accurately as possible.[5] The quote which opens this chapter highlights how the act of *témoignage*, or bearing witness, remains one of the organisation's pillars. But it is a tricky proposition, considering how multiple actors have instrumentalised MSF's public messages; the self-righteous directives levelled at states over what they should or should not do; the sterile rhetoric of indignation;[6] and the worry that the organisation is seen as awarding itself *"a licence to adopt positions on every topic in the name of some hypothetical universal moral doctrine"*.[7]

Leaving these pitfalls aside, what exactly does bearing witness entail? A restrictive but highly concrete definition would be similar to a legal

DOI: 10.4324/9781003542247-14

interpretation, i.e. the fact of being an eyewitness, particularly when no one else is present.[8] From this perspective, there have only been a few instances in MSF's history when it has been an eyewitness, *"such as Kibeho in Rwanda and Srebrenica, or the Brazzaville massacres in '98. Because MSF had a physical presence on the ground, and there were no journalists or human rights NGOs."*[9]

In 1995, the first international meeting mobilising the entire MSF movement resulted in an agreement on the core principles that underpin the organisation's identity. Article 2 stipulates that *"the presence of volunteers with people in danger as they provide medical care which implies being near and listening"* must constitute the basis for *témoignage*. It also mentions the *"duty to raise public awareness about these people"*, as well as the possibility of denouncing breaches of international conventions.[10] The text thus offers a clear definition of what is involved in bearing witness, an act that must not be *ex nihilo*, but, rather, requires humanitarian assistance and the presence of staff in its provision.

However, both the notion of *témoignage* and the environment in which MSF operates have changed significantly since the organisation was founded in 1971. It is now rare for MSF to be the only humanitarian organisation present, or the only entity in a position to raise awareness or even denounce events. What is more, the rise of social media makes it possible for the people directly impacted by crises to bear witness themselves. The fact that the organisation no longer seeks to limit itself to relaying the testimonies it collects, but wants to convey stories in collaboration with the individuals affected, represents a major shift. However, the act of bearing witness is based on procedures essentially designed and implemented by MSF – such as identifying the regions and social groups concerned, and prioritising certain types of crises – which, therefore, lessens participation by people at the heart of events.

Despite the existence of an institutional definition of *témoignage*[11] and the omnipresence of the term in MSF's internal perceptions and discourse, there are many different interpretations and multiple ways of bearing witness. While there are those who systematically combine *témoignage* with speaking up publicly to expose and denounce a situation, others prefer to embed the act of bearing witness within advocacy work seeking to influence the structural causes of a crisis.[12] This chapter examines some of the ethical issues raised by the concept of *témoignage*: the unequal relationship between aid worker and aid recipient, the need to protect the dignity of those being photographed, and new forms of collaboration centring on advocacy challenges. It will also look at notable changes the notion has undergone over recent decades.

I Bearing Witness: An Unequal Relationship?

Every component of an MSF operation can constitute a testimony, whether it is the journey of patients fleeing their homes due to fighting, an ambulance driver's account of being arrested by armed groups, photographs taken during a rescue at sea, or medical data showing a rise in the number of patients who are survivors of sexual violence. However, delivering medical care and relaying witness accounts do not necessarily coexist easily, particularly in the case of individual experiences. The fact is that the relationship between aid provider and recipient is unequal, which may lead people to believe that their testimony is a prerequisite for assistance.

This observation raises many questions. To what extent is providing testimony affected by an individual's dependence on an organisation? The issue of free and informed consent comes into play and cannot be evaded:

> *A fundamental principle of ethical storytelling is informed consent. When NGOs and journalists talk to people [...], film them, record them, photograph them, participants should have a clear understanding of why they are being interviewed, where their content will end up, and have the right to withdraw consent at any time.*[13]

Speaking on behalf of the people the organisation assists runs the risk of reducing the agency of communities often presented as powerless victims and passive recipients of aid.[14] In MSF's case, *témoignage* is partly rooted in a neocolonial heritage reflected in some of its practices and a historical concentration of power in its European headquarters, as well as an iconography that at times draws on the white saviour myth:[15]

> *It is not a simple matter of resemblance – how contemporary humanitarian action appears to echo the patterns and ambitions of earlier imperial "projects" – but that the two phenomena are ultimately bound together in a series of mutually constituting histories, in which the ideas and practices associated with imperial politics and administration have both been shaped by and have in themselves informed developing notions of humanitarianism.*[16]

Therefore, the process for collecting and using testimonies, particularly the choice of who decides their purpose and application (ultimately determined by MSF), can contribute to the perpetuation of certain stereotypes. This, in turn, can further exacerbate the existing inequalities in relationships the organisation has with the people it seeks to assist.[17]

There are ways of reducing the dependency characterising this relationship. Since the act of providing care falls under medical and patient confidentiality, it is preferable for individual accounts to be collected by non-medical staff or, in certain cases, medical staff operating outside the caregiving context. This creates a distance between a consultation and the process of gathering testimonies, conveying to the person a clear message that they can refuse without it affecting their treatment by the organisation.

However, it is unlikely that these precautions can guarantee truly free consent, particularly in cases where participants suffer from major physical or psychological vulnerability.[18] When an NGO gives bearing witness a central role, it does not follow that each and every dramatic account should be related at all costs, at the risk of re-traumatising victims or even endangering the very people the organisation is meant to help. On the other hand, it is also important not to fall into a form of paternalism that takes away their right to decide whether they are capable of sharing their experiences or not.

The unequal relationship that exists between the person gathering testimony and the person giving it is magnified by the use MSF makes of the stories and images it collects, the life journeys people share, and the situations it sometimes witnesses first hand. The question arises of how the quality and power of an account are assessed within MSF. A number of fundamental criteria are applied, which are, at least theoretically, objective: the reliability of the story, how singular it is, and the organisation's legitimacy in expressing itself on the subject.

The 2015 air strike on the MSF-run hospital in Kunduz in Afghanistan, which led to the death of patients and staff, meets the criteria of a direct and, therefore, dependable witness account, since the facts were related by staff present during the attack.[19] The degree of trust placed in the truthfulness of a report often differs according to how credible the source is and how close they are to operations. Data collected by MSF through its activities, or testimony from somebody employed by the organisation, for example, meet both criteria. Other types of information may be considered reliable to varying degrees, such as patients' statements to MSF staff that can be corroborated by medical data.

It is possible to see this scale of values as tainted by condescension. And it is true that the credibility accorded to stories shared by patients, especially women, is often tentative and fragile; a measure of scepticism is not unusual within MSF. This was recently the case in Chad when testimonies from women who had experienced sexual violence in Sudan were gathered from the survivors themselves:[20] "*Is this not just anecdotal? Do they really know who the attacker is? Can we trust them, do they have another motive?*" And when the reliability of people's words is not challenged, then the use made of them and the value of their consent are questioned: "*She certainly didn't realise what the risks were when she agreed to her story being made public.*"[21]

What is more, the organisation's editorial choices are shaped by how decision-makers assess the "value" or relevance of a testimony, along with its reliability and the risks associated with its use.[22] However, while these decision-makers now hail from a greater variety of places, men still hold most of these positions.[23] As a result, women from the Global South – who remain under-represented in managerial positions, particularly in MSF field operations – are at the intersection of several forms of discrimination.

Scepticism about people's motivations and the truthfulness of testimonies collected is particularly acute when it concerns accounts from MSF employees working in their home country.[24] It is clear that individuals recruited locally have a different relationship with the societies in which MSF operates than their international colleagues do. However, making a radical distinction between two types of employees is, to some extent, misguided. The teams work within a shared set of forces and constraints, and this approach can prove discriminatory inasmuch as it presupposes that locally hired staff may lack objectivity when it comes to their own society, or that they cannot fully embody the organisation's core principles.[25] Keeping a certain distance from country-specific political and social dynamics is surely crucial to MSF's ability to operate, and this mindset does not apply only to international employees. Consequently, the existence of an implicit hierarchy between different types of stories, often intersecting with gender or racial stereotypes and suggesting mistrust of people thought to be too directly affected by ongoing crises, remains a problem.[26]

II Speak Up or Stay Silent? Associated Risks

Bearing witness, especially when it involves speaking out about injustice or discrimination, or even atrocities, often means accepting some degree of risk, namely the possibility of reprisals, first and foremost for the people concerned.

Assessing the risks faced by communities and MSF staff is just as subjective as the process of evaluating the relevance of a story, and will influence the use made of the testimonies collected. An accusation targeting authorities, whether a state or a non-state armed group, will almost inevitably have repercussions. On the other hand, it does not typically result in long-term and widespread loss of access to populations or endangerment of MSF teams and people receiving humanitarian aid. However, the worst-case scenario is often envisaged – expulsion or a major security risk – and this underpins the choice to stay silent.

This assessment of the danger seems to be specifically linked to communication and can sometimes create conditions that will exacerbate a number of risks. In several countries where the state apparatus is particularly powerful and restrictive, MSF tends to limit its communications, thereby failing to occupy the public space:

> *In Ethiopia, after staying silent for years, we denounced abuses committed by government forces when the war broke out in Tigray. We could never have eliminated the risks associated with speaking out, but we could have prepared the ground by communicating beforehand about who we are, our medical activities. Making sure that the public knew about us would no doubt have helped to check the rumours, and possibly even to obtain a degree of support from the population.*[27]

An example of a state instrumentalising the organisation's policy of *témoignage* occurred a few years ago in the wake of a media scandal in West Africa. In late 2022, Reuters published a detailed report revealing that the Nigerian Army had run a secret abortion programme for ten years, allegedly involving over 10,000 women. The women, some of them in their eighth month of pregnancy, came from areas of Nigeria held by Boko Haram and *"liberated"* by the army.[28] The Nigerian government launched an internal investigation while arguing that if the accusations had any truth to them, MSF, which was present in the refugee camps, would have denounced the situation. The organisation has since reviewed medical data, testimonies, and context analyses produced at the time without finding any evidence that it could have known about the abuses, and thus was not in a position to flag them. It is highly unlikely that the army would have authorised, much less organised, the transportation of victims of a secret programme to health centres run by MSF. But what the Nigerian authorities revealed by basing their argument on MSF's silence is a well-founded understanding of the principles underpinning humanitarian testimonies and the ability to manipulate public projections and expectations of the organisation's actions for their own purposes.

Fear of losing access to a community or region stems from a presumption that is particularly important within MSF: that the organisation plays an essential role by offering significant medical and humanitarian aid to people who would receive none otherwise. When the care provided can seem insufficient or even derisory, given the scale of the needs, and/or when MSF is not the only actor present, the question arises of reviewing our risk assessment:

> *It is often the case that our operations can only be extremely limited and cannot meet all the most urgent needs of a group of people. Systematically choosing to stay silent for fear of losing access or, even worse, in the hope of obtaining it by basing the decision on this presumption is often misguided.*[29]

Nevertheless, it is worth noting recent efforts to include the people concerned in the decision-making process, particularly patients and their communities, as well as locally recruited staff members.[30] These are the people who are the first to suffer the consequences of speaking out: consequences that are not always immediate or obvious, but which can emerge over the long term when the organisation is no longer present, including threats, extortion, bribery, and bureaucratic hindrances. Although commendable, such efforts may have often seemed superficial, serving to support a decision already taken or creating the impression that the voices of people concerned are used to endorse directives discussed elsewhere.[31] The choice to make public a testimony is, therefore, occasionally perceived as arbitrary or contingent on an individual or decision-making group, meaning that it is steeped in contradictions. Depending on the person relaying people's stories and the position they want to support, Rohingya in open-air prisons in Myanmar or migrants imprisoned in Libya "*absolutely do not want us to compromise the continuity of our operations*" or, conversely, want to speak out.[32]

The organisation has an undeniable responsibility towards the patients and their families who trust it to use their testimonies dutifully. It must take all possible precautions to minimise potential risks to people after they have spoken out, by obtaining their informed consent regarding how their story or image is used and guaranteeing to protect their anonymity where necessary. Although speaking out has only rarely led to a lasting loss of access to people in need, it remains a challenging and often uncomfortable decision, and one for which the organisation has to take full responsibility.[33] Lastly, assessing risks that locally hired staff are exposed to is a tricky task, particularly when incidents occur within the private or family sphere, and because very few are reported to the organisation.

III Representing Suffering: From Passive Victim to Active Collaboration

> *The idea that photographs are an effective means to raise collective awareness is so deeply rooted in the sector's culture that displaying shocking images of human suffering is part of a vow to "tell it as it is" encapsulated in MSF's conception of* témoignage.[34]

Images, photojournalism, and documentary photography have always been intrinsic to humanitarian testimonies. An image is itself a way of relating a story, since it illustrates what has been witnessed and experienced. Moreover, it lends credibility to personal narratives.[35] Humanitarian photography is thus a form of "object as witness" that cannot easily be challenged.

Over the past 50 years, MSF has documented a great many crises all over the world and produced thousands of images, sometimes in partnership with journalists, making photography a key element of its identity. However, it is crucial to deconstruct, at least partially, what the organisation means by "visual *témoignage*" and, in particular, distortions that may be present between photographer and subject, as well as the moral assumption that justifies the use of images of suffering to prompt a predominantly Western audience to protest or take action.[36] While multiple interpretations of a visual *témoignage* exist within MSF, the ethical and political motivations that underpin the concept are clear and acknowledged: MSF has a duty to show things as they really are, to illustrate reality, in order to inform, alarm, arouse empathy, and, at times, shock. This aim of shocking the audience has become the focus of numerous ethical discussions over what constitutes a dignified representation of the people photographed or filmed:

> *Such images have a catalysing effect on international solidarity, while also creating a specific regime of representation [...]. Suffering human bodies are seen alongside pictures of health-care professionals in action, contributing to the notorious construct of the imaginary ideal of the western saviour – or "white saviour" – committed to science-based action, asserting neutrality in aid interventions.*[37]

Faced with the need to communicate, it may be tempting to hide behind the concept of bearing witness to sideline all ethical considerations as well as the organisation's responsibility within this process. The directive to *"tell it like it is"* could reach its limits when it conflicts with the imperative to avoid dehumanising and stigmatising the people being photographed, usually from the Global South.[38] The challenge today, then, is to produce new representations that continue to alert the public without systematically reducing the people whom MSF assists to suffering bodies who need to be saved.

IV Institutional Wake-up Call

While images can inspire emotions, they also influence how the world is perceived, especially when focused on communities rarely represented in the media. By collecting and sharing a large volume of images, MSF has played a part in shaping not only the sector's standards but also the way we visualise a humanitarian crisis and the people it affects. Some of these images, due to their widespread exposure, have become deeply entrenched stereotypes. On the other hand, a number of authors believe that representation of suffering can be justified if it leads to action, such as fundraising, or conveys a strong enough moral message.[39]

For the purposes of bearing witness or raising funds, MSF and numerous other organisations have published images of extreme suffering – naked, starving bodies and emaciated faces, labelled in the early 1980s as a form of social pornography.[40] The Ethiopian famine of 1984 gave rise to a multiplication of shocking images, marking a turning point in raising awareness of the need to use more dignified portrayals.[41] In recent years, the entire humanitarian sector has delved deeper into a critical exploration of the issue of representing the people it helps and the power relations inherent to the production of images.[42]

As an organisation, the first step has been to deconstruct the image creation process and the motivations behind it. In 2021, MSF launched an extensive review of its audiovisual database with the goal of identifying problematic images, adding warning notices, or removing them from usage, depending on criteria such as protecting minors, extreme suffering, stereotypes, and "white saviourism", i.e. images of mainly Western aid workers alongside victims from the Global South.[43] Over 10,000 photos were flagged and the process was presented internally to raise awareness among MSF staff. The organisation then reviewed its ethical guidelines for employees, as well as for the journalists it works with.

Adopting a new epistemological starting point is, therefore, crucial: just as bearing witness does not occur in a neutral system, so there is no one way to relate a reality. The aestheticisation of poverty and suffering has likely contributed to their normalisation and to entrenching fixed categories of people. While some authors believe that introducing beauty into a disaster scene can combat stereotypes,[44] the hoped-for wave of indignation tends to recede in response to representations that often arouse weariness or even pity. One of the underlying challenges lies in the fact that *"it is an easy, well-trodden path to photograph victims as evidence of an injustice. It's much harder to think about how to photograph an unjust system."*[45]

Fundamentally, while the aim is not to denounce all the structural causes of a crisis, NGOs have a duty to put the images in context to prevent the people represented serving as symbols of a far larger and more complex problem. This depoliticisation of suffering often means that the participants are reduced to their hardships, offering an incomplete picture of their social and political conditions.[46] In doing so, it has at times strengthened discrimination and assumptions, running counter to the advocacy objectives and the reasons why the images were collected in the first place. For example, photographs of African men crowded on to makeshift rafts in the middle of the Mediterranean raised awareness of the violence of European migratory policies in some people, while fuelling xenophobia in others.[47]

V Re-adjusting the Focus?

How can we continue to bear witness in such a complex environment without falling into the trap of sensationalism? Prioritising respect for consent, along with the dignity and safety of the person at the centre of the image, could feasibly set a shift in motion. This would mean giving the photographic impact less importance, in favour of concerns around the contributor's well-being. This shift in focus requires a clear-sighted rethink of MSF's roles and expectations in relation to the photographer–subject–audience triangle.

In concrete terms, people photographed or filmed would need to become collaborators rather than passive subjects, through closer involvement in the production process and editorial decision-making. The humanitarian sector is responding to this need by exploring alternative approaches to visual narrative in collaboration with the communities it assists. Certain initiatives, inspired by educator Paulo Freire's research,[48] remained confined to specific regions for many years. One example is Central America in the 1990s and 2000s, where disposable cameras were distributed to street children cared for by MSF, so that they could capture images from their environment. These initiatives are now being revived. In 2024, MSF developed two projects giving contributors the role of photographer and creative director. Texas, a Sudanese teenager, used a camera to document his daily life in a camp in Calais, northern France. He wanted to show the challenges facing a young person living on the streets, transforming the experience of violence, poverty, and exile into poetry.

The second project took place in Chocó, in the Pacific region of Colombia. Photographer Fernanda Pineda and the MSF community engagement team worked with communities of African descent to document, in an artistic manner, the impact of armed conflict and institutional shortcomings in basic services. Women healers used traditional medicine to symbolically treat photographs of places marked by fighting, armed incursions, and assassinations, highlighting their desire to remain on their lands.

The key value of these initiatives lies in the personal aspect of the photographs, far removed from the dominant representations usually seen in the press. This does not mean that MSF is sanitising suffering or no longer showing it: rather, the goal is to present challenging situations in various ways, with a focus on understanding complex individual or collective stories.

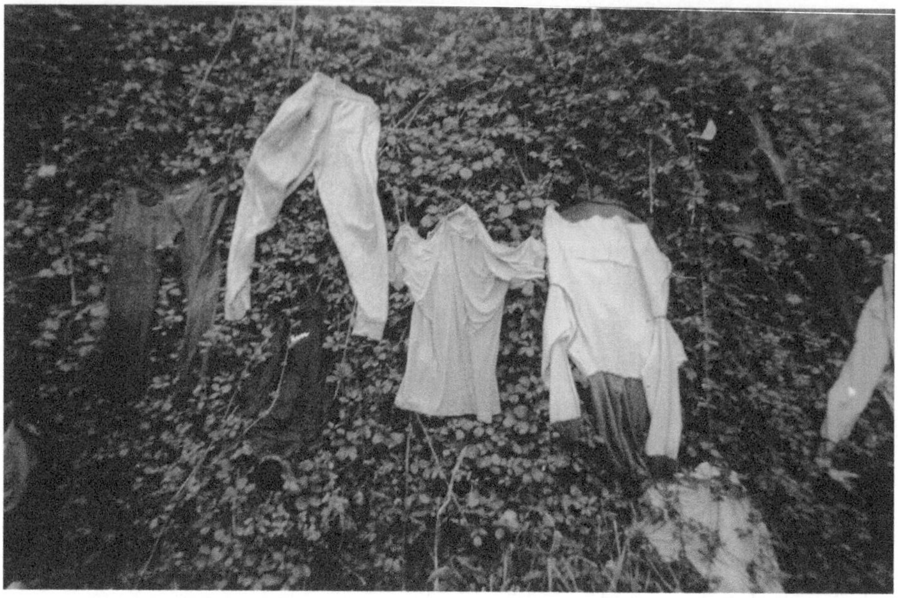

Figure 7.1 Just-washed clothes drying in the trees. © Texas/Projet Calais Darkroom/MSF

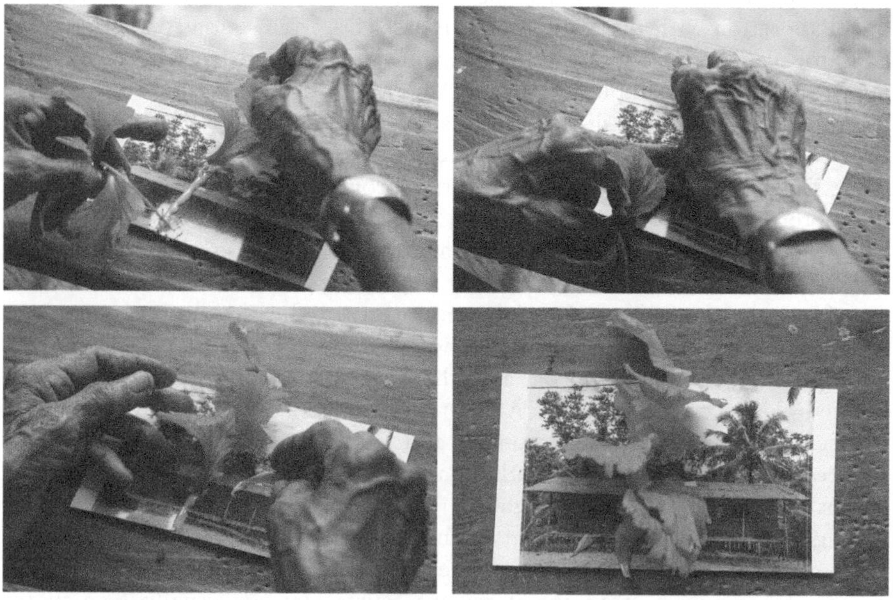

Figure 7.2 Teolinda Castro heals the photograph of her community with a *resucito* flower, which she uses as an infusion to treat headaches and stomach aches. © Yazury Dumaza/Fernanda Pineda/MSF.

The organisation is now using discussion groups with patients and MSF staff from affected communities to examine the factors motivating contributors to take part in audiovisual projects, and to solicit feedback on a selection of photographs presented to the group. While it is still too early to draw any conclusions, the process has already revealed differences rooted in the degree of dependency on MSF. For example, the gratitude felt by survivors of rescue operations in the Mediterranean towards MSF influences their desire to have their photo taken. But they also cite a wish to tell their story to the public as another motivation, in what some authors term a *"continuum of choice"*.[49] People's aspirations, therefore, often overlap, and decisions need to be taken on a case-by-case basis.

It is worth noting that the goal is not to offer a new definition of visual *témoignage*, which is constantly evolving, nor to diminish the legitimacy of the power of images. Representations of suffering can still play an important role, though they should be produced and shared thoughtfully and cautiously, always protecting the dignity of the participants. The biggest change is needed on the other side of the camera, questioning the process of collecting images, reviewing the methodologies currently in use, and thinking of the people filmed or photographed as collaborators in their own right. This means that MSF should, in some cases, simply play the role of facilitator, leaving the individuals concerned to choose how the images and stories collected should be produced.[50]

VI Advantages and Drawbacks of Silent Advocacy

The notion of bearing witness at MSF has often been perceived collectively as a cry of indignation, capable of bringing about change by raising awareness. It is rooted in the idea that shedding light on a tragic situation could result in public demands for leaders to live up to their responsibilities.[51] Currently, traditional means for pressurising Western governments are becoming less effective, while other actors, primarily China and Russia, extend their spheres of influence.

MSF has adapted to this process by adding a diplomatic component and more in-depth and sophisticated bilateral actions to its engagement strategies. This means that the organisation is developing subtler, less visible advocacy initiatives which, in the long run, have sometimes proved more effective than public denunciations. For example, in al-Hol in north-eastern Syria, where families were held after fleeing during the fall of Deir ez-Zor, the last stronghold of the Islamic State group, in 2019, MSF advocated for the repatriation of children and their detained mothers. The organisation supported efforts undertaken by other actors and addressed the governments concerned directly, relaying the extreme harshness of the living conditions observed.[52]

Assessing the impact of these actions is a central issue. MSF's testimony and advocacy undeniably helped to keep media attention on al-Hol and highlight the danger faced by minors. In Ethiopia, the UN Special Rapporteur on violence against women and girls partly relied on MSF's testimony to denounce the widespread use of rape in the Tigray conflict.[53] However, did these denunciations deliver justice and reparation for survivors? It is difficult to reach any objective conclusions, but MSF's *témoignage* is a crucial link in the chain of advocacy efforts.

It is worth noting that there is a strong temptation to exclusively opt for low-profile advocacy initiatives with the implicit aim of gaining only the benefits of bearing witness (exposing a crisis, expressing solidarity with people affected) while avoiding the risks (compromising access to communities or the organisation's reputation). Nevertheless, an approach where back-channel diplomacy in embassies replaces speaking out would not only undermine the original purpose of *témoignage* at MSF, which is closely tied to public denunciation, but would alter its essentially time-limited nature. The fact is that advocacy as practised by MSF relies on the organisation's proximity to a given situation, generally aiming to bring about rapid change to improve the lives of those affected by a specific crisis.

A humanitarian organisation's goals are almost always temporary, or should adhere to an *"interim ethic"*, to use David Rieff's expression.[54] Long-term ambitions, such as bringing about changes in laws and altering sociocultural norms, are not considered to be within the realm of legitimate action for humanitarian aid organisations like MSF. Aside from a handful of exceptions in the health field – such as the decisive role MSF played via its operations in Nigeria and patient testimonies to ensure that the gangrenous disease noma was added to the World Health Organization's list of neglected tropical diseases[55] – MSF helps to move certain issues forward but does not supplant the states and organisations whose responsibility it is to do so. The desire to embrace a policy for bringing about long-term change must remain limited if the organisation wants to maintain its capacity to respond to the most urgent humanitarian emergencies. The majority of advocacy efforts combine private and public components, and their goals evolve according to the needs identified during medical and humanitarian operations. For instance, after the Islamic State group withdrew from Rakka in Syria, testimonies from teams and patients injured by anti-personnel mines and other explosive devices – as well as medical data illustrating the extent of the phenomenon – were instrumental in the development of an advocacy strategy in favour of demining homes, hospitals, and other civilian buildings.[56] This strategy centred on public efforts (reports and articles) and private actions (bilateral actions targeting governments, information-sharing and coordination with humanitarian demining actors) to support the initiatives run by other organisations. Although this type of advocacy has a limited time frame, it may have a lasting and useful impact: the efforts undertaken in this case led to increased attention on civilian demining.[57]

More recently, a public report detailed the scale of sexual violence committed by armed groups in Sudan, accompanied by an engagement strategy targeting actors in the conflict and their state backers. While the report and strategy did not result in an end to these crimes, they did help draw attention to the issue.[58] In Cox's Bazar, Bangladesh, where nearly a million Rohingya have been exiled, MSF has increased the active participation of the people it assists. Rohingya colleagues who had previously worked with MSF in Myanmar and now find themselves, along with their families, among the refugees are documenting acts of violence or discrimination targeting displaced people. They are familiar with the organisation and share the daily lives of the camp's residents, who know and respect them, yet their active participation in the use made of these testimonies is not sought out. A policy for *témoignage* that is truly rooted in the spirit of collaboration should at least partially include the people affected in deciding how their stories are used. It would also mean integrating the different demands that can coexist within the Rohingya community, which may require the organisation to accept that collected testimonies serve objectives it does not necessarily share; in doing so, MSF would need to assume the associated political or reputational risks.

This concern is becoming increasingly significant as MSF continues to adjust the scope of its operational model by collaborating with local organisations in a growing number of contexts. Some of these organisations may adopt more partisan positions than MSF, which seeks to align itself with the viewpoints of affected people rather than pressing for specific political demands. The challenge lies in finding the balance between potentially divergent interests while also protecting the integrity of all actors involved. It is also worth noting that demands emanating from within a given community are often diverse, and reflect the specific aspirations of several groups. The organisation must be mindful to take this heterogeneity into account when designing its practices of *témoignage*.

VII Conclusion

"Throughout their history, humanitarian actors have worked in many conflicts deeply marked not only by the clash of metal and bodies, but also by the din of conflicting words, claims and narratives."[59] The proliferation of social media has made it more difficult to speak out in contexts where MSF tries to implement actions inextricably linked to *témoignage*: violations of the duty to protect hospitals, criminalisation of humanitarian operations, and disinformation campaigns make access to affected populations increasingly fragile. It is hard to hear the voices of the most disadvantaged and oppressed people in a saturated media landscape. In this context, it is particularly important to take the time to express nuanced testimonies in response to an ever-faster consumption of information and images, described by some authors as the fruit of "attention capitalism".[60] At the time of writing, very few journalists and barely any human rights organisations have access to Sudan, the scene of one of the deadliest wars in recent memory. The very worst abuses are being committed with total impunity behind this wall of silence.

Bearing witness always has a clear, relevant, and urgent goal: to bring about change in a situation, for the well-being of the people affected by it. This is not a mandate assumed by MSF, but rather a means of accomplishing the task it has set itself: saving lives, alleviating suffering, and restoring dignity and humanity through medical and humanitarian aid.[61] In recent decades, MSF has diversified and new entities have been created, with a renewed commitment and dedication to the notion of *témoignage*, but also claiming the right to reinvent it by introducing greater equality and inclusivity. The goal is to ensure that bearing witness is rooted in the involvement of patients, communities, and employees throughout the process and in a spirit of collaboration. Lastly, it is crucial for MSF to maintain a critical understanding of its practices so that they can be updated in a constantly shifting environment. Indeed, this imperative could also be extended to the entire aid sector, especially at a time when humanitarian aid is seeing its relevance and freedom to act questioned more than ever.[62]

Notes

* Translated from French by Philippa Bowe.

1 MSF, 2006: La Mancha Agreement, approved by the MSF International Council on 25 June 2006 after over a year of discussion and debate.

2 Brauman, 2012, p. 1525.

3 See Brauman, 2005; Desgrandchamps, 2011, pp. 95–108; Desgrandchamps, 2018.

4 Binet and Saulnier, 2019, p. 198–201.

5 Benoît, 2019.

6 Brauman, 2005.

7 MSF France President's Report 2000–2001, cited by Soussan, 2008, p. 36. Translated from French by Philippa Bowe.

8 See Guilhaumou, 1999, pp. 138–40.

9 Brauman, 2008. Translated from French by Philippa Bowe.

10 MSF, 1997.

11 MSF, 2020, p. 9.

12 *"Advocacy is something that came from the human rights community, with an idea of addressing some of the underlying causes, very much the Anglo-American approach. Whereas the francophone approach was much more grounded in the* cri du cœur, *a moral outrage being expressed."* (Marc DuBois in Gorin, 2021, p. 29).

13 Roberts, 2024.

14 *"[There is] no need to hear your voice, when I can talk about you better than you can speak about yourself ... I want to know your story. And then I will tell it back to you in a new way. Tell it back to you in such a way that it has become my own. Rewriting you, I write myself anew. I am still author, authority. I am still the coloniser, the speaking subject."* (hooks, 1989, p. 22).

15 "*MSF adopted medical practices rooted in the colonial era (mobile medicine, mass vaccinations, training for health workers, etc.) because they provided a suitable technical response to its objectives.*" (Brauman, 2005). Translated from French by Philippa Bowe. See also Bancel, 2005; Cole, 2012; Neuman, 2017.

16 Skinner and Lester, 2013, cited by Davey, Borton, and Foley, 2013.

17 Plowright, 2024, pp. 112–21.

18 Arnsten, 2009, pp. 410–22.

19 Rasmussen, 2015.

20 MSF, 2024b; Duroch et al., 2024.

21 Private communication with managers from the Operations and Medical departments, MSF Netherlands and MSF Belgium, January–July 2024. Translated from French by Philippa Bowe.

22 See the collection of case studies exploring the organisation's actions and decision-making processes during crises which have led it to speak out. Available online at https://www.msf.org/speakingout.
23 In 2023, 38.5% of MSF international mobile staff were women (compared to 46% in 2018) and very few of them had operational decision-making roles (21% mission heads and 31% project coordinators). (MSF, 2024a).
24 In 2023, locally hired staff represented 91.1% of project teams. *Ibid.*
25 Healy, 2021; Davey, 2024.
26 Davey et al., 2023, pp. 89–90.
27 Private communication with a communications advisor, MSF Netherlands, April 2023. Translated from French by Philippa Bowe.
28 Carsten et al., 2022.
29 Private communication with a medical department director, MSF Netherlands, October 2024.
30 Weissman, 2023.
31 Private communication with MSF teams in Malaysia, March 2025; Davey et al., 2023, p. 181.
32 Private communication with heads of mission, June 2021 and November 2023.
33 See the collection of case studies exploring the organisation's actions and decision-making processes during crises which have led it to speak out. Available online at https://www.msf.org/speakingout.
34 Duroch and L'Homme, 2022.
35 *"The status of witness effectively assumed by the photograph is based on this personal experience. From a symbolic viewpoint, it embodies the external agent who has personally witnessed what is related by the NGO (directly concerned by the story)."* (Contreras-Gama, 2016, p. 270). Translated from French by Philippa Bowe.
36 Campbell, 2003, pp. 69–96.
37 Martínez, 2024, p. 66.
38 Chouliaraki and Stupart, 2025, pp. 306–21.
39 Calain, 2013, pp. 278–85.
40 Lissner, 1981.
41 *"For some, this shift was not only motivated by a concern to avoid representations of death or suffering but also a desire to positively brand their organisation and to display its effectiveness. Efforts to reframe humanitarian imagery thus continued to raise questions about the ethical implications of picturing people in situations of vulnerability."* (Duroch and L'Homme, 2022).
42 Jacobs and Garms, 2022.
43 MSF, 2022b.
44 Campbell, 2003, pp. 69–96.
45 Garms, 2024, p. 16. See also Jacobs and Garms, 2022, pp. 14–6.
46 Dauphinée, 2007, pp. 139–55.
47 Healy and Russell, 2021, pp. 28–39.
48 See Contreras-Gama, 2016, p. 201.
49 Foster and Minwalla, 2018, pp. 53–64.
50 Roberts, 2024, p. 28.
51 MSF, 2020.
52 MSF, 2022a.
53 OHCHR, 2021.
54 Rieff, 2003.
55 WHO, 2023; MSF, 2023.
56 MSF, 2018.
57 See https://www.mineactionreview.org/country/syria.
58 MSF, 2024b.

59 Healy and Russell, 2021, p. 29.
60 Citton, 2014.
61 See, e.g. Gorin, 2021.
62 Rambaud, 2009, pp. 723–56.

References

Arnsten, Amy F. T. (2009), 'Stress Signalling Pathways That Impair Prefrontal Cortex Structure and Function', *Nature Reviews Neuroscience*, vol. 10, n° 6, pp. 410–422. doi:10.1038/nrn2648.

Bancel, Nicolas (2005), 'Le colonialisme, un projet humanitaire?'. [https://msf-crash.org/fr/rencontres-debats/le-colonialisme-un-projet-humanitaire].

Benoît, Avril (2019), 'Telling It like It Is: Why We Speak Out', *Médecins Sans Frontières*. [https://www.doctorswithoutborders.org/latest/telling-it-it-why-we-speak-out].

Binet, Laurence, and Martin Saulnier (2019), 'Médecins Sans Frontières, Evolution of an International Movement: Associative History 1971–2011'. [https://www.msf.org/sites/default/files/2022-06/msf-associative-history-evolution-of-an-international-movement.pdf].

Brauman, Rony (2005), 'MSF et les limites de l'action humanitaire', *Centre de réflexion sur l'action et les savoirs humanitaires*. [https://msf-crash.org/fr/acteurs-et-pratiques-humanitaires/msf-et-les-limites-de-laction-humanitaire].

Brauman, Rony (2008), 'Témoignage: il est nécessaire d'avoir une approche dépassionnée', *Centre de réflexion sur l'action et les savoirs humanitaires*. [https://msf-crash.org/fr/acteurs-et-pratiques-humanitaires/temoignage-il-est-necessaire-davoir-une-approche-depassionnee].

Brauman, Rony (2012), 'Médecins Sans Frontières and the ICRC: Matters of Principle'. *International Review of the Red Cross*, vol. 94, n° 888, pp. 1523–1535. doi:10.1017/S1816383113000283.

Calain, Philippe (2013), 'Ethics and Images of Suffering Bodies in Humanitarian Medicine', *Social Science & Medicine*, vol. 98, pp. 278–285. doi:10.1016/j.socscimed.2012.06.027.

Campbell, David (2003), 'Salgado and the Sahel: Documentary Photography and the Imaging of Famine', in François Debrix and Cynthia Weber (eds), *Rituals of Mediation: International Politics and Social Meaning*, Minneapolis: University of Minnesota Press.

Carsten, Paul, Reade Levinson, David Lewis, and Libby George (2022), 'Nigerian Military Ran Secret Mass Abortion Program in War against Boko Haram', *Reuters*. 7 December. [https://www.reuters.com/investigates/special-report/nigeria-military-abortions/].

Chouliaraki, Lilie, and Richard Stupart (2025), 'Between Morality and the Market: The Circulation of Humanitarian Photography', *International Journal of Communication*, vol. 19, pp. 306–321.

Citton, Yves (2014), 'L'attention, un bien précieux', *CNRS Le Journal*. [https://lejournal.cnrs.fr/articles/lattention-un-bien-precieux].

Cole, Teju (2012), 'The White-Savior Industrial Complex', *The Atlantic*. [https://www.theatlantic.com/international/archive/2012/03/the-white-savior-industrial-complex/254843/].

Contreras-Gama, Rosana (2016), 'Comprendre les dispositifs photo-humanitaires: être journaliste dans l'humanitaire, faire de l'humanitaire avec des photographies', Université de Lorraine. [https://theses.hal.science/tel-01508553v1/file/DDOC_T_2016_0271_CONTRERAS_GAMA.pdf].

Dauphinée, Elizabeth (2007), 'The Politics of the Body in Pain: Reading the Ethics of Imagery', *Security Dialogue*, vol. 38, n° 2, pp. 139–155.

Davey, Eleanor (2024), 'The road from La Mancha: Narratives of failure and institutional reform', *Centre de réflexion sur l'action et les savoirs humanitaires*. [https://msf-crash.org/en/humanitarian-actors-and-practices/road-la-mancha-narratives-failure-and-institutional-reform].

Davey, Eleanor, John Borton, and Matthew Foley (2013), 'A History of the Humanitarian System: Western Origins and Foundations', Overseas Development Institute, HPG Working Paper. [https://odi.org/en/publications/a-history-of-the-humanitarian-system-western-origins-and-foundations/].

Davey, Eleanor, Lioba Hirsch, Myfanwy James, and Molly Naisanga (2023), 'In Service of Emergency: Understanding Power and Inequality in MSF', Médecins Sans Frontières.

Desgrandchamps, Marie-Luce (2011), 'Revenir sur le mythe fondateur de Médecins sans frontières: les relations entre les médecins français et le CICR pendant la guerre du Biafra (1967–1970)', *Relations internationales*, vol. 146, n° 2, pp. 95–108. doi:10.3917/ri.146.0095.

Desgrandchamps, Marie-Luce (2018), 'Le Biafra et le mythe du nouvel ordre humanitaire', *Campus*. [https://www.unige.ch/campus/numeros/134/dossier4/].

Duroch, Françoise, and Maelle L'Homme (2022), 'Ethical Considerations around the Use of Humanitarian Imagery', *Humanitarian Alternatives*, n° 21, pp. 92–105. [https://www.alternatives-humanitaires.org/en/2022/11/29/ethical-considerations-around-the-use-of-humanitarian-imagery/].

Duroch, Françoise, Nelly Staderini, Pamela Were, and Clémence Chbat (2024), 'Les blessures intimes des réfugiées soudanaises au Tchad', *Médecins Sans Frontières*. [https://www.msf.ch/nos-actualites/articles/blessures-intimes-refugiees-soudanaises-au-tchad].

Foster, Johanna E., and Sherizaan Minwalla (2018), 'Voices of Yazidi Women: Perceptions of Journalistic Practices in the Reporting on ISIS Sexual Violence', *Women's Studies International Forum*, vol. 67, pp. 53–64. doi:10.1016/j.wsif.2018.01.007.

Garms, Juliette (2024), 'Re-Adjusting the Focus', MSF Internal Report.

Gorin, Valérie (2021), 'Witnessing and Témoignage in MSF's Advocacy', *Journal of Humanitarian Affairs*, vol. 3, n° 2, pp. 28–33. doi:10.7227/JHA.063.

Guilhaumou, Jacques (1999), 'Renaud Dulong, Le témoin oculaire. Les conditions sociales de l'attestation personnelle', *Mots. Les langages du politique*, vol. 59, n° 1, pp. 138–140.

Healy, Sean (2021), 'Neutrality: Principle or Tool?', *Humanitarian Practice Network*. [https://odihpn.org/publication/neutrality-principle-or-tool/].

Healy, Sean, and Victoria Russell (2021), 'The Critical Risk of Disinformation for Humanitarians – The Case of the MV Aquarius', *Journal of Humanitarian Affairs*, vol. 3, n° 1, pp. 28–39. doi:10.7227/JHA.056.

hooks, bell (1989), 'Choosing the Margin as a Space of Radical Openness', *Framework: The Journal of Cinema and Media*, n° 36, pp. 15–23.

Jacobs, Jean-Marc, and Juliette Garms (2022), 'Re-Adjusting the Focus: Our Responsibility towards People We Photograph', MSF International Activity Report 2022. [https://www.msf.org/international-activity-report-2022/our-responsibility-towards-people-we-photograph].

Lissner, Jorgen (1981), 'Merchants of Misery', *New Internationalist*. [https://newint.org/features/1981/06/01/merchants-of-misery].

Martínez, Cristina García (2024), 'Is It Possible to Communicate Differently? (De)Colonisation of Visual Humanitarian Communication', Groupe URD. [https://www.urd.org/en/review-hem/is-it-possible-to-communicate-differently-decolonisation-of-visual-humanitarian-communication/].

Mine Action Review, 'Syria'. [https://www.mineactionreview.org/country/syria].

MSF, 'Speaking Out Case Studies'. [https://www.msf.org/speakingout].

MSF (1997), 'Chantilly Principles'. [https://www.msf.org/sites/default/files/Principles%20Chantilly%20EN.pdf].

MSF (2006), 'La Mancha Agreement', 25 June. [https://www.msf.org/sites/default/files/La%20Mancha%20Agreement%20EN.pdf].

MSF (2018), 'Syrie: à Rakka, les engins explosifs continuent de faire des victimes', 13 April. [https://www.msf.fr/actualites/syrie-a-rakka-les-engins-explosifs-continuent-de-faire-des-victimes].

MSF (2020), 'Telling It as It Is: MSF Public Communications Framework', MSF Internal Document.

MSF (2022a), 'Between two fires: Danger and desperation in Syria's Al-Hol camp'. [https://www.msf.org/danger-and-desperation-syria%E2%80%99s-al-hol-camp-report-msf].

MSF (2022b), 'MSF International President responds to photo ethics concerns'. [https://www.doctorswithoutborders.org/latest/msf-international-president-responds-photo-ethics-concerns].

MSF (2023), 'Noma Included by WHO in Neglected Tropical Diseases List'. [https://www.msf.org/noma-included-who-neglected-tropical-diseases-list].

MSF (2024a), '2023 Staff Data and Trends Report', MSF Internal Report.

MSF (2024b), 'A war on people: The human cost of conflict and violence in Sudan'. [https://www.msf.org/war-people-human-cost-conflict-and-violence-sudan].

Neuman, Michaël (2017), 'Dying for humanitarian ideas: Using images and statistics to manufacture humanitarian martyrdom', *Centre de réflexion sur l'action et les savoirs humanitaires*. [https://msf-crash.org/en/humanitarian-actors-and-practices/dying-humanitarian-ideas-using-images-and-statistics-manufacture].

OHCHR (2021), 'Tigray conflict: UN experts call for urgent action to stop violence against women', 3 December. [https://www.ohchr.org/en/2021/12/tigray-conflict-un-experts-call-urgent-action-stop-violence-against-women].

Plowright, William (2024), 'The Imperial Past and Decolonised Future of Humanitarian Action', *Humanitarian Alternatives*, n° 25, pp. 112–121. [https://www.alternatives-humanitaires.org/en/2024/03/20/the-imperial-past-and-decolonised-future-of-humanitarian-action/].

Rambaud, Elsa (2009), 'L'organisation sociale de la critique à Médecins sans frontières', *Revue française de science politique*, vol. 59, n° 4, pp. 723–756. doi:10.3917/rfsp.594.0723.

Rasmussen, Sune Engel (2015), 'Kunduz Hospital Attack: How a US Military "Mistake" Left 22 Dead', *The Guardian*, 21 October. [https://www.theguardian.com/world/2015/oct/21/kunduz-hospital-attack-even-in-20-years-we-wont-get-such-a-hospital-again].

Rieff, David (2003), *A Bed for the Night: Humanitarianism in Crisis*, New York: Simon & Schuster.

Roberts, Henry (2024), 'Decolonisation – the media challenge', International Broadcasting Trust. [https://ibt.org.uk/reports/decolonisation-the-media-challenge/].

Skinner, Rob, and Alan Lester (2012), 'Humanitarianism and Empire: New Research Agendas'. *The Journal of Imperial and Commonwealth History*, vol. 40, n° 5, pp. 729–747. doi:10.1080/03086534.2012.730828.

Soussan, Judith (2008), 'MSF et La Protection: Une Question Réglée? Discours et Pratiques Autour de La "Protection Des Civils"', *Centre de réflexion sur l'action et les savoirs humanitaires*. [https://msf-crash.org/sites/default/files/2017-06/97590daa8b1b115332a0d77bc14d9113.pdf].

Weissman, Fabrice (2023), 'The patient-centered approach: We need an independent Ombudsman', *Centre de réflexion sur l'action et les savoirs humanitaires*. [https://msf-crash.org/en/blog/medicine-and-public-health/patient-centered-approach-we-need-independent-ombudsman].

WHO (2023), 'WHO officially recognizes noma as a neglected tropical disease', 15 December. [https://www.who.int/news/item/15-12-2023-who-officially-recognizes-noma-as-a-neglected-tropical-disease].

Part III

Challenging Adaptations

8 Liberal vs. Critical

Diverging Paths in Humanitarian Aid and Global Health

*Patricia Nayna Schwerdtle**

I How Did We Get Here?

The humanitarian aid sector is deeply rooted in the principles of philosophical liberalism and humanism. Philosophical liberalism, with its focus on defending individual freedom, rights, and equality, laid the foundation for the belief in universal human dignity and the duty to help those in need. Humanism, valuing the inherent worth of all people and universal rights, aims to address social inequalities and injustices to build a more equitable society.

The convergence of these ideals has shaped "Liberal Social Justice" (LSJ), a framework for advancing justice and equality. While LSJ was not solely responsible for all social justice progress, liberal ideas underpinned many successful global movements. In India, LSJ values of equality and rights were key to Mahatma Gandhi's struggle for independence. Martin Luther King Jr used LSJ principles in his *I Have a Dream* speech to champion racial equality and justice, inspiring the civil rights movement and achievements like the Civil Rights Act of 1964. LSJ also helped affirm that women and racial and sexual minorities have the same moral right to access what society has to offer.[1]

LSJ has also underpinned global health and humanitarian assistance, advocating for human rights, alleviating suffering, and promoting justice and dignity for all, regardless of nationality, race, religion, or politics. Humanitarians can take pride in this history and philosophy, which guides their compassionate, empathetic, and supportive efforts for people in crisis worldwide. However, LSJ has not solved all inequalities, and this shortcoming has sparked frustration. In response, a new set of intellectual and cultural ideas has emerged as an apparent alternative to LSJ, becoming dominant in Western, industrialised democracies.

These ideas, known as "Critical Social Justice" (CSJ), are rooted in identity-based theories primarily developed in the United States (US), reflecting their unique social and intellectual history. Progressive frameworks are now split between CSJ, which emphasises group identity and oppressive power structures theorised in a US context, and LSJ, which champions universal principles and values viewpoint diversity. Originating in postmodern deconstructionism, CSJ is sceptical of the objective, evidence-based epistemology favoured by LSJ, prioritising instead the subjective "lived experience".[2] Consequently, CSJ rejects

DOI: 10.4324/9781003542247-16

the LSJ notion of pluralistic freedom of speech and critique as tools for refining objective truth, instead viewing LSJ's emphasis on freedom as a means to uphold an inherently biased status quo. This belief often leads CSJ proponents to dismiss critiques of their ideas as bigotry or attempts to preserve unequal power structures rather than seeing them as legitimate observations. As a result, CSJ tends to favour utopian radicalism over the incremental, consensus-driven social change preferred by LSJ.

While both LSJ and CSJ share the goal of promoting equality, diversity, and inclusion, they differ significantly in their views on the root causes of social issues, as well as on visions for change and approaches to addressing inequality. From 2020 to 2022, a collision of these worldviews created tensions in global health, international development, humanitarian aid, philanthropy, and within MSF itself. What made CSJ ideas appealing in these fields?

First, CSJ's focus on social change and tackling systemic inequalities resonates with many humanitarians passionate about equity. Second, its emphasis on group identity and collective action fosters solidarity among marginalised communities and their allies. International non-governmental organisations, long challenged by structural inequalities, see CSJ as offering a seemingly new and promising lens. Third, CSJ simplifies the complexities of structural inequalities and power dynamics, reducing confusion and frustration. Concepts like "privilege", "intersectionality" and "microaggressions" are widely recognised in Western academia and offer intellectual and moral appeal. Lastly, CSJ's relevance to contemporary issues of race, gender, sexuality, and economic inequality makes it an engaging perspective for activists, scholars, and policymakers.

A more complex reason for CSJ's rise in popularity lies in the unique historic moment the West is experiencing. Liberalism, though not fully victorious, has achieved significant success in a short time. For instance, some people today remember when homosexuality was illegal, whereas now, hate speech against it is prosecutable in many countries. Not long ago, women were excluded from elite universities, but today they are over-represented in higher education across the West. Liberalism has become the status quo. Yet progressives still seek causes to fight for, because challenging the system is central to the left's identity. This inadvertently leads them to weaken the principles that allowed the status quo to become liberal in the first place. As a result, liberals who try to preserve the gains represented by a fairly liberal status quo appear conservative, while CSJ proponents present themselves as progressive, despite their regressive ideas that replay identitarian notions, undermining liberal gains.[3]

Some argue that CSJ's peak influence has waned, while others believe it has successfully embedded itself in institutions. Regardless, there is consensus that the fervour has diminished, creating an opportunity to reflect and situate these ideas within a broader intellectual tradition. This chapter provides that reflection by defining the origins and assumptions of LSJ and CSJ, with examples of their presence in global health, humanitarianism, philanthropy, and MSF, and assessing their impact. This chapter is not a combative one, but it intends to show that CSJ is not synonymous with "social justice" (the aim for a just society) and must be debated alongside other approaches. Applying CSJ universally in global health and humanitarianism may distort complex realities. Uncritical acceptance of CSJ has led to questionable analysis in the science underpinning global health. Additionally, this chapter warns scholars, activists, and practitioners of the risks in overextending the decolonisation metaphor favoured by CSJ, conflating it with human emancipation.[4] This can undermine the agency of formerly colonised populations, crowd out analysis and action on proximal causes of inequity, and provide cover for authoritarian regimes violating universal human rights.

Most humanitarians, whether they favour LSJ or CSJ, do not need reminders of humanitarianism's core values, just as most people do not need lessons on liberalism or humanism to recognise their role in historical progress. However, over time, we begin to take these first principles for granted, viewing them as ever-present, obvious, and even dull. When they fade from view, we may be drawn to something that seems like an exciting evolution but ultimately betrays those principles. This chapter seeks to remind readers of the radical potential of liberal values, particularly LSJ, and the need for each generation to defend them against intolerance and authoritarianism. To fully understand the distinctions between these two worldviews, it is necessary to clearly define the foundational principles and assumptions that underpin LSJ and CSJ approaches.

Philosophical Liberalism and Liberal Social Justice

"Philosophical liberalism" is often misunderstood, so it is important to clarify its meaning here. In this context, "liberalism" does not refer to economic, political, or historical liberalism, but to a set of pre-political first principles embraced by people of various political, economic, religious, and philosophical views. Liberalism, favouring ongoing reform, should be seen not as a finished project but as an evolving practice of making society more liberal through the consistent application of these principles. While critiques of economic, political, and historical liberalism are relevant to humanitarian aid, they are not the focus of this chapter.

Sometimes called "modernity", philosophical liberalism and LSJ rest on first principles that defend individual freedom (individualism), tolerate and appreciate difference (pluralism and freedom of speech), and value shared humanity (humanism). LSJ views it as a moral duty to ensure that everyone enjoys the same rights, freedoms, and responsibilities (universalism).[5] This means treating people as fellow humans, not based on immutable characteristics or identities.

Philosophical liberalism and LSJ acknowledge historical oppression and advocate for distributing resources, privileges, and opportunities based on need rather than equally, in pursuit of social justice. LSJ favours reforms within existing liberal institutions and systems (incrementalism), aiming to improve social conditions and extend rights to marginalised groups, such as education for girls or healthcare for migrants. These goals of reforming systems to create fairer, more equitable societies are shared by human rights campaigners globally, showing that liberal principles are not exclusively Western-centric.

Postmodernism and Critical Social Justice

CSJ originates from postmodernism, a mid-twentieth-century philosophical movement characterised by scepticism towards universal truth, objective reality, and grand narratives. Postmodernism challenges the validity of overarching explanations and ideologies, emphasising the relative and subjective nature of knowledge, truth, and meaning. It focuses on deconstructing established structures, norms, and assumptions, revealing how they are shaped by power dynamics, historical contexts, and cultural discourses.

The CSJ framework emerged when postmodern deconstruction techniques were applied to identity issues, a shift known as the "applied postmodern turn".[6] Modern CSJ scholarship includes fields like postcolonial theory (decolonisation), queer theory, critical race theory, intersectionality, third-wave feminism, and gender studies, along with disability and fat studies.[7] The CSJ worldview is based on the notion that society is structured by intersecting systems of power and privilege, perpetuating oppression based on race, gender, sexuality, and class (intersectional identitarianism). Members of these groups are considered to share values, beliefs, and experiences (especially of oppression) which are only truly understood by fellow group members (essentialism). Expressions that counter this belief are censored as inherently violent (censorship). CSJ centres the voices and experiences of marginalised groups (lived experience) while critiquing dominant narratives and institutions, even those involving empirical or scientific facts. CSJ advocates aim to dismantle these systems through radical activism and social change initiatives (radicalism).

Although both LSJ and CSJ focus on social justice, clear tensions exist between the two frameworks, and these have impacted on the humanitarian aid sector and MSF. The next section of this chapter will examine how these tensions have manifested across five domains where LSJ and CSJ are in opposition: empiricism vs. lived experience; free speech vs. censorship; individualism vs. intersectional identitarianism; universalism vs. essentialism; and incrementalism vs. radicalism.

II LSJ and CSJ in the Humanitarian Sector

Empiricism vs. Lived Experience: Is Progress Possible?

LSJ, rooted in Enlightenment ideals, values evidence-based inquiry, believing progress comes from understanding problems through empirical research and recognising the complex causes of social phenomena. In contrast, CSJ, influenced by postmodern deconstructionism, emphasises the relativity of truth based on historical, cultural, and identity contexts, often prioritising the lived experiences of marginalised groups over empirical evidence. CSJ contends that truth claims reflect power hierarchies, with frameworks advocating that those marginalised voices be elevated above requests for data. Hirsch articulated this position most clearly when she argued for the reform of global health so that "*[people of colour's] demands and experiences will not be met by ever-increasing demands for more proof and more data and more surveys*".[8]

Listening to lived experiences can reveal systemic inequalities that liberal frameworks might overlook, and has the potential to improve global aid efforts. For example, during the 2018–19 Ebola outbreak in the Democratic Republic of the Congo (DRC), the International Federation of Red Cross and Red Crescent Societies and DRC Red Cross implemented an effective safe and dignified burials service. This approach incorporated lessons learned and the first-hand accounts of local actors from previous Ebola outbreaks, resulting in burial teams managed by community actors and supported by, but not owned by, humanitarian organisations. This integration of local knowledge ensured culturally sensitive and efficient burial practices, crucial for controlling the virus spread.[9] Disregarding local expertise is widely considered poor practice. Local knowledge should not have a lower standing than international expertise, because the most beneficial insights and policies arise from combining the best propositional and experiential knowledge from whatever source.[10]

CSJ tends to rely on a power lens for analysis and, therefore, risks conflating disparities, injustices, and power abuses, which are three overlapping but distinct realities that require evidence to distinguish, for true progress and accountability. Similarly, the CSJ worldview often attributes all inequalities to power imbalances, claiming that even benevolent acts are covers for oppressive power systems. An MSF open letter from 2020 exemplifies this: signed by over 1,000 past and present MSF employees in the wake of the Black Lives Matter (BLM) movement in the US, the letter appeared in board packs across the organisation and was picked up by mainstream media outlets like *The New Humanitarian* and *The Guardian*. It argued that emergency medical assistance itself perpetuates oppression: "*We see no commitment to dismantle the humanitarian 'virtue signal' behind which acts of discrimination and oppression have continued unchecked.*" The letter suggested that racism is not just a problem MSF must address but a central aspect of its identity – "*It is racism and white supremacy that shape the culture and mindset that still defines our organisation*" – criticising past responses as lacklustre and performative. The letter also called for a transformative overhaul of MSF's approach to humanitarian action; independent assessments of racism; internal audits of hiring processes; and comprehensive anti-racism training and policy reviews.[11]

Similar CSJ themes appear in the MSF Netherlands Power Analysis,[12] and in the *Dignity at MSF* report, which claims that MSF exploits and discriminates to maintain systemic inequalities.[13] The view that global aid is irredeemably white supremacist is echoed in MSF discourse – "*Humanitarianism is still structurally racialised and gendered and, even when best intentions are assumed, is a mirror image of the powers in the 'imperialist white supremacist capitalist patriarchy'*"[14]; and it is reflected in the broader global health literature – "*Ours is a discipline that holds within itself a deep contradiction – global health was birthed in supremacy, but its mission is to reduce or eliminate inequities globally.*"[15]

Supporters of an LSJ framework might argue that the evolution of global health – from supporting colonialism to developing a depoliticised model and aiming to tackle health disparities – is not best explained by the strategic confusion or racial supremacy described above. Instead, it may be seen as evidence of historical progress.[16] The consequences of viewing everything solely through a CSJ power lens, and denying liberal principles' achievements, are exemplified by the closure of the Lankelly Chase charitable trust in the UK. After 30 years of challenging injustice, the trust, which distributed £13 million annually to charities focused on social, racial, and climate justice, sought "*bold new alternatives*" to what it called philanthropy's "*cult of benevolence*". The CEO explained this decision with the following rationale:

Philanthropy is a function of colonial capitalism, it has been shaped by it, is being driven by it, and yet philosophically it tries to position itself as somehow a cure for the ills of colonial capitalism, and that contradiction needs to stop.[17]

Viewing philanthropy (and global health/humanitarian assistance) as deeply flawed and in need of drastic reform, dismantlement, or defunding could result in abolishing both the good and the bad. This perspective unintentionally provides a rationale to divest and withdraw already fragile support for global health and philanthropy. Will marginalised people truly benefit from the closure of Lankelly Chase and the services it funded, either in the short or long term? The Lankelly Chase board has called for a "*radical reimagining*", but there has been no public update on what that means in practice.[18]

The MSF open letter provided little empirical evidence for its accusations, yet called for a "*radical reimagination of our approach to humanitarian action*". However, the proposed actions, such as audits and diversity training, rely on conventional procedural approaches that are unlikely to dismantle systemic power dynamics or achieve the sweeping change the letter demands. The claim that "*MSF's humanitarianism still suppresses indigenous voices, overlooks indigenous knowledge, denies individual and community agency, and makes a mockery of solidarity*" is typical of CSJ analysis, offering no concrete examples.[19] While demanding transparency, accountability, and action against white supremacy, the letter's proposals for diversity audits, anti-racism training, and policy changes have been shown to yield limited benefits in improving workplace equality and representation.[20] Additionally, research suggests that identity-based hiring practices are often unpopular with the minority groups they aim to support.[21] CSJ's approach can turn cynical, denying progress by asserting claims like "*MSF still has a problem with racism*" without clearly defining what success would entail or acknowledging improvements. This risks prioritising moral posturing over the pursuit of actionable solutions.

The open letter, despite being filtered through an ideological lens, acknowledges real issues within MSF, such as favouritism towards international staff with European ties, leading to unequal pay, benefits, recruitment, and expatriation opportunities. Other legitimate concerns include ongoing experiences of racism; discrimination; limited access to training; and the need for more representative governance. While CSJ often identifies genuine problems, which partly explains its appeal, it applies a rigid ideological framework that rejects accurate diagnoses of root causes. This approach frequently employs the "motte-and-bailey" fallacy, where defensible positions like the power of language to influence social interactions are used to justify more extreme claims, such as labelling certain terms or questions as microaggressions that cause real harm.[22] Similarly, while critical examination of colonialism is widely accepted, CSJ proponents take a radical stance, arguing that humanitarian aid is inherently colonial, and must dismantle invisible power systems like whiteness or toxic masculinity. This rhetorical tactic complicates discussions on social justice and hinders constructive change. As former MSF France president Jean-Hervé Bradol noted in 2020, rejecting CSJ's framework does not equate to indifference to racism:

> *I think it is entirely fair that MSF USA has thrown its weight behind the BLM movement. [...] But I don't think it relevant for the directors of MSF, whether in America or elsewhere, to accept the concepts or the analytical table of certain currents of left-wing thinking that are intolerant to other people's positions. I am thinking here of such ideas as: MSF – a racist institution; white fragility; white privilege; white supremacy; an organisation that is necessarily racist when its anti-racism is not defined by this fraction on the left, etc.*[23]

Advocates of LSJ and CSJ frameworks share a commitment to addressing issues of inequality. A collaboration between the epistemological rigour promoted by LSJ frameworks and the insights into lived experience and power provided by CSJ framing has the potential to make great strides towards that goal. But this requires mutual recognition of shared good intentions and empirical honesty. CSJ's radically critical worldview should not be regarded as synonymous with "caring" about an issue, just as articulating the view that things have improved at MSF should not be misconstrued as denying ongoing problems. Crucially, collaboration is only possible where both approaches are recognised as legitimate and proponents of each viewpoint feel free to express their views.

Free Speech vs. Censorship: Viewpoint Diversity, Knowledge Production, and Moral Orthodoxy

The LSJ focus on evidence-based epistemology leads to another core liberal principle, often in tension with CSJ approaches: freedom of speech and viewpoint diversity. LSJ recognises that conflicting ideas must be openly debated in order to refine our understanding of truth. For this reason, LSJ opposes censorship, even of ideas considered heretical or offensive, advocating instead for these ideas to be robustly critiqued in public view. CSJ, influenced by Herbert Marcuse's doctrine of "repressive tolerance", takes an alternative stance.

Marcuse argued that liberal tolerance maintains the status quo by empowering oppressive voices while silencing marginalised ones. He advocated for selective intolerance, where social justice is pursued by censoring views deemed harmful.[24] As a result, CSJ approaches tend to discourage critique, treating divergent opinions as inherently oppressive and supporting their censorship.

This censorious aspect of the CSJ approach caused tensions at the MSF Australia and New Zealand biannual meeting in 2020. Some members strongly opposed a proposal to debate institutional racism in MSF, an effort intended to hear diverse views on how to address the issue. Instead, they called for a "racism listening session" where members with "privileged" identities would remain silent while those with "oppressed" identities spoke. This approach defined groups primarily by skin colour, despite many members in both groups sharing similar socio-economic and educational backgrounds. Likewise, the MSF open letter was based on the belief that discussing the nuance or empirical basis of its claims would be seen as denying the problems or reinforcing oppressive practices.

This hyper-moralistic and identity-focused aspect of CSJ frequently provokes an antagonistic mindset, triggering a fight-or-flight response in those targeted. CSJ encourages people to identify with a specific group, often framed as being in competition with another, such as "privileged" versus "oppressed", "people of colour" versus "white people", or "settler" versus "colonised", in other contexts. This can reduce social justice to a zero-sum power struggle, where the goal is to impose CSJ beliefs and advocate for one's group at the expense of other, potentially more effective, approaches. Consequently, some MSF sections (for instance, Australia, Canada, and South Africa) invested donor money on external consultants to scrutinise their boards and policies for evidence of systemic racism and white supremacy. However, it is unclear whether these investigations effectively addressed the underlying issues or led to meaningful progress. While disparities and inequities exist within MSF, rigidly applying a CSJ framework that disregards diverse viewpoints and constructive dissent may steer MSF further from objective analysis and viable solutions – especially in an organisation that fosters a culture of debate as a means of moving forward. Instead, performative adherence to CSJ beliefs replaces the hard work of refining ideas into effective policies. Take the MSF Spain statement of 2022:

> *[W]e hereby issue our sincere apology to all our colleagues who are Black and Indigenous People, People of Colour and from other racialised groups. We have failed to fulfil our role as a "Responsible Employer". In MSF, we should provide a working environment that is free of discrimination, yet we have failed to protect our colleagues from acts of racism and micro-aggression. As a result, we acknowledge we perpetuated a racist culture over the last five decades.*[25]

While CSJ adherents may see MSF Spain's apology as a necessary act of symbolic atonement for historical wrongs, others might argue that it did little to benefit racial minorities within the organisation. Pressured by the Decolonise

MSF movement, the leadership felt compelled to apologise to avoid accusations of oppressive behaviour. However, the CSJ framework driving the movement did not require MSF to address the practical challenges of reducing inequality within a rapidly evolving global organisation. As Bradol noted in 2020, "*I think the leaders of our international movement are letting themselves be intimidated too easily, thereby showing 'political fragility', even a kind of 'jumping on the bandwagon'.*"[26] MSF, historically known for encouraging robust debate, pluralism, and constructive dissent,[27] should be wary of any framework claiming moral infallibility while dismissing alternative approaches. While aspects of a CSJ worldview can highlight important inequities, if taken to extreme it risks stifling collaboration, narrowing viewpoint diversity, and fostering divisive rather than constructive debate.

Individualism vs. Intersectional Identitarianism: Western-centric Stereotyping and Elite Ideas

CSJ uses identity categories like race, gender, sexuality, and other immutable features to understand society, often resulting in policies based on group membership that assume shared experiences of social disadvantage rooted in identity. In contrast, LSJ encourages identity-neutral policies, promoting equality by understanding disadvantage as stemming from the unfair distribution of resources, privileges, and opportunities, which may overlap with, but are not necessarily defined by, identity. While LSJ's individualist approach can overlook historical inequalities, CSJ's focus on identity can exacerbate divisions, foster resentment, and lead to tokenism (superficial or symbolic efforts, without genuinely addressing underlying inequalities) or legal challenges. LSJ advocates for recognising group identity but prioritising individual rights, as seen in civil rights, women's rights, and gay rights movements. An excessive focus on group identity can undermine liberalism's emphasis on individual rights and universal dignity, and identity is not always the best indicator of disadvantage.[28]

Within MSF, CSJ-informed identitarianism has increasingly shaped the organisation's culture, practices, and policies in recent years, with some sections, such as MSF Canada, reportedly holding racially segregated meetings. Other DEI recommendations include mandating all employees to actively engage in anti-racism work, enforcing race- and gender-based quotas, and removing individuals resistant to anti-racism measures.[29]

The narratives assigned to identity categories in CSJ models are highly Western-centric, rooted in North American race relations and the Western civil rights movement. In the context of humanitarian aid, which deals with global human diversity, these simplistic categorisations often lack explanatory power and overlook differences within and between identity groups. This can be unhelpful for humanitarians navigating complex local identities, cultures, and histories. For example, applying the oppressor–oppressed framework to complex crises like the Rwandan Genocide or the Israeli–Palestinian conflict oversimplifies and distorts reality, leading to misguided advocacy, false solutions, and compromising impartiality and neutrality.[30]

Critics argue that CSJ is a Western-centric worldview primarily serving academic and cultural elites rather than the disadvantaged populations it claims to assist. These "elite" or "luxury" ideas are often embraced by affluent, educated groups, reflecting their values without addressing the practical needs of less privileged communities.[31] In global health, terms like decolonisation have been criticised as vague and co-opted by elite institutions, benefiting elites more than the disadvantaged.[32] The African philosopher Olúfẹ́mi Táíwò's critique of epistemic deference[33] shows how privileged members of marginalised groups can dominate political agendas, sidelining the truly disadvantaged.[34] CSJ's focus on complex and abstract concepts makes them less accessible to those without a specialised education, creating intellectual gatekeeping. Terms like "deconstruction", "epistemic violence", and "intersectionality" require academic training, limiting practical application and often overlooking material conditions such as economic inequality and healthcare needs. Thus, CSJ theories can inadvertently fail to assist, and may even harm, the populations they aim to help, by prioritising ideological considerations over tangible results.

Elite capture[35] occurs when privileged members of marginalised groups dominate political agendas, sidelining the truly disadvantaged. In the aid sector, including organisations like MSF, this can happen when decision-making roles are held by individuals from marginalised groups who have more access to education or global networks. These elites may push policies reflecting their own experiences, such as identity politics or decolonisation, rather than addressing the concrete needs of communities in project locations. At MSF, elite capture can shift focus from immediate needs like healthcare to more abstract debates. This risks misaligning aid efforts and prioritising ideology over practical effectiveness, potentially undermining the humanitarian mission.

Advocates of CSJ are right to urge proponents of LSJ to deal sensitively with experiences like racism, sexism, and homophobia that are informed by identity. Equally, people working in the global context of humanitarian assistance would be wise to be aware of elite ideas and not to take for granted the narratives ascribed to identity by Western-centric CSJ models.

Universalism vs. Essentialism: The Unintended Consequences of Decolonisation Narratives

In 1947, the American Anthropological Association (AAA) criticised the United Nations' efforts to draft a Universal Declaration of Human Rights, calling it "ethnocentric" and an attempt to impose a Western worldview on oppressed peoples. However, in 1999, the AAA retracted its statement, accepting that basic human rights are universal, not culturally or ethnically relative.[36] The Universal Declaration of Human Rights exemplifies LSJ's belief in universalism, asserting that fundamental rights, such as freedom from torture and freedom of conscience, are not mediated by identity. Universalism holds that people from different backgrounds share essential human qualities and should work towards mutual understanding across superficial differences. While liberal philosophy has previously fallen short of this ideal, LSJ proponents would advocate to action historical shortcomings by strengthening universalist ideals in the present. Universalism is also central to humanitarianism, reflecting the belief that all humans share common rights and dignity, including the right to life and health.

CSJ critiques of universalism favour a form of essentialism, viewing individuals primarily through the lens of group identity, typically in a binary of "oppressed" or "oppressor". These categories are often based on a superficial reading of power relations between identity groups. The decolonisation movement, a CSJ metanarrative, embodies this dualism, framing art, international relations, and even science as a struggle between Western colonial oppressors and virtuous indigenous cultures. Other examples include dark-skinned (oppressed) vs. light-skinned (oppressor), and cisgender (oppressor) vs. transgender (oppressed). These strict "in-groups" and "out-groups" deny the possibility of universal human nature, impeding mutual understanding across identity lines. While being part of an "in-group" can foster solidarity, it can also obscure the humanity of the "out-group". Unlike LSJ, which emphasises commonality to encourage collaboration, CSJ can amplify competitive and confrontational aspects of human behaviour.

CSJ narratives often reject universal systems of knowledge, such as science or mathematics, claiming that "indigenous ways of knowing", like spirituality or inherited wisdom, are equally valid for deriving objective facts. During the COVID-19 pandemic, some governments undermined Western knowledge under the guise of decolonisation to avoid criticism and gain support for expedient but ineffective policies.[37] Denying scientific knowledge based on identity opens the door to political demagoguery. Humanity has a long history of politicising science, with devastating consequences. For example, South African president Thabo Mbeki invoked anti-colonial sentiment to justify his denial of the viral causes of AIDS and the efficacy of antiretroviral drugs. While there is some validity to the claim that Western pharmaceutical companies were capitalising on the illness of people living in sub-Saharan Africa, essentially profiting from suffering, the Mbeki government's opposition contributed to more than 330,000 people dying prematurely from HIV/AIDS over five years.[38] The overextension of "decolonisation" narratives must also bear some responsibility for the 35,000 babies born with preventable HIV infection under Mbeki's rule.[39]

Táíwò, in his book *Against Decolonisation: Taking African Agency Seriously*, criticises the modern use of decolonisation as an all-encompassing grand narrative. He argues that the term has drifted from its original purpose of ending Western political and economic domination over Africa and now stifles African intellectual growth and denies African agency. Táíwò critiques its blanket application to fields like literature, sociology, psychology, and medicine, claiming that it has become more focused on cataloguing historical wrongs than fostering meaningful scholarship and progress in Africa. He argues that conflating modernity[40] with coloniality leads to a wholesale rejection of modern advancements that could benefit African societies. This approach, Táíwò contends, infantilises African thinkers and imposes external values, undermining the movement's own goals.[41] Right-wing elites have particularly profited from CSJ's rejection of universalism and embrace of identitarian essentialism. If universal human rights are dismissed as products of Western colonialism, their rejection can be framed as radical decolonisation – casting off oppressive Western norms[42] – rather than a regressive excuse for authoritarian governments to abuse citizens' rights. Indian prime minister Narendra Modi has used this tactic effectively, rejecting Western concepts of human rights and freedom of speech to impose authoritarian control over civil society under the guise of "decolonisation" and returning to Indian roots.[43] The "decolonise aid" and "decolonise global health" movements have similarly extended the concept of decolonisation to reject universalist principles and to critique global health and aid systems as inherently colonial.

Critics of LSJ frameworks argue that promoting universal human rights undermines cultural diversity and indigenous values. However, liberals are not dismissive of cultural diversity; they view it within the broader context of human evolutionary history. Aware of the dangers of in-group/out-group bias, LSJ approaches emphasise avoiding actions that trigger this mentality. Leading liberal thinkers advocate for expanding our in-group to be as inclusive as possible, embracing differences while recognising shared humanity.[44] The humanitarian sector has a duty to ensure that the CSJ theme of "decolonisation" is not overextended and used to justify authoritarian regimes.

Incrementalism vs. Radicalism: Revolution or Lasting Change?

LSJ has been heavily criticised by CSJ advocates for its commitment to incrementalism. LSJ proponents favour reform over revolution, recognising that social change gains broader support when introduced gradually. A key example is the advancement of women's rights, for example in India, Rwanda, and Kenya. Early reforms, like granting women the right to vote and access to education, paved the way for more comprehensive changes. Over time, these steps have led to legal protections against domestic violence, greater political representation, and improved healthcare access. This gradual approach allows societies to adapt, embedding changes deeply within the social and legal fabric, ensuring that they are sustainable.

Supporters of CSJ argue that incrementalism is inherently limited and often inadequate for addressing deep-rooted systemic injustices, even suggesting that LSJ preserves inequalities inherent in the status quo. In contrast, the CSJ worldview is radical, advocating for revolution over reform. A recent example is the BLM movement, which calls for a national defunding of the police to solve racial inequalities in policing.[45] After the 2020 BLM protests, the state of Oregon moved towards this radical policy by shutting down its gun violence reduction unit, accused of systemic racism. However, the policy was reversed after a significant rise in shooting deaths.

The radical nature of CSJ is deeply embedded in decolonisation literature in global health, drawing on Herbert Marcuse's doctrine of "repressive tolerance"

(See "Free Speech vs. Censorship" section above), as well as Frantz Fanon's ideas and assertion that *"decolonisation is always a violent phenomenon"*.[46] CSJ advocates for dismantling theorised oppressive systems through confrontational means like protest, direct action, and civil disobedience. Writing in *The Lancet*, Hirsch, who co-authored MSF Netherlands' Power Analysis,[47] exemplifies this revolutionary stance, stating, *"So, although I am not advocating violence, I am advocating anger and revolution."* This is justified, in her view, because of the *"inherent violence of colonialism"* that she extends to global health as a field of research and practice. She doubts that structural change can be achieved by *"working through channels that were set up within structures that uphold white supremacy"*, and calls for people of colour to *"dismantle the current system"*.[48] In the CSJ worldview, oppressed people's actions can, at times, be justified without moral critique. This view suggests that oppression absolves such groups from moral accountability, even for actions that would be condemned if committed by others.[49]

CSJ's distaste for practical or incremental solutions is evident in Smith's critique of pragmatism in global health:

> *The promotion of pragmatism alone will be the death of global health, if it has not killed it already. Currently, pragmatism in global health is pervasive and unchecked, which enables conservative positioning and reformist, incremental change processes that typically serve to preserve the status quo.*[50]

CSJ proponents often advocate for a destructive revolutionary mindset, calling to disrupt, defund, and dismantle global health[51] – yet these calls rarely include alternative solutions. For instance, in 2022, leading decolonisation thinkers suggested that global health's obliteration might be beneficial, without offering a replacement: *"If the future is a radical transformation, decolonization should obliterate global health. That might not be a bad outcome."*[52]

The effectiveness of the CSJ approach in improving conditions for minorities is debatable, while incremental, evidence-based strategies advocated by LSJ have consistently shown positive results. A key example within MSF are the 83 project teams' proposals, based on discussions facilitated by the MSF France Association in December 2020 about racism, discrimination, and inequality.[53] The talks revealed empirical evidence of favouritism towards international staff or those with European ties, leading to unequal pay, health policies, and opportunities. From these findings, the 83 suggestions proposed practical actions like fairer remuneration, reducing salary gaps between headquarters and programme staff, and harmonising benefits, all in line with LSJ principles of equal rights and responsibilities. In contrast, the MSF open letter takes a more radical, ideological stance, emphasising institutional racism, neocolonialism, and systemic oppression. It criticises MSF for failing to adequately address racism and suggests that the organisation is morally compromised without fundamental transformation. The 83 suggestions take a more practical, incremental approach, focusing on specific issues like favouritism, unequal pay, and limited access to training. Rather than radical systemic change, they propose addressing these operational inequalities through reforms in human resources policies, communication, and governance, to ensure fairness and representation.

The liberal tradition has a long history of successfully opposing the status quo when it constrains certain groups and erects barriers to their access to the rights, opportunities, and freedoms enjoyed by dominant groups.[54] LSJ offers a powerful approach to challenging authoritarianism by the state and other influential forces in society. The humanitarian sector is better served by LSJ's approach of principled yet gradual transformation to sustainably reduce inequality, rather than the destructive radicalism of CSJ.

In Summary

CSJ and LSJ represent contrasting worldviews because they diverge on key philosophical, ideological, and practical principles. As outlined under the five dichotomies above, their differences extend to their vision for societal change, their understanding of the root causes of social issues, and their approaches to addressing inequality. As a result, their coexistence is contentious and fraught with conflict. While CSJ may provide some valuable insights, it resists allowing its core tenets to be critiqued or compared with alternative explanations.

When the stark differences between CSJ and LSJ encounter each other in an organisation, it often leads to polarising rhetoric and ideological conflict. Advocates of each worldview may demonise the other as being either too radical or too complacent, resulting in a lack of dialogue and understanding. This polarisation can create ideological echo chambers where individuals are only exposed to perspectives that align with their own thinking, reinforcing tribalism and exacerbating conflict. This is fuelled by our current unhealthy information environment and the compartmentalised feeds controlled by algorithms that further exploit our tribal instincts by driving us towards more and more content that confirms our existing biases.

Another way in which these worldviews are antithetical is that they have incompatible policy agendas. Attempts to implement policies that align with one worldview may be perceived as undermining the principles of the other. For example, a CSJ approach to diversity and inclusion training might start with our public identification as belonging to certain social groups (POC/BIPOC[55] or white). This conflicts with LSJ's commitment to seeing people first as fellow humans and also as unique individuals. This type of practical incompatibility can lead to gridlock and paralysis in decision-making processes, as well as heightened tensions between advocates of CSJ and LSJ.

III A Way Forward

CSJ and the postmodern philosophy underlying it recently broke the boundaries of academia and gained great cultural power in Western society. The identitarian symptoms of postmodernism are easily recognisable but the ethos underlying them is poorly understood. This set of ideas, while not new, has recently taken an applied turn, and has entered the mainstream in such a way that it has significantly influenced thought, culture, policy, and practice in global health, philanthropy, humanitarian aid and, therefore, inevitably, MSF.

These ideas have not been tested or proven effective in the humanitarian field, nor have they been extensively critiqued. This lack of critique is partly due to the nature of these concepts, which are often intolerant to criticism, and because they portray themselves as either synonymous with social justice or a new and improved version of social justice. Consequently, critiquing these ideas risks being perceived as opposing social justice itself. This presents a significant challenge in evaluating their true efficacy and impact in humanitarian contexts.

To avoid being reactionary and catastrophising, it is important to accept that postmodern ideas and CSJ are an interesting analytical frame which can help us understand complex issues around inequity. Further, no ideas should be censored, silenced, or chilled in an open and liberal institution like MSF. However, when this intellectually interesting set of ideas shifts to become an explanatory framework – a "paradigm" – and is applied to complex problems, it tends to simplify and misdiagnose their causes, leading to false solutions. For example, conflating colonisation with modernity and prescribing decolonisation as a universal remedy risks neglecting specific, contextually relevant strategies that could foster upward mobility and address inequities more effectively. Similarly, framing science as a tool of Western oppression can undermine the evidence base that underpins global health action, weakening trust in science and the often fragile support for international humanitarian assistance. Additionally, viewing gender disparities in health outcomes strictly through the lens of patriarchal structures can lead to interventions that overlook other significant determinants of health. And when the paradigm is broadly applied in policy and practice, it can become a "regime" with the power to demoralise and destabilise the organisation by subverting important norms and values. If left unchecked, postmodernism and CSJ have the potential to impose artificial constraints on MSF's medical humanitarian operations; the risk being a slow, steady infiltration into the institution, undermining empiricism in favour of subjectivity, suppressing robust debate through the chilling effect of censorship, and prioritising intersectional identitarianism over each person's unique individuality and collective humanity. These changes risk fracturing the movement along identity lines and diminishing the essential role that universalism plays in upholding humanitarian principles. Finally, a growing impatience with incremental and sustainable change in favour of untested, potentially destructive radicalism could further destabilise MSF's core mission.

As MSF continues its work in international medical humanitarian assistance, it is important to distinguish between those trends that help preserve and renew its core principles, ethos, norms, and values,[56] and those that risk subverting them.

Notes

* *This chapter was written in early 2024, prior to a renewed wave of conservative activism, particularly in the United States, that has since emerged in opposition to Critical Social Justice. These developments are therefore not included in the analysis. However, the chapter does anticipate and warn of such dynamics before they became visible.*

1 Pluckrose, 2024.
2 Casey, 2023, pp. 282–97.
3 Pluckrose, 2017.
4 Táíwò, 2022.
5 Mill, 1985; Pluckrose, 2024.
6 Pluckrose and Lindsay, 2020.
7 Key concepts of CSJ include decolonisation (Fanon, 1961 and 1952; Mbembe, 2001), Western hegemony (Foucault, 1977; Said, 1978; Spivak, 1988; Lyotard, 1984; Derrida, 1976), intersectionality (Crenshaw, 1991), and white privilege (DiAngelo, 2016; Kendi, 2019).
8 Hirsch, 2021, pp. 189–90.
9 Warsame et al., 2023.
10 Hellowell and Nayna Schwerdtle, 2022.
11 MSF Open Letter, 25 June 2020.
12 Davey et al., 2024.
13 Majumdar and Mukerjee, 2021.
14 Aloudat, 2021.
15 Pai, 2021.
16 Hellowell and Nayna Schwerdtle, 2022.
17 Butler, 2023.
18 Nayna Schwerdtle, 2023.
19 MSF Open Letter, 25 June 2020.
20 Dobbin and Kalev, 2018, pp. 48–55.
21 Harris, 2024.
22 Shackel, 2005, pp. 295–320.
23 Bradol, 2020.
24 Marcuse, 1965.
25 MSF Spain Governing Body, 2022a.
26 Bradol, 2020.
27 Fox, 2015.
28 For example, during the COVID-19 pandemic, some US states distributed vaccines based on race, to address historical disadvantages. However, the primary risk factors for mortality proved to be age, socio-economic status, comorbidities, and essential worker status. Epidemiological modelling showed that race-based vaccine distribution would result in more fatalities overall, including among minority groups. In 2021, the Office for Civil Rights issued federal guidance to reverse these state policies. See https://www.hhs.gov/civil-rights/for-providers/civil-rights-covid19/guidance-federal-legal-standards-covid-19-vaccination-programs/index.html.
29 MSF Spain Governing Body, 2022b.
30 In humanitarian assistance, the principles of impartiality and neutrality are foundational to ensuring that aid reaches those in need without bias or taking sides in

political or social conflicts. In simple terms, impartiality means that aid is given based on need alone, regardless of identity, while neutrality requires that humanitarian actors do not take sides in conflicts or political disputes. When applying CSJ frameworks, which tend to simplify conflicts into binary categories of oppressors and oppressed, based on identity, these principles can be compromised because such frameworks inherently assign moral value to one side over the other. This can lead to biased advocacy or humanitarian interventions that favour certain groups while marginalising others.

31 Storr, 2021.
32 Krugman, 2023.
33 Epistemic deference refers to the tendency of individuals, particularly in progressive circles, to defer to the views and experiences of members of marginalised groups on the assumption that they hold superior insight into issues of injustice: Táíwò, 2020.
34 *Ibid.*
35 Elite capture refers to the process by which the most privileged members of marginalised groups dominate political agendas and discourse, sidelining the interests and needs of the broader, less privileged members of their communities. *Ibid.*
36 Engle, 2001, pp. 536–59.
37 Hellowell and Nayna Schwerdtle, 2022.
38 Vandormael, 2007, pp. 217–33.
39 Nayna Schwerdtle, 2022.
40 In the context in which Olúfẹ́mi Táíwò uses it, modernity refers to the intellectual, social, political, and economic advancements and systems that emerged in the post-Enlightenment era, characterised by values such as scientific progress, democracy, individual rights, industrialisation, and rationalism.
41 Táíwò, 2022.
42 Nanda, 2001.
43 Lewis and Lall, 2024, pp. 1471–88.
44 Christakis, 2019; Pinker, 2011.
45 See https://blacklivesmatter.com/actions/act-now-to-defund-the-police-and-invest-in-communities/.
46 Fanon, 1961.
47 Davey et al., 2024.
48 Hirsch, 2021, pp. 189–90.
49 Walzer, 2023.
50 Smith et al., 2023.
51 Gichane and Wallace, 2022; Pai, 2021; Fofana, 2021, pp. 1155–66; Mukerjee and Majumdar, 2021.
52 Pai, 2021; Abimbola and Pai, 2020, pp. 1627–28.
53 MSF France Association, 2020.
54 Fawcett, 2015; Gopnik, 2019; Dunt, 2021.
55 People of Colour/Black, Indigenous, People of Colour.
56 Fox, 2015.

References

Abimbola, Seye, and Madhukar Pai (2020), 'Will Global Health Survive Its Decolonisation?' *The Lancet*, vol. 396, n° 10263, pp. 1627–1628. doi:10.1016/S0140–6736(20)32417-X.

Aloudat, Tammam (2021), 'Who Gets to Decolonise Humanitarianism?', *Centre for Humanitarian Action.* [https://www.chaberlin.org/en/blog/who-gets-to-decolonise-humanitarianism-2/].

Black Lives Matter, 'Act Now to Defund The Police and Invest in Communities'. [https://blacklivesmatter.com/actions/act-now-to-defund-the-police-and-invest-in-communities/].

Bradol, Jean-Hervé (2020), 'From bureaucratic inertia to "policy fragility"', *Centre de réflexion sur l'action et les savoirs humanitaires*. [https://msf-crash.org/en/publications/humanitarian-actors-and-practices/bureaucratic-inertia-policy-fragility].

Butler, Patrick (2023), 'UK Charity Foundation to Abolish Itself and Give Away £130m', *The Guardian*, 11 July. [https://www.theguardian.com/society/2023/jul/11/uk-charity-foundation-to-abolish-itself-and-give-away-130m].

Casey, Patrick J. (2023), 'Lived Experience: Defined and Critiqued', *Critical Horizons*, vol. 24, n° 3, pp. 282–297. doi:10.1080/14409917.2023.2241058.

Christakis, Nicholas A. (2019), *Blueprint: The Evolutionary Origins of A Good Society*, New York: Little, Brown Spark.

Crenshaw, Kimberle (1991), 'Mapping the Margins: Intersectionality, Identity Politics, and Violence against Women of Color', *Stanford Law Review*, vol. 43, n° 6, pp. 1241–1299. doi:10.2307/1229039.

Davey, Eleanor, Lioba Hirsch, Myfanwy James, and Molly Naisanga (2024), 'In Service of Emergency: Understanding Power and Inequality in MSF', Médecins Sans Frontières. doi:10.13140/RG.2.2.13972.31361.

Derrida, Jacques (1976), *Of Grammatology*, Baltimore: Johns Hopkins University Press.

DiAngelo, Robin (2016), 'WHITE FRAGILITY.', *Counterpoints*, vol. 497, pp. 245–253.

Dobbin, Frank, and Alexandra Kalev (2018), 'Why Doesn't Diversity Training Work? The Challenge for Industry and Academia', *Anthropology Now*, vol. 10, n° 2, pp. 48–55. doi:10.1080/19428200.2018.1493182.

Dunt, Ian (2021), 'Defending EU Liberalism', in Toby Buckle (ed.), *What Is Freedom? Conversations with Historians, Philosophers, and Activists*, New York: Oxford University Press. doi:10.1093/oso/9780197572214.003.0011.

Engle, Karen (2001), 'From Skepticism to Embrace: Human Rights and the American Anthropological Association from 1947–1999', *Human Rights Quarterly*, vol. 23, n° 3, pp. 536–559. doi:10.1353/hrq.2001.0034.

Fanon, Frantz (1952), *Black Skin, White Masks*, New York: Grove Press.

Fanon, Frantz (1961), *The Wretched of the Earth*, New York: Grove Press.

Fawcett, Edmund (2015), *Liberalism: The Life of an Idea*, revised edition, Princeton: Princeton University Press.

Fofana, Mariam O. (2021), 'Decolonising Global Health in the Time of COVID-19', *Global Public Health*, vol. 16, n° 8–9, pp. 1155–1166. doi:10.1080/17441692.2020.1864754.

Foucault, Michel (1977), *Discipline and Punish: The Birth of the Prison*, New York: Pantheon Books.

Fox, Renée C. (2015), *Doctors Without Borders: Humanitarian Quests, Impossible Dreams of Médecins Sans Frontières*, reprint edition, Baltimore (MD): Johns Hopkins University Press.

Gichane, Margaret W., and Deshira D.Wallace (2022), 'Dismantling and Reimagining Global Health Education', *Global Health Action*, vol. 15, n° 1. doi:10.1080/16549716.2022.2131967.

Gopnik, Adam (2019), *A Thousand Small Sanities: The Moral Adventure of Liberalism*, first edition, New York: Basic Books.

Harris, Thomas (2024), 'The EDI Tax: How Equity, Diversity and Inclusion Is Hobbling British Businesses', *The Free Speech Union*. [https://freespeechunion.org/the-edi-tax-how-equity-diversity-and-inclusion-is-hobbling-british-businesses/].

Hellowell, Mark, and Patricia Nayna Schwerdtle (2022), 'Powerful Ideas? Decolonisation and the Future of Global Health', *BMJ Global Health*, vol. 7, n° 1. doi:10.1136/bmjgh-2021–006924.

Hirsch, Lioba A. (2021), 'Is It Possible to Decolonise Global Health Institutions?', *Lancet*, vol. 397, n° 10270, pp. 189–190. doi:10.1016/S0140–6736(20)32763-X.

Kendi, Ibram X. (2019), *How to Be an Antiracist*, New York: One World.

Krugman, Daniel W. (2023), 'Global Health and the Elite Capture of Decolonization: On Reformism and the Possibilities of Alternate Paths', *PLOS Global Public Health*, vol. 3, n° 6. doi:10.1371/journal.pgph.0002103.

Lewis, Alexandra, and Marie Lall (2024), 'From Decolonisation to Authoritarianism: The Co-Option of the Decolonial Agenda in Higher Education by Right-Wing Nationalist Elites in Russia and India', *Higher Education*, vol. 87, n° 5, pp. 1471–1488. doi:10.1007/s10734–10023–01074–0.

Lyotard, Jean-François (1984), *The Postmodern Condition: A Report On Knowledge*, Minneapolis: University Of Minnesota Press.

Majumdar, Arnab, and Monica Mukerjee (2022), 'Research as Agitation: Generative Activism in the Age of Resistance', *PLOS Global Public Health*, vol. 2, n° 1. doi:10.1371/journal.pgph.0000142.

Marcuse, Herbert (1965), *Repressive Tolerance*, in Robert Paul Wolff, Barrington Moore, Jr., and Herbert Marcuse, *A Critique of Pure Tolerance*, Boston: Beacon Press. [https://www.marcuse.org/herbert/publications/1960s/1965-repressive-tolerance-fulltext.html].

Mbembe, Achille (2001), *On the Postcolony*, Berkeley: University of California Press.

Mill, John Stuart (1985), *On Liberty (1859)*, London: Penguin Books Limited.

MSF France Association (2020), 'Racism, Discrimination and Inequalities within MSF: Observations and Proposals from the Field', MSF internal forum.

MSF Spain Governing Body (2022a), 'Agora Statement – Walk the Talk: An Overdue Apology for Racism in MSF and a Call for (More) Action', MSF internal forum.

MSF Spain Governing Body (2022b), Anti-racism Committee, 'DEI Action Plan'.

Mukerjee, Monica, and Arnab Majumdar (2021), "Dignity at MSF: A Report by Decolonise MSF on Abuse and Discrimination at Doctors Without Borders". [https://decolonisemsf.univer.se/dignity-at-msf].

Nanda, Meera (2001), 'We Are All Hybrids Now!', *Journal of Peasant Studies, vol. 28, n ° 2, pp. 162–86.* doi:10.1080/03066150108438770.

Nayna Schwerdtle, Trish (2022), 'The Problem with "Decolonizing" Global Health', *Persuasion.* [https://www.persuasion.community/p/the-problem-with-decolonizing-global].

Nayna Schwerdtle, Trish (2023), 'Conscience Over Consequences: Reassessing the Drive To End Philanthropy', *Discourse.* [https://www.discoursemagazine.com/p/conscience-over-consequences-reassessing-the-drive-to-end-philanthropy].

'Open Letter to Senior Management and Colleagues in MSF: Beyond Words to Anti-Racist Action' (2020), 25 June. [https://decolonisemsf.univer.se/2020-open-letter].

Pai, Madhukar (2021), 'Decolonizing Global Health: A Moment To Reflect On A Movement', *Forbes.* [https://www.forbes.com/sites/madhukarpai/2021/07/22/decolonizing-global-health-a-moment-to-reflect-on-a-movement/].

Pinker, Steven (2011), *Better Angels of Our Nature: The Decline of Violence in History and Its Causes*, first edition, London: Viking Adult.

Pluckrose, Helen (2017), 'How French "Intellectuals" Ruined The West: Postmodernism And Its Impact, Explained', *Areo Magazine*, 27 March.

Pluckrose, Helen (2024), *The Counterweight Handbook: Principled Strategies for Surviving and Defeating Critical Social Justice—at Work, in Schools, and Beyond*, Durham, NC: Swift Press.

Pluckrose, Helen, and James Lindsay (2020), *Cynical Theories: How Activist Scholarship Made Everything about Race, Gender, and Identity—and Why This Harms Everybody*, Durham, NC: Pitchstone Publishing.

Said, Edward W. (1978), *Orientalism*, New York: Pantheon Books.

Shackel, Nicholas (2005), 'The Vacuity Of Postmodernist Methodology', *Metaphilosophy*, vol. 36, n° 3, pp. 295–320. doi:10.1111/j.1467–9973.2005.00370.x.

Smith, James, Ezekiel Boro, Edwin Jit Leung Kwong, and Megan Schmidt-Sane (2023), 'Resisting Unchecked Pragmatism in Global Health', *The Lancet Global Health*, vol. 11, n° 8, pp. e1176–1177. doi:10.1016/S2214–2109X(23)00208–00205.

Spivak, Gayatri C. (1988), 'Can the Subaltern Speak?', in Cary Nelson and Lawrence Grossberg (eds.), *Marxism and the Interpretation of Culture*, London: Macmillan.

Storr, Will (2021), *The Status Game: On Human Life and How to Play It*, London: William Collins.

Táíwò, Olúfẹ́mi (2020), 'Being-in-the-Room Privilege: Elite Capture and Epistemic Deference', *The Philosopher*, vol. 108. [https://www.thephilosopher1923.org/post/being-in-the-room-privilege-elite-capture-and-epistemic-deference].

Táíwò, Olúfẹ́mi (2022), *Against Decolonisation: Taking African Agency Seriously*, London: Hurst.

US Department of Health and Human Services (2021), 'Guidance on Federal Legal Standards Prohibiting Race, Color and National Origin Discrimination in COVID-19 Vaccination Programs'. [https://www.hhs.gov/civil-rights/for-providers/civil-rights-covid19/guidance-federal-legal-standards-covid-19-vaccination-programs/index.html].

Vandormael, Alain (2007), 'The TAC's "Intellectual Campaign" (2000–2004): Social Movements and Epistemic Communities', *Politikon*, vol. 34, n° 2, pp. 217–233. doi:10.1080/02589340701725306.

Walzer, Michael (2023), 'Even the Oppressed Have Obligations', *The Atlantic*. [https://www.theatlantic.com/ideas/archive/2023/11/oppression-palestine-israel-hamas/675907/].

Warsame, Abdihamid, Gwendolen Eamer, Alaria Kai, Lucia Robles Dios, Hana Rohan, Patrick Keating, Jacques Katshishi, and Francesco Checchi (2023), 'Performance of a Safe and Dignified Burial Intervention during an Ebola Epidemic in the Eastern Democratic Republic of the Congo, 2018–2019', *BMC Medicine*, vol. 21, n° 1. doi:10.1186/s12916–12023–03194-x.

Zoom-in: Reflecting on Diversity, Equity, and Inclusion in MSF

Meg Adhiambo Otieno

While it may seem obvious that humanitarian organisations are not immune to societal shifts, the recent movement against racial discrimination in the United States (US) has had a marked and lasting impact on MSF. By examining both internal and external factors, this zoom-in will give a brief history of how MSF came to affirm commitments and develop initiatives related to diversity, equity and inclusion (DEI).[1] Based on her observations as DEI lead at MSF Switzerland, the author will then touch upon internal reactions to staff concerns around discrimination and structural racism,[2] finally focusing on the challenges in implementing significant changes in policies and practices.

MSF's DEI Journey

While basic good practice adaption can be gleaned from multiple contexts in which MSF is operational, there are some key dates to keep in mind. As early as 2006, a major reform process within MSF culminated with the La Mancha Agreement, which explicitly recognised the key role played by locally recruited staff, as well as the *"urgent need to address any issues of discrimination"* and to offer *"fair employment opportunities for all staff"*.[3] In June 2017, a series of motions and recommendations related to workforce diversity, racism, abuse of power, and harassment were approved during MSF USA's general assembly. The motion titled "Unpacking Racism, Prejudice, and Privilege in MSF" was later submitted to MSF's annual International General Assembly (IGA). Instead of holding a vote, the IGA asked all institutional members and the executive to *"take all necessary steps to address and prevent discrimination from occurring"*.[4] In October, the international executive leadership of MSF acknowledged concerns about *"current policies and/or practices [being] experienced as exclusive, discriminatory and abusive"* and committed to restoring trust with *"individuals that are an integral part of [the organisation]"*.[5]

In the following year, several statements, surveys, and initiatives, such as a project on the inclusion of persons with disabilities, discussions on workforce development and mobility, and the adoption of a more equitable global grid for the remuneration of international staff, indicated that the issue was being actively addressed across the MSF movement. In 2019, the Swiss section

DOI: 10.4324/9781003542247-17

integrated inclusion and diversity as guiding principles in its new strategic plan, aiming to *"improve our understanding of and adaptation to the contexts we operate in and our connection with the populations we serve"*.[6]

The death of George Floyd in May 2020 and the worldwide shock that followed reignited debates about structural racism in MSF.[7] In the wake of yet another example of police brutality against Black people, protests erupted across the US, with millions demanding police reform and an end to racial inequalities.[8] The resulting widespread media coverage and public outcry drew global attention to the Black Lives Matter movement, which served as a catalyst for change and awareness about racial discrimination. Rallies of support were held around the world. Within MSF, personal accounts and reflections on racism were shared on internal forums, soon followed by an open letter signed by 1,000 current and former staff members calling for the urgent recognition of institutional racism in MSF.[9] Just a few months later, the IGA passed a motion to "actively dismantle racism and oppression by adopting an 'equity, diversity and inclusion in everything' approach".

After 50 years of providing emergency medical assistance across continents to those most in need, MSF would have to grapple with the legacy of its roots and operational set-up – in essence, a Eurocentric NGO headquartered in the North, far from where aid is delivered, despite over 90% of staff being hired locally[10] – and address historical shortcomings in terms of recognising and valorising the diversity of its workforce.[11]

Organisational Shock

For an organisation used to internal debate and reflection, such as MSF, self-criticism comes naturally. Yet this instance was different, sparking feelings of shock, disbelief, confusion, and sometimes anger amongst staff: MSF, a well-recognised humanitarian actor striving to provide healthcare to the most vulnerable, was labelled racist and condemned for actions viewed as discriminatory. This cuts deeper, as the organisation's mission is profoundly intertwined with why people choose to work there. The dissonance could be sensed across several associative discussions: it was argued that nepotism or favouritism, rather than racism, was the appropriate term to describe discrimination in MSF;[12] some instead spoke of situations perceived as *"unjust"*;[13] while others firmly believed that the organisation had *"normalized institutional racism within its systems and organizational culture"*.[14]

In silent corners, many started asking questions such as, "I am white, does that make me a racist?" "Am I privileged because of the colour of my skin?" "What happens now that this is how the world views me and the organisation I work for?" The inevitable pain that follows such introspection leaves a lasting impression. Some attempted to find solutions, while others argued that the discussion was theoretical and derailing, at best. Distinct historical contexts and experiences, such as those between the US and Europe, led to different perspectives on how to best address racial inequality. Applying the US-inspired approach, which focuses on racial identity, was sometimes considered unsuitable, particularly in countries where the concept of universalism is prevalent. While people could be willing to reflect on their biases, they rejected the idea of identification based on race or ethnicity.[15]

From Pledge to Progress – Challenges and Successes

In many ways, diversity, equity, and inclusion have very different meanings and evoke different emotions. Due to the wide interpretation or misunderstanding about DEI, some individuals were reluctant or sceptical about its intentions. Others believed that DEI would solely target racism instead of encompassing all forms of discrimination. In some instances, there was satisfaction because an issue which used to be swept under the rug was now out in the open for discussion and potential actions that would kick-start the wheels of change.[16] Project teams in countries of intervention were also part of the process and put forward concrete proposals.[17] Key movement-wide platforms agreed to establish common actions that would be rolled out across the organisation. This move did evoke some sense of direction on how MSF could then navigate this new terrain. At around the same time, DEI experts were brought in to help clarify strategies that would improve staff engagement.

Laying the Groundwork

Compared to other organisations, MSF was relatively inexperienced when it came to DEI – not necessarily a new topic, but a new approach with limited historical precedent or internal expertise. The question of focus was repeatedly raised. Because MSF sections have the freedom to develop their own strategies, various DEI proposals and interpretations emerged. During the author's interview for the DEI lead position, a cautious approach to the subject was evident, as well as the need to properly understand and address concerns. Implementing change in an organisation of this size and nature requires time, especially given that DEI touches not only on policy, but on behaviour and practices.

Viewing DEI as a behavioural approach rather than an additional "task", it was important for the author to create open spaces for people to share their experiences. DEI trainings and workshops are now well under way in both HQ and project locations, with simple but effective guidelines that ensure staff engagement and ownership of the initiatives: all employees are invited to the sessions, from the head of mission to the guard, and local languages are used. The sessions foster safe spaces for staff to openly share their perspectives on DEI and connect these discussions to their specific contextual realities. The workshops provide a foundational introduction to DEI terminology and concepts, enriched by techniques that emphasise practical, real-life examples to facilitate meaningful learning and engagement. However, project teams can sometimes struggle to appreciate the relevance of, and make time for, a "new priority from HQ", amidst an already heavy workload.

Paving the Way and Spotting the Roadblocks

Even though expectations are high, DEI initiatives will not cover all gaps at once; thus the need to focus on actionable priorities. In 2025, MSF Switzerland's gender balance campaign aims to overcome obstacles that hinder women from joining or advancing within the organisation, one particular issue being the decline of female international staff (from 46.2% in 2018 to 38.5% in 2023) and the persistently low percentage of women in its locally hired personnel (around 32%). In countries where gender inequality is rife, women are *de facto* less represented in the workforce, meaning that some of MSF's international teams are made up entirely of men.[18] The lack of female representation amongst MSF staff, notably in managerial positions, is a glaring example of how discrimination can linger and become intractable. By raising awareness and striving for greater gender balance in its teams, MSF hopes to create a safer environment for patients and staff while also improving access to healthcare for women in its projects.

Implementing a DEI lens in recruitment can serve as a powerful tool to address historical imbalances in team composition. But despite seemingly obvious benefits, significant barriers and resistance can persist in certain countries with long-standing rivalries, tensions, or competition between communities. More often than not, efforts to ensure effective representation of all social and cultural backgrounds in a project team help gain acceptance and trust amongst a community. However, cooperation between staff from different regions or ethnic backgrounds can be challenging, sometimes leading to discrimination against, or ill-treatment of, specific team members. Sometimes, the practical application of diversity and inclusion principles stops outside MSF gates: staff members may conform to expected behaviour in order to secure their job rather than to embrace inclusivity goals. In introducing such values, MSF will always face a delicate balance between idealism and pragmatism, as some individuals may disagree with them or view the organisation as entitled.

While DEI initiatives no doubt have the potential to bring about positive change, their impact will be less meaningful if consistent progress-tracking is still a limitation. Ideally, perceptions as well as statistics would be collected and measured (how people feel before and after the workshop, where their priorities lie). Though this should be feasible in HQ, it is less so in projects, due to high turnover of staff. DEI trainings include a section during which participants can share their fears and concerns, openly or anonymously. Such fears and concerns often stem from perceptions about management practices and equitable treatment within the organisation. While many staff members raise issues during training sessions, it is crucial to establish a robust mechanism that enables these frustrations to be addressed beyond the country offices. Implementing a well-structured feedback system would not only address these issues more effectively but also reassure staff that their voices are genuinely being heard and valued. Information needs to be communicated from the top down as well as from the bottom up, otherwise participants might question the relevance of their contributions.

Some Final Thoughts

Making systems equitable, changing perceptions, and increasing awareness all take time, knowing, as well, that not all unequal outcomes are due to systemic discrimination. There are limitations to what can be achieved, even if expectations are high. The complexity of behaviour change, coupled with important evaluation challenges, can create a misalignment between approach and reality. What is more, even the most well-intentioned DEI initiatives will always face constraints, in that they do not necessarily align with personal beliefs and values. Policies implemented by MSF, an employer, on moral and political issues that can be sensitive (individual views on women's role in society or sexual orientation) can be problematic in certain countries where MSF operates.

However, a lot of good has come out of discussions and engagement with staff. Policies have been put in place that now enable MSF employees to aim for opportunities and advance in their careers. There are also sustained efforts to ensure a safe working environment through prevention courses at project level and the improvement of reporting tools for discrimination, sexual abuse, and harassment. And while staff may still experience confusion if the path to inclusion is unclear, in organisations where DEI is central to the strategy and seen as a vehicle for delivering objectives, benefits abound, as there is room to learn and try out new ways of approaching work.

Notes

1 Diversity refers to observable and non-observable attributes (such as ethnicity, gender, disability, values, cultural perspectives, and sexual orientation) and suggests that diverse people work together in a way that harnesses those differences. Equity is defined, by different sources, as the fair treatment, access, opportunity, and advancement for all people, while striving to identify and eliminate barriers that have prevented the full participation of some groups. Inclusion refers to the practice of allowing each employee to feel welcomed, respected, supported, and valued to fully participate in processes, activities, development opportunities, and decision-making within the organisation.

2 "*A system in which public policies, institutional practices, cultural representations, and other norms work in various, often reinforcing ways to perpetuate racial group inequity.*" (Aspen Institute, n.d.).

3 MSF, 2006. Also see Davey, 2024.

4 MSF International General Assembly, 2017.

5 MSF Full Executive Committee, 2017.

6 MSF Operational Centre Geneva, "Strategic Plan 2020–2023".

7 On 25 May 2020 in Minneapolis, George Floyd, a Black man, was arrested and died as he was pinned to the ground and a police officer knelt on his neck.

8 Buchanan, Bei, and Patel, 2020.

9 MSF Open Letter, 25 June 2020.

10 In 2023, locally hired staff represented 91.1% of the total programme staff (full-time equivalents): MSF, 2024.

11 Some might argue that MSF's legacy lies more in the political convictions of its founders around international solidarity and the anti-colonialism movement.

12 Associative debate held in Niger.

13 Associative debate held in Haiti.
14 In its "BLM & Racism within MSF – Time for Action" statement, the MSF East Africa Association (2020) mentions, among others, the lack of accountability following individual acts of racism, policies that favour international staff over locally hired personnel, and bias from management when handling grievances and disciplinary issues.
15 For instance, in 2018, France's National Assembly voted to remove "race" from the Constitution, underlining the scientific precept that recognises only one human species: Bessone, 2021, pp. 367–82.
16 See the Decolonise MSF movement at https://decolonisemsf.univer.se.
17 MSF France Association, 2020.
18 MSF, 2024.

References

Aspen Institute, 'Glossary for Understanding the Dismantling Structural Racism/Promoting Racial Equity Analysis'. [https://www.aspeninstitute.org/wp-content/uploads/files/content/docs/rcc/RCC-Structural-Racism-Glossary.pdf].

Bessone, Magali (2021), 'Critical Race Theory and the removal of the word "race" from the French Constitution: An exercise in translation?', *Droit et société*, vol. 108, n° 2, pp. 367–382. doi:10.3917/drs1.108.0367.

Buchanan, Larry, Quoctrung Bui, and Jugal K. Patel (2020), 'Black Lives Matter May Be the Largest Movement in U.S. History', *The New York Times*, 3 July. [https://www.nytimes.com/interactive/2020/07/03/us/george-floyd-protests-crowd-size.html].

Davey, Eleanor (2024), 'The road from La Mancha: Narratives of failure and institutional reform', *Centre de réflexion sur l'action et les savoirs humanitaires*. [https://msf-crash.org/en/la-mancha/road-la-mancha-narratives-failure-and-institutional-reform].

Decolonise MSF movement. [https://decolonisemsf.univer.se].

MSF (2006), 'La Mancha Agreement', 25 June. [https://www.msf.org/sites/default/files/La%20Mancha%20Agreement%20EN.pdf].

MSF (2024), '2023 MSF Staff Data and Trends Report', MSF Internal Report.

MSF East Africa Association (2020), 'BLM & Racism within MSF – Time for Action', MSF internal forum.

MSF France Association (2020), 'Racism, Discrimination and Inequalities within MSF: Observations and Proposals from the Field', MSF Internal Forum.

MSF Full Executive Committee (2017), '"People at the Centre": People, People and People', MSF internal forum, 18 October.

MSF International General Assembly (2017), 'Statement from the IGA: Diversity and Inclusion', 1 July.

MSF Operational Centre Geneva, 'Strategic Plan 2020–2023', MSF Internal Document.

'Open Letter to Senior Management and Colleagues in MSF: Beyond Words to Anti-Racist Action' (2020), 25 June. [https://decolonisemsf.univer.se/2020-open-letter].

9 Absorbed into the War Machine

What Is Independence When Everything Is Connected?

Martin Searle and Beatrice Lau

While the digital age has significantly improved the efficiency and effectiveness of humanitarian services, it simultaneously exposes such organisations to entirely new risks. These risks are not only technological; they threaten a very core principle upon which impartial relief work is founded – independence. Independence is often fundamental to the ability of humanitarian organisations to negotiate access to populations in need. Nonetheless, independence has long been contested, with some arguing that its maintenance is more the exception than the rule across the history of humanitarian work. But in MSF's experience, when independence is compromised – or more precisely, when it is perceived as compromised – trust gets eroded, and with it the ability to deliver aid directly to those who need it.

To explore this issue, the chapter first introduces the so-called capability–vulnerability paradox in the cyber domain, which holds that technological advancements both improve the efficiency and effectiveness of humanitarian services and expose humanitarian organisations to new risk. It then examines existing international legal frameworks protecting humanitarian data and identifies gaps, particularly in relation to cyber reconnaissance. Finally, the chapter discusses the need for a broader, multilayered approach to address cyber technologies' challenge to humanitarian independence that goes beyond legal measures to include operational and technical safeguards. Through this analysis, the authors aim to highlight the critical necessity for humanitarian organisations to reassess their cybersecurity strategies – including, a priori, a paradigm shift that recognises malicious cyber activities as not "merely" an information and communications technology (ICT) problem but a direct threat to core operational values.

I The Capability–Vulnerability Paradox – Risks Involved in the Digitalisation of Humanitarian Information

As humanitarian organisations become more present in cyberspace, they increase both their operational abilities and their exposure to risk of operational compromise. Military and smart-city analysts call this the capability–vulnerability paradox.[1] In essence, the more connected an entity is to

DOI: 10.4324/9781003542247-18

cyberspace, the greater the attack surface available in that space to target them. Humanitarians may have little choice on whether to digitise, but they can still choose the extent and content of their digitisation and so make an informed decision on the size of the attack surface they are willing to present.

MSF and other humanitarian groups have expanded their presence in cyberspace for several operational purposes. As a result, they produce ever more data about the people they support and the places they work. Data consolidation and aggregation tools (such as digital health information systems), AI-driven diagnosis, geospatial analysis, digitised epidemiology and needs assessments, chatbots, telemedicine, and cyber-based social network analysis often create personal identifiable information (PII) and demographically identifiable information (DII). Internet of Things (IoT) technology – which gives any physical object a corresponding identity in cyberspace, and which some groups use to improve the efficiency of their stock management and logistics distribution – can also create DII. If logistics items each carry such an identity, it becomes possible to track, for example, what drugs and other materials are going where, and so infer actionable conclusions about the populations in the area. Such expanded data production comes with a well-documented tendency to over-collect and sluggishly destroy data. Finally, all this data necessarily creates significant metadata (data about data) too. Today, humanitarians almost exclusively store, process, analyse, and communicate all data in a digital form and through cyber means, including cloud services.

Hacking Humanitarians – A Worrying Trend

There is a clear and arguably growing willingness to exploit this expanded attack surface. In 2022, the International Committee of the Red Cross (ICRC) suffered a highly sophisticated cyberattack.[2] This was perhaps the first time a high-profile humanitarian victim chose to go public. But there are indications that such incidents are more widespread than commonly acknowledged. The US, British, and Chinese states, as well as allegedly private entities, have reportedly used cyber-based methods to garner information from NGOs like Médecins du Monde and several UN agencies, including the World Health Organization.[3] A similar range of attacks have been documented in Syria, Greece, and elsewhere, targeting NGOs, activists, civil society organisations and displaced peoples themselves.[4]

The simplest and most invasive of these attacks allow perpetrators to record all user activity on any machine on a compromised network and transmit it to an external receiver. This means that it is not only data produced by these new cyber-based activities that are vulnerable; *all* information collected, stored, analysed, processed, or transmitted during the course of conducting humanitarian activities (humanitarian information activities) can be exposed.[5] These may include the results of needs assessments (as well as the raw data gathered as part of the process), feedback recorded from aid recipients about the assistance they have received and the programmes delivering it, and even digitised personal records of offline meetings. For a medical service provider like MSF, it further contains large amounts of PII and DII collected through medical consultations. And as an organisation often working in insecure, conflict-affected settings, it includes information and insights gathered from offline interactions and channels that are critical for our situational awareness. While, in practice, intruders will likely use more targeted methods to limit the data transmitted externally and so evade detection, in principle *any* stored digital data could be accessed.

Why Should We Care about Lost Control of Data?

The most urgent implication of such loss of data control is the risk of actively doing harm. For example, humanitarian organisations might share PII with actors who have political or other interests in the data subjects. Data on the Rohingya refugee population in Bangladesh produced by the United Nations High Commissioner for Refugees (UNHCR) was reportedly ultimately shared with Myanmar's State Administrative Council: the entity accused of ethnically cleansing them.[6] Former recipients of humanitarian aid have reportedly been denied loans based on algorithms built, in part, on datasets that track recipients of aid. Those models seemingly detected a correlation between having received aid and repayment default, connecting these humanitarian information activities to a private, profit-based agenda. Similarly, people have been overlooked or excluded from aid distributions administered using AI because the training data underlying those models ignored certain groups systematically.[7]

Meanwhile, the use of AI in any decision-making process raises the plausible risk of training datasets being deliberately "poisoned" to skew the determinations that any AI trained on that data ultimately makes.[8] This risk comes on top of the more commonly discussed "bias" that can arise when training data inadvertently produces skewed results because its training dataset is not sufficiently representative. MSF is currently experimenting with AI-enabled diagnosis of several diseases, including tuberculosis, mpox, and cervical cancer, and with other areas, such as electrocardiogram reading, patient triage, outbreak response, and migration-related medical operations. The ethical reviews of these projects have been rightly extensive. But those reviews and the risk mitigation in place are forced to address a fundamentally new risk that did not exist before. Imagine a model trained on data deliberately and surreptitiously altered to misdiagnose disease, as a means of sabotaging a healthcare system, or even to misdiagnose based, in part, on an irrelevant variable, like ethnicity, to further some political agenda.

Beyond harm, loss of control over data quickly becomes an issue of independence and instrumentalisation, too. Sometimes this is through third-party partnerships that create conflicts of interest. Palantir, a US software company that specialises in Big Data analytics, presumably gained access to both open and closed data sources held by UNHCR as part of its contracted work to develop a unified interrogable tool for data management. While that data itself is no doubt legally protected, Palantir can freely develop products for its other clients – which include the US Central Intelligence Agency – using insights acquired from that project and the data accessed as part of it. MSF has experienced a private contractor refusing to surrender intellectual property derived from the testing and diagnosis of a particular medical sample. That company can now use that property to develop products for the market.

Other times, humanitarian information may simply be expropriated. As militaries increasingly rely on probabilistic modelling to identify targets, they require a growing volume of diverse data to test and refine predictive accuracy, and to train targeting models. Preoccupied with correlation rather than causation, data gatherers now collect any available data and test whether it can inform their operations. This is exemplified in the US National Security Agency's terrorist "Kill Lists".[9] When MSF runs one of a very limited number of clinics in an opposition-held area, any military analyst might plausibly hypothesise that attending an MSF clinic – perhaps to receive treatment or to bring a family member for treatment – is a useful variable to include in a model predicting whether an individual belongs to an enemy group. Who knows what the conclusion of the test of that hypothesis may have been, given the proximity of MSF clinics to precisely the areas being targeted by, for example, the US in Pakistan and Afghanistan, or by Israel's Gospel platform, an AI system that is used extensively to recommend targets in Gaza?[10]

Similarly, MSF necessarily maintains contact with precisely the arms-bearers that may become targets for the opposing side in a conflict. That communication is, presumably, encrypted. However, a military analyst may be drawn to unencrypted, unprotected metadata produced by MSF's communication and look for clues that can help identify and locate targets. Governments are now seemingly prepared to select targets based on such metadata.[11]

Independence, Trust, and Why They Matter

Independence often underpins humanitarians' ability to negotiate access to contested areas. In such contexts, demonstrating autonomy from any opponent (whether the national government or otherwise) and its various international backers remains essential to convince authorities (*de jure* and *de facto*) who could potentially block aid to instead grant it safe passage. As such, perception of independence can be at least as important as actual independence.

What is so convincing about independence? Independence helps resist instrumentalisation: *"the blatant abuse and distortion of relief operations to achieve political objectives that are often antithetical to humanitarianism ... [and] more subtle manipulations arising from the convergence of [aid agencies' and others'] interests"*.[12] Independence – and, as importantly, the perception of independence – is jeopardised when humanitarian aid is instrumentalised to serve such non-humanitarian agendas.

Yet, cyberspace's capability–vulnerability paradox exposes humanitarian actors more to the risk of instrumentalisation. This process is not necessarily driven by the *agency* of the organisation themselves; they do not (we presume) knowingly permit their data to be used for non-humanitarian purposes. Rather, it is due to the *structures* to which humanitarians inevitably bind themselves as they insert themselves deeper into cyberspace. The capability–vulnerability paradox is inherent to those structures: since any expansion of an organisation's cyber presence automatically increases the attack surface available to potential perpetrators, the risk of instrumentalisation systematically grows. As that structural risk of instrumentalisation grows, independence erodes, both in perception and in reality, and with it trust.[13] Trust is crucial for humanitarian groups like MSF to negotiate access to the places they are most needed.

II Possible Frameworks to Safeguard Independence?

Faced with these challenges, how can humanitarian organisations safeguard their digitised humanitarian information activities and mitigate their risks?

Legal frameworks could be one source of protection, but which ones? The interconnectedness of the cyber domain and the transnational nature of ICT operations, coupled with the reality that state or state-sponsored actors are often involved in cyber operations, mean that domestic legal frameworks may be insufficient. Rules at the international level seem more promising, both as predictors of states' behaviour and in shaping the development of domestic frameworks governing cyber activities.

At this time, we know of no international treaty developed specifically to govern behaviour in cyberspace. Indeed, divergent views exist as to whether specific rules or principles of international law tailored for cyberspace are even necessary.[14] Notwithstanding this, several multilateral, regional, and bilateral initiatives have developed agreements on how existing international law applies in the cyber context.[15] At the international level, the UN's twin tracks – the Group of Governmental Experts (GGE)[16] and the Open-ended Working Group on developments in the field of information and telecommunications in the context of international security (OEWG)[17] – have fostered significant consensus in this regard. Similarly, this chapter proceeds with the understanding that international law is applicable within the ICT environment, and will examine three different domains: the law on privileges and immunities, international humanitarian law (IHL), and human rights law.[18]

Notion of Privileges and Immunities

Humanitarian organisations that qualify as international organisations (IOs) enjoy certain privileges and immunities (P&Is) granted by states.[19] However, most humanitarian groups do not qualify, as they are private or non-governmental organisations (NGOs) rather than IOs. Rare exceptions exist: the ICRC – a private association established under Swiss law – holds a treaty-based mandate from states[20] and is accorded P&Is in most places it operates.[21] MSF has also concluded bilateral agreements with 12 states that secure certain P&Is.

How Do P&Is Help Protect Humanitarian Information?

P&I provisions in bilateral status agreements between humanitarian organisations and host states generally mirror those found in the Vienna Convention on Diplomatic Relations[22] (VCDR) and the Convention on the Privileges and Immunities of the United Nations (P&I Convention).[23] These P&Is include the *"inviolability of premises"*,[24] *"inviolability of archives and documents"*,[25] *"freedom of communications without any interference"*,[26] and respect for the confidentiality of correspondence.[27] In the case of the ICRC, there is a specific undertaking not to divulge the content of their reports and correspondence to anyone other than the intended recipient.[28]

Nevertheless, unless explicitly addressed in a bilateral agreement, the applicability of these P&Is to the ICT activities of a humanitarian organisation – even if granted IO-equivalent status – remains uncertain. The work of the GGE and the OEWG has not yet considered the application of this diplomatic law in cyberspace.

In contrast, the non-binding *Tallinn Manual 2.0*[29] affirms for the first time that the VCDR *"substantially reflect[s] customary international law"*,[30] and that those notions above apply to ICT activities concerning diplomatic missions.[31] However, the *Manual* explicitly indicates that *"the law that governs international organisations is not specifically addressed"*.[32]

Additionally, commentaries to existing rules suggest that, even if they do apply to the ICT activities of humanitarian organisations, their protection may be inadequate. For example, it is forbidden to physically violate premises. However, a remote intrusion into the cyber infrastructure or disruption or alteration of data is not considered such a violation unless the cyber infrastructure is located physically inside the mission[33] or the intrusion results in physical consequences therein.[34]

Conversely, the International Group of Experts (Experts) agreed an expansive scope of protection under the rule concerning electronic archives, documents, and correspondence, highlighting that the purpose of Rule 41 is to ensure confidentiality.[35] Protected materials include *"external hard drives, flash drives, and other media on which electronic documents are stored"*,[36] documents and their drafts *"preserved [...] in the course of their activities"*, emails, and other messages that relate to a mission or the functions thereof.[37] This protection includes freedom from seizure, enforcement, judicial action, cyber espionage, and other forms of interference by a state.[38] However, there was no conclusion amongst the Experts on the prohibition of electronic surveillance by third states,[39] and the Rule is not applicable to the actions of private entities unless they are attributable to a state.[40]

Rule 42 on free communication, meanwhile, may create a positive obligation to take *"all appropriate steps"* to *protect* official communications (i.e. relating to the functions of the mission) from interruption by others.[41] This includes taking reasonable measures to terminate an attempt to hack a mission's official website or block its cyber communications. But, again, it is unclear if such a duty applies to IOs, given that relationships between IOs and states lack the reciprocity of those between states and other states.

Protection of Humanitarian Missions under IHL

After years of controversies,[42] there is now general agreement that IHL applies to ICT during armed conflicts.[43] Nevertheless, meaningful realisation of IHL-derived protection depends on the transposition of *how* these rules and principles apply to the cyber context. This question remains unsettled. Much has been written on the interpretive difficulties and diverse perspectives surrounding this application.[44] Two outstanding areas are of particular relevance: (i) the notion of "attack" for the purpose of IHL in the cyber context; and (ii) digital data as "object". The lack of international agreement on these two issues leaves the application of IHL protections to humanitarian information activities uncertain.

Divergent views exist regarding whether *"a cyber operation that results in a loss of functionality without causing physical damage"* qualifies as *"an attack"*[45] that activates IHL protection premised on the principle of distinction. Even in the broadest sense, however, the deletion of, or tampering with, humanitarian data only amounts to an "attack" if it renders the humanitarian infrastructure dysfunctional or causes significant disruption to the organisation's ability to deliver essential services.[46] Cyber espionage alone almost certainly is not an "attack" in this sense.[47] Unauthorised access, such as hacking or surveillance of humanitarian data, remains outside the scope of this protection.

A more fundamental challenge lies in whether digitised civilian data – including medical data, biometrics, or other digital information collected in the course of humanitarian operations – qualifies as a "civilian object". The issue is less whether the nature of the data is civilian and more whether data, in its digital form, can be considered an "object".[48] According to the Experts and some states, "objects" are, by definition, *"visible and tangible"*; therefore, data cannot be a civilian object for the purpose of IHL.[49] To the minds of the authors, an interpretation suggesting that the fundamental protection afforded to civilian objects, as reflected in Article 48 of Additional Protocol I, should be removed or diminished merely because the data exists in digital rather than physical form could not be a good-faith application of the rules.[50] Nonetheless, it is unclear how ongoing international deliberations will settle this question.

Other Possible Avenues?

According to the ICRC,[51] the protection of humanitarian – and particularly medical – electronic data can also be achieved through transposing IHL principles that specifically protect medical missions[52] and humanitarian relief operations.[53] For example, humanitarian data could be protected as objects indispensable to the survival of the civilian population, at least if the humanitarian assistance in question were indeed so indispensable.[54] Additionally, the obligations to facilitate and protect humanitarian relief actions[55] translate to a prohibition of cyber operations that are *"designed or conducted to interfere unduly"*[56] with humanitarian assistance. Similarly, even if a cyber operation does not amount to an "attack", the obligation to respect and protect medical facilities "*must be understood as extending to digitalised medical data belonging to those facilities*" regardless of whether electronic data itself is considered as an "object".[57] These avenues may avoid some of the interpretative complexities discussed earlier.

Notable Protection Gaps under the Framework of IHL

Humanitarian groups, including MSF, increasingly rely on third-party cloud services to store data in servers based elsewhere. Does a cloud server, or a part thereof, enjoy special protection under IHL solely by virtue of hosting medical data relevant to humanitarian work?[58] What if neither the third-party service provider nor the state hosting the cloud server is a party to the conflict?

While existing rules may protect humanitarian and medical data from cyber operations that would *"negatively affect"*[59] or *"interfere unduly"*[60] with medical or humanitarian functions, they do not appear to prohibit other forms of unauthorised access. Cyber reconnaissance, or copying or extracting data without altering or deleting it, do not materially impact the delivery of medical or humanitarian assistance, and so remain compliant. This leaves a crucial protection gap, given the risks stemming from such actions to core humanitarian principles discussed above.

Furthermore, the interconnectedness of cyber networks may render the precise contours of the specific protection of medical or humanitarian missions extremely nebulous. Recall that such protection can be lost if any part of the protected object is *"being used to commit, outside their humanitarian functions, acts harmful to the enemy"*.[61] This raises questions about whether, and at which point, protection will be forfeited if the medical or humanitarian data is *"stored in the same data centre, server, or computer as military data"* or military communication will pass through the *"same web and communication networks"*, *"undersea fibre-optic cables, satellites, routers or nodes"* as those used by humanitarian missions.[62]

Finally, even if adequate protection were to exist under IHL, it would only cover cyber operations carried out during armed conflict. Therefore, a significant portion of cyber incidents fall outside its scope.[63]

Bridging the Gap? Protection under Human Rights Law

Human rights law may help address this protection gap for at least three reasons. First, it applies both in peacetime and in times of armed conflicts,[64] and there is clear consensus that international human rights enjoyed "offline" are also protected "online".[65] Second, while cyber espionage is not unlawful under international law per se,[66] it nonetheless remains *"subject to [an] applicable human rights law obligation to respect the right to privacy"*.[67] Third, derogation from, or limitation to, the right to privacy is allowed only if specific criteria and conditions are met.[68] This restrains interference, at least as a matter of law, even if it is purportedly done for national security or counterterrorism, which are considered as legitimate reasons for surveillance or cyber reconnaissance.[69]

The Experts of the *Tallinn Manual* more ambitiously assert that an obligation to protect exists under the human rights framework that includes a *"duty of States to safeguard individuals from human rights abuses that are initiated in cyberspace, but may affect their rights offline"*.[70] This appears to put a duty to protect on the host state, as the breach of these individuals' right to privacy in cyberspace has a direct effect on their rights of life, liberty, and security in physical space.[71]

Nonetheless, the human rights framework presents its own set of shortcomings. Notably, private hackers, as non-obligation-bearers under international human rights law, are not directly bound. States also retain significant discretion in interpreting the necessity and proportionality required for derogation – justifying measures, such as lawful surveillance, which would pose the same threat to humanitarian information. Furthermore, proportionality can be a double-edged sword that could justify rather than prevent the hacking of humanitarian information if it is deemed *"the least intrusive means"*[72] to protect national security.[73] The practical effectiveness in invoking the protection is also questionable if the author of the cyber intrusions is the state concerned.

For our purposes, the greatest deficiency arguably lies in human rights law's primary focus on the protection of individual(s): as such, it cannot directly safeguard humanitarian organisations from instrumentalisation or lost independence due to malicious cyber activities. To the contrary, the right to privacy obliges humanitarian organisations to exercise sufficient due diligence to fulfil their duty of care towards the individuals from or upon whom they have collected data or information.[74]

Finally, attribution of responsibility in cyber incidents is notoriously difficult. When perpetrators use certain tactics like proxy servers, spoofing IP addresses, or mobilising botnets or zero-day exploits, or when states "sponsor" non-state actors to conduct attacks on their behalf, or attackers employ a multistage process that can appear to involve several different actors, it can be extremely difficult to determine the source of an attack.[75] From a legal perspective, reliable attribution is a necessary prerequisite for any legal measure to offer actual protection. From a political perspective, incorrect attribution can sour relations, escalate tension, and bring independence into question.

Fundamentally, no existing legal framework satisfactorily addresses our concerns about the implications of cyber-based technologies on humanitarian independence.

III A Call to Go beyond Legal Protection

Too often, data protection is perceived as "merely" a technical ICT issue, detached from the fundamental operational principles that underpin humanitarian action. However, as this discussion has demonstrated, the principle of independence – a cornerstone of humanitarian operations that enables trust, access, and informed consent – is at risk in the digital domain.

Recognition and Awareness – A Necessary Paradigm Shift

Addressing this challenge requires a fundamental shift in the way humanitarian actors perceive and approach cybersecurity. The safeguarding of humanitarian information should no longer be viewed solely as a technical or administrative function, but rather as an integral component of operational security and risk management. This paradigm shift must translate into tangible changes in the way resources and attention are allocated. Just as rigorous security measures are applied in the physical sphere to protect staff, aid recipients, and operations, an equivalent – if not greater – level of vigilance must be dedicated to cybersecurity.

This includes ensuring that the infrastructure used to store and process humanitarian data, as well as the engagement of third-party service providers, is subject to stringent scrutiny and oversight. Additionally, contractual agreements governing data-sharing must clearly articulate control mechanisms to safeguard humanitarian information. By embedding cybersecurity considerations into the core of humanitarian operations, organisations can better protect their independence, ensure operational integrity, and maintain the trust of those they serve in an increasingly digitalised world.

Taking Responsible Technical Measures

Hitherto, most critical literature on responsible data management in humanitarian settings has, understandably, focused on the risks of violating privacy and causing harm. This has been MSF's focus too. While the concerns raised in this chapter are different, many of the technical- and principle-based recommendations made in that literature towards responsible data management can also help address this threat to independence. For instance, improving the robustness of security software and implementing the "Professional Standards for Protection Work" formulated and agreed by the ICRC, MSF, and others (particularly those related to data minimisation) will inevitably make it harder for any attack to succeed.[76] While humanitarians' resources for this are limited compared to at least some likely state and non-state attackers, and the political, military, and economic motivations for mounting an attack outlined in this chapter may often be extremely strong, humanitarians should already be motivated to do all they reasonably can to stop attacks from succeeding by the principle to do no harm. All efforts to respect this principle will also help mitigate risks of instrumentalisation and lost independence. Such efforts will at least ensure that humanitarian groups know if a breach has occurred, so they can make informed decisions about how to respond and mitigate both harm and lost trust.

But given this mismatch in resources, existing literature recognises that a successful protection of data against a truly determined attacker is difficult.

This assessment is the root of several other best practices, such as data protection impact assessments.[77] Conventionally, such assessments focus on the potential risk of a data-processing activity causing harm to the individuals whose data is being handled. However, the process could expand to consider additional risks to the independence (or perception of independence) of the humanitarian organisations handling the data.

Based on the outcome of that assessment, several further technical steps could help. These include minimising how much data is collected, how long data is stored, and how much data is shared.[78] While this was intended to limit the risk of losing control mostly of PII data, the loss of which could cause harm to individuals, the same principle would reduce the risk of losing control of other forms of data that could serve non-humanitarian agendas, too. A data protection impact assessment done to cover, first and foremost, potential harm to individuals, but also the potential impact on perceptions of independence if control of certain data is lost, could help determine whether certain data is worth keeping.

For the data that remains, existing literature counsels anonymisation to the greatest degree, with due recognition that this will still be insufficient to address many problems.[79] Indeed, by definition, anonymisation is only possible with PII, and so only of partial use to mitigate the challenges raised in this chapter. One analogous technique that could be considered for both PII and non-PII data is the creation of so-called synthetic data.[80] Such data is artificially generated but mimics the relationships held in real-world data, allowing for the same analysis to be conducted while the real-word data is deleted. This certainly helps prevent PII being lost and may also help protect against other data being co-opted to serve non-humanitarian agendas. That said, if the military, political, or economic value of that data lies in the relational properties within the dataset, then this technique will offer little protection against the perceived or actual loss of independence.

Finally, the ICRC wisely counsels humanitarian groups to adopt context-specific standards for the different places they work.[81] These standards will vary based on prevailing domestic law, cultural practices, and operational considerations, the last of which are likely to include the particular alternative agendas for which the data that humanitarians are collecting could be used and the various stakeholders (both local and non-local) who are pursuing those agendas.

As with the legal protections reviewed, it is clear that these technical and procedural measures cannot alone ensure that humanitarian groups continue to operate separately from the non-humanitarian agendas of others. Humanitarians will need to retain much data to continue providing quality services. Some of that data could potentially benefit the military, political, or economic objectives of other stakeholders who are active in the same setting.

Sensitisation and Engagement

In the absence of sufficient legal and technical protection, the most likely recourse is a political solution. The ICRC has invested significantly here through its Delegation to Cyberspace. MSF and other humanitarian groups could do more to pool experience and reflections and feed them into these efforts to socialise how hacking humanitarian organisations undermines their ability to provide aid. To a great degree, the nature of cyberspace levels the playing field between state and non-state actors.[82] Quite apart from the practice of states sponsoring non-state actors to conduct cyberattacks on their behalf in ways that are then deniable, non-state actors of the type operating in places humanitarian organisations intervene are also no doubt conducting cyber operations of their own. The barriers for such activities are far lower than those for kinetic warfare. The nature of MSF's work brings it into contact with such groups, presenting an opportunity to further this socialisation among groups that have been seemingly ignored until now. The ICRC, for example, has been advocating *"operational dialogue"* with state and state-sponsored attackers,[83] and has issued *"guidelines"* for civilian hackers.[84]

MSF's second added value is a corollary of the first. As an impartial humanitarian organisation acting in accordance with IHL, MSF engages with all parties – *de jure* and *de facto* – exercising effective control of a territory. Such engagement is operationally necessary to reach populations in need within that territory. Without adequate socialisation on the implications of conducting cyber operations against humanitarian groups with all actors – state or non-state alike – MSF could find its operations being targeted for precisely the reasons of military or political expediency raised in this chapter. As noted throughout this piece, such attacks would function to erode the independence and, fundamentally, undermine the trust of those in *de facto* control of the territory. To reiterate our earlier concern, why would any political or military leader allow a humanitarian organisation access to their territory if that organisation cannot prevent itself from becoming a source of strategically valuable intelligence for their opponents?

IV Conclusion

The more humanitarian organisations insert themselves into cyberspace, the more they are confronted by a capability–vulnerability paradox. Cyber-based technology is dramatically improving the effectiveness of humanitarian information activities. But it is also increasing the quantity and quality of data and analysis that could further various political, economic, or even military agendas. Meanwhile, reliance on cyberspace heightens humanitarians' vulnerability to being hacked by anyone pursuing such non-humanitarian agendas. The subsequent risk of harming the people that humanitarians are trying to help has understandably been the focus of the growing critical literature on the responsible use of cyber-based technology. But as MSF and other humanitarian organisations consider their fitness for the future, they must understand how this capability–vulnerability paradox also impacts the operational principles on which they have historically relied to carry out their work. This has not received the same level of attention. Foremost among these impacts is the impact on the principle of independence. This is not a matter of *agency*; it is not about humanitarians deciding to support one or another agenda. Instead, this is about humanitarians tying themselves into *structures* that can result in them supporting one or another agenda regardless of what they consciously decide to do.

Essentially, maintaining independence depends on keeping actionable information away from those who would use it for non-humanitarian ends. We find the legal regimes in place (IHL and human rights law-based) and the technical tools and protocols available to be insufficient to achieve this. However, several tools and best practices could, at the minimum, mitigate risk.

But ultimately, humanitarian independence will depend on a political solution. The ICRC has taken a strong lead in this regard. Others, like MSF, must do more in support. On at least two issues – engagement with non-state actors and respect for information produced within territories held by *de facto* authorities – MSF must take up this call to engage, if we wish to see our position on aid delivery brought forward into the emerging, cyber-enabled world.

Notes

1 Schneider, 2016; Kitchin and Dodge, 2017, pp. 1–19.
2 ICRC, 2022.
3 Byrne, 2014; Ball and Hopkins, 2013; Gilman, 2014.
4 Byrne, 2014; Maitland and Bharania, 2017.
5 Campo et al., 2018, p. 8.
6 Rahman, 2021.
7 Beduschi, 2022.
8 Paracha et al., 2025.
9 Obama, 2020.
10 Davies, McKernan, and Sabbagh, 2023.
11 Badalič, 2023.
12 Donini, 2012, p. 2.
13 On the agency/structure debate and its application to organisational theory, see Heugens and Lander, 2009, pp. 61–85; Reed, 2003, pp. 289–309; Koster, 2020, pp. 45–67.
14 Akande et al., 2022, pp. 7–8. See also UN General Assembly, 2021b.
15 Moynihan, 2019, fn. 265.
16 The first GGE, established in 2004, focused on "Developments in the Field of Information and Telecommunications in the Contexts of International Security". In 2018, by Resolution 73/266, the UN General Assembly established a 25-member new GGE on "Advancing responsible State behaviour in cyberspace in the context of international security". See dedicated webpage of the GGE at https://disarmament.unoda.org/group-of-governmental-experts/.
17 First established in December 2018 through UN General Assembly Resolution 73/27. In 2020, pursuant to General Assembly Resolution 75/240, a new five-year OEWG on security of and in the use of information and communications technologies was established. See dedicated webpage of the OEWG at https://disarmament.unoda.org/open-ended-working-group/.
18 UN Doc. A/AC.290/2021/CRP.2 (UN General Assembly, 2021c), para. 7, 10 March 2021.
19 Schermers and Blokker, 2018, para. 33. See also Debuf, 2015, p. 322.
20 Debuf, 2015, p. 320. See also Article 2(2) of the ICRC Statutes (ICRC, 2018).
21 The bilateral status agreements between the ICRC and the host state are negotiated through confidential dialogue and, therefore, the existence or content of such

agreements are generally not disclosed. According to the ICRC, it has concluded bilateral status agreements granting it legal status similar to that of an IO with 95 countries. See Debuf, 2015, p. 327.

22 UN, 1961. Ratified by 193 states, entered into force on 24 April 1964.

23 UN General Assembly, 1946. Ratified by 162 states, entered into force on 17 September 1964.

24 VCDR, Article 22(3); P&I Convention, section 3.

25 VCDR, Article 24; P&I Convention, section 4.

26 VCDR, Article 27(1); P&I Convention, section 9. See also rights relating to correspondence in P&I Convention, section 10, and VCDR, Article 27(2) and (3).

27 P&I Convention, section 10. See also VCDR, Article 27(2) and (3).

28 Debuf, 2015, p. 339.

29 Schmitt, 2017.

30 *Ibid*, section 7, para. 1. See also ICJ, 1980, paras. 62 and 69.

31 See Schmitt, 2017, Rules 39, 41, and 42.

32 *Ibid*, section 7, para. 5.

33 Diplomatic law parlance but analogous to the usage in the humanitarian sector.

34 Schmitt, 2017, Commentary to Rule 39, para. 3 and 4.

35 Schmitt, 2017, Commentary to Rule 41, para. 1.

36 *Ibid*, para. 3.

37 *Ibid*.

38 *Ibid*, para. 1.

39 *Ibid*, para. 9.

40 *Ibid*, para. 2.

41 Schmitt, 2017, Commentary to Rule 42, paras. 4 and 6.

42 See, e.g. Väljataga, n.d.; Sukumar, 2017. In the context of the OWEG, see submissions of Iran on the Initial 'Pre-draft' of the United Nations General Assembly. See also submissions of China, Cuba, and the Russian Federation, available at https://disarmament.unoda.org/open-ended-working-group/.

43 See UN General Assembly, 2021a, para. 71(f), adopted by consensus at the UN General Assembly pursuant to Resolution 76/19; Resolution 341C/24/R2, adopted by consensus in the International Conference of the Red Cross and Red Crescent, 2024, which includes the participation of 196 states party to the Geneva Conventions. See also the interpretation by the Experts, Schmitt, 2017, Rule 80.

44 Mačák, 2021, pp. 411–28; ICRC, 2019; Mačák and Gisel, 2022; Rodenhäuser and Mačák, 2021; Schmitt, 2017, chapter 17.

45 See Mačák and Gisel, 2022, p. 147; ICRC, 2019, p. 7. Reportedly, states that subscribe to the broader view to include loss of functionality under the notion of "attack" – which is also the interpretation of the ICRC – include Ecuador, France, Germany, Guatemala, Italy, Japan, and New Zealand. On the contrary, Denmark, Israel, and Peru hold the narrower view that physical damage is required. See national positions at Cyber Law Toolkit, 2025. Rule 92 of the Tallinn Manual defines cyberattack in the narrow sense, with the majority of the Experts accepting that interference with functionality can qualify as damage if *"restoration of functionality requires replacement of physical components"*: see Schmitt, 2017, Commentary to Rule 92, para. 10.

46 See Schmitt, 2017, Commentary to Rule 92, para. 14.

47 *Ibid*. This is the case unless the means or methods by which it is conducted causes consequences that qualify the act as an attack.

48 Such as in Denmark, Chile, and Israel. See Mačák, 2021, pp. 422–3; ICRC, 2019, p. 8.

49 Mačák, 2021, p. 422. Schmitt, 2017, Commentary to Rule 100, para. 6.

50 ICRC, 2019, p. 8. Schmitt, 2017, Commentary to Rule 100, para. 7.

51 Mačák, 2021, p. 421.

52 See ICRC, Customary IHL Rules 25, 26, 28, and 29.

53 See ICRC, Customary IHL Rules 31 and 32.
54 See ICRC, Customary IHL Rules, Rule 54, API, Article 54(2); Schmitt, 2017, Rule 141.
55 See API, Article 70 and APII, Article 18(2).
56 Schmitt, 2017, Rule 145. Noting the divergent views on the application of this rule in non-international armed conflicts, see Commentary to Rule 145, para. 2.
57 Mačák and Gisel, 2022, p. 148; ICRC, 2019, p. 8. See also Schmitt, 2017, Rule 132 and the accompanying Commentary, para. 1.
58 For a good discussion on the challenges with respect to third-party service and technology providers, see Marelli, 2020.
59 Schmitt, 2017, Commentary to Rule 132, para. 3.
60 *Ibid*, Rule 145.
61 See ICRC, Customary IHL Rules, API, Article 13; APII, Article 11, Rules 25 and 28; Schmitt, 2017, Rule 134.
62 See Schmitt, 2017, Commentary to Rule 132, para. 4; ICRC, 2019, pp. 6–7.
63 According to the ICRC, cyber incidents in the past few years took place primarily outside armed conflicts. See Mačák and Gisel, 2022, p. 144; Mačák and Lawson, 2021.
64 See jurisprudence of the International Court of Justice, cases 95 and 131 (ICJ, 1996). See also HRC, 2004, para. 11.
65 See UN Resolution 75/176, 16 December 2020, recalling the same affirmation in four other resolutions in relation to the right to privacy in the digital age, in 2013, 2014, 2016, and 2018; UN General Assembly, 2015, para. 13(e). The Tallinn Manual (Schmitt, 2017) also notes similar agreements in regional bodies, including Council of the European Union, 2014, para. 6, and Shanghai Cooperation Organization, 2009, Article 4, para. 1.
66 Schmitt, 2017, Rule 32. See also Commentary, para. 5.
67 Universal Declaration of Human Rights (UDHR) (UN General Assembly, 1948), Article 12; International Covenant on Civil and Political Rights (ICCPR) (UN General Assembly, 1966), Article 17; Convention on the Rights of the Child (CRC) (UN General Assembly, 1989), Article 16; Convention on the Rights of Persons with Disabilities (UN General Assembly, 2006), Article 22; Schmitt, 2017, Commentary to Rule 35, para. 15; See UN Resolutions 75/176, 68/167, 69/166, 71/199, and 73/179 on the right to privacy in the digital age.
68 As a general matter, states' obligations in international human rights law can be temporarily suspended according to the conditions provided for in a treaty (i.e. derogation), or limited if the right concerned does not qualify as an "absolute right", such as freedom from torture and slavery. Pursuant to Article 4(2) of the ICCPR, the right to privacy is not a non-derogable right. It is also generally considered not as an absolute right. As a reference of principles, see ICCPR, Articles 4, 12, and 19; HRC, 2001, Article 4. In the specific context relating to ICT activities, see Schmitt, 2017, Rule 37.
69 Noting, for example, that the Experts regard that monitoring of online communications for a counterterrorism purpose does not violate the right to privacy. See Schmitt, 2017, Commentary to Rule 37, para. 5.
70 *Ibid*, Commentary to Rule 36, para. 7.
71 UDHR, Article 3; ICCPR, Articles 6 and 9.
72 Schmitt, 2017, Commentary to Rule 37, para. 7. See also HRC, 2011, Article 19, para. 34, affirmed also by the ICJ in its Advisory Opinion, 2004, p. 136.
73 Hollis has put forward a provocative proposition of *"a duty to hack"*, albeit in the context of proportionality in IHL: Hollis, 2015.
74 See, e.g. the Signal Code of the Harvard Humanitarian Initiative, which identifies five human rights relevant to the data and ICT activities of humanitarian actions and how the respective international standards translate into the humanitarian context: Greenwood et al., 2017. Other humanitarian guidelines on responsibility include IASC, 2023; OCHA, 2021; Marelli (ed.), 2024. See also discussions by Schmuck et al., 2023, pp. 41–63.

75 Finlay and Payne, 2019, pp. 202–6.
76 ICRC, 2024c; IASC, 2023.
77 Marelli (ed.), 2024.
78 Greenwood et al., 2017.
79 Campo et al., 2018.
80 Zwitter and Gstrein (eds), 2023.
81 ICRC, 2024a.
82 Rid, 2013.
83 Marelli, 2020, pp. 385–6.
84 ICRC, 2024b.

References

Akande, Dapo, Antonio Coco, and Talita de Souza Días (2022), 'Drawing the Cyber Baseline: The Applicability of Existing International Law to the Governance of Information and Communication Technologies', *International Law Studies*, vol. 99, n° 1. [https://digital-commons.usnwc.edu/ils/vol99/iss1/2].

Badalič, Vasja (2023), 'The Metadata-Driven Killing Apparatus: Big Data Analytics, the Target Selection Process, and the Threat to International Humanitarian Law', *Critical Military Studies*, vol. 9, n° 4, pp. 619–639. doi:10.1080/23337486.2023.2170539.

Ball, James, and Nick Hopkins (2013), 'GCHQ and NSA Targeted Charities, Germans, Israeli PM and EU Chief', *The Guardian*, 20 December. [https://www.theguardian.com/uk-news/2013/dec/20/gchq-targeted-aid-agencies-german-government-eu-commissioner].

Beduschi, Ana (2022), 'Harnessing the Potential of Artificial Intelligence for Humanitarian Action: Opportunities and Risks', *International Review of the Red Cross*, vol. 104, n° 919, pp. 1149–1169. doi:10.1017/S1816383122000261.

Byrne, Rory (2014), 'Trends in Intelligence Gathering by Governments', *Global Interagency Security Forum*. [https://gisf.ngo/resource/trends-in-intelligence-gathering-by-governments/].

Campo, Stuart R., Caitlin N. Howarth, Nathaniel A. Raymond, and Daniel P. Scarnecchia (2018), 'The Signal Code: Ethical Obligations for Humanitarian Information Activities', Signal Program on Human Security and Technology: Harvard Humanitarian Initiative. [https://hhi.harvard.edu/publications/signal-code-ethical-obligations-humanitarian-information].

Council of the European Union (2014), 'EU Human Rights Guidelines on Freedom of Expression Online and Offline'.

Cyber Law Toolkit (2025), 'Attack (International Humanitarian Law)'. [https://cyberlaw.ccdcoe.org/wiki/Attack_(international_humanitarian_law)].

Davies, Harry, Bethan McKernan, and Dan Sabbagh (2023), '"The Gospel": How Israel Uses AI to Select Bombing Targets in Gaza', *The Guardian*, 1 December. [https://www.theguardian.com/world/2023/dec/01/the-gospel-how-israel-uses-ai-to-select-bombing-targets].

Debuf, Els (2015), 'Tools to Do the Job: The ICRC's Legal Status, Privileges and Immunities', *International Review of the Red Cross*, vol. 97, n° 897–8, pp. 319–344. doi:10.1017/S181638311500051X.

Donini, Antonio (ed.) (2012), *The Golden Fleece: Manipulation and Independence in Humanitarian Action*, Sterling, VA: Kumarian Press.

Finlay, Lorraine, and Christian Payne (2019), 'The Attribution Problem and Cyber Armed Attacks', *AJIL Unbound*, vol. 113, pp. 202–206. doi:10.1017/aju.2019.35.

Gilman, Daniel (2014), 'Cyber-Warfare and Humanitarian Space', *Global Interagency Security Forum*. [https://gisf.ngo/resource/cyber-warfare-and-humanitarian-space/].

Greenwood, Faine, Caitlin Howarth, Danielle Escudero Poole, Nathaniel A. Raymond, and Daniel P. Scarnecchia (2017), 'The Signal Code: A Human Rights Approach to Information During Crisis', Harvard Humanitarian Initiative. [https://hhi.harvard.edu/publications/signal-code-human-rights-approach-information-during-crisis].

Heugens, Pursey P. M. A. R., and Michel W. Lander (2009), 'Structure! Agency! (And Other Quarrels): A Meta-Analysis Of Institutional Theories Of Organization', *Academy of Management Journal*, vol. 52, n° 1, pp. 61–85. doi:10.5465/amj.2009.36461835.

Hollis, Duncan B. (2015), 'Re-Thinking the Boundaries of Law in Cyberspace: A Duty to Hack?', in Jens David Ohlin, Kevin Govern, and Claire Finkelstein (eds), *Cyber War: Law and Ethics for Virtual Conflicts*, Oxford: Oxford University Press, pp. 129–174. doi:10.1093/acprof:oso/9780198717492.003.0008.

HRC (1999), 'CCPR General Comment No. 27: Article 12 (Freedom of Movement)'. [https://www.refworld.org/legal/general/hrc/1999/en/46752].

HRC (2001), 'CCPR General Comment No. 29: Article 4: Derogations during a State of Emergency'. [https://www.refworld.org/legal/general/hrc/2001/en/30676].

HRC (2004), 'General Comment No. 31 [80], The Nature of the General Legal Obligation Imposed on States Parties to the Covenant'. [https://www.refworld.org/legal/general/hrc/2004/en/52451].

HRC (2011), 'General Comment No. 34, Article 19, Freedoms of Opinion and Expression'. [https://www.refworld.org/legal/general/hrc/2011/en/83764].

IASC (2023), 'Operational Guidance on Data Responsibility in Humanitarian Action'. [https://interagencystandingcommittee.org/operational-response/iasc-operational-guidance-data-responsibility-humanitarian-action].

ICRC, 'Customary IHL Rules'. [https://ihl-databases.icrc.org/en/customary-ihl/v1].

ICRC (2018), 'Statutes of the International Red Cross and Red Crescent Movement'. [https://www.icrc.org/en/document/statutes-international-committee-red-cross-0].

ICRC (2019), 'International Humanitarian Law and Cyber Operations during Armed Conflicts', ICRC Position Paper. [https://www.icrc.org/sites/default/files/document/file_list/icrc_ihl-and-cyber-operations-during-armed-conflicts.pdf].

ICRC (2022), 'Cyber-Attack on ICRC: What We Know'. [https://www.icrc.org/en/document/cyber-attack-icrc-what-we-know].

ICRC (2024a), 'Data Protection Standards for Humanitarian Organizations and Partners'. [https://www.icrc.org/sites/default/files/2024-11/Track%201%20-%20WS%201%20%28WG%201%29%20-%20Data%20Protection%20standards%20for%20humanitarian%20organizations%20and%20partners.pdf].

ICRC (2024b), 'Eight rules for "civilian hackers" during war, and four obligations for states to restrain them'. [https://www.icrc.org/en/article/8-rules-civilian-hackers-during-war-and-4-obligations-states-restrain-them].

ICRC (2024c), 'Professional Standards for Protection Work: By Humanitarian and Human Rights Actors During Armed Conflict and Other Violence'. [https://shop.icrc.org/professional-standards-for-protection-work.html].

ICJ (1980), *United States Diplomatic and Consular Staff in Tehran (United States of America v. Iran)*. [https://www.icj-cij.org/case/64].

ICJ (1996), *Legality of the Threat or Use of Nuclear Weapons*. [https://www.icj-cij.org/case/95].

ICJ (2004), *Legal Consequences of the Construction of a Wall in the Occupied Palestinian Territory*, Advisory Opinion. [https://www.icj-cij.org/case/131].

International Conference of the Red Cross and Red Crescent (2024), Resolution 341C/24/R2, Protecting Civilians and Other Protected Persons and Objects against the Potential Human Cost of ICT Activities during Armed Conflict.

Kitchin, Rob, and Martin Dodge (2017), 'The (In)Security of Smart Cities: Vulnerabilities, Risks, Mitigation, and Prevention', *Journal of Urban Technology*, vol. 26, n° 2, pp. 47–65. doi:10.1080/10630732.2017.1408002.

Koster, Ferry (2020), 'Organizing for Autonomy. A Combined Contingency and Agency Perspective', *Dynamic Relationships Management Journal*, vol. 10, n° 2, pp. 45–67. doi:10.17708/DRMJ.2021.v10n02a01.

Mačák, Kubo (2021), 'Unblurring the Lines: Military Cyber Operations and International Law', *Journal of Cyber Policy*, vol. 6, n° 3, pp. 411–428. doi:10.1080/23738871.2021.2014919.

Mačák, Kubo, and Laurent Gisel (2022), 'The Legal Constraints of Cyber Operations in Armed Conflict', *ORF and Global Policy Journal*. [https://www.orfonline.org/research/future-warfare-and-technologies-issues-and-strategies].

Mačák, Kubo, and Ewan Lawson (2021), 'Avoiding Civilian Harm during Military Cyber Operations: Six Key Takeaways', *Humanitarian Law & Policy Blog*. [https://blogs.icrc.org/law-and-policy/2021/06/15/avoiding-civilian-harm-military-cyber-operations/].

Maitland, Carleen, and Rakesh Bharania (2017), 'Balancing Security and Other Requirements in Hastily Formed Networks: The Case of the Syrian Refugee Response', *Social Science Research Network*. doi:10.2139/ssrn.2944147.

Marelli, Massimo (2020), 'Hacking Humanitarians: Defining the Cyber Perimeter and Developing a Cyber Security Strategy for International Humanitarian Organizations in Digital Transformation', *International Review of the Red Cross*, vol. 102, n° 913, pp. 367–387. doi:10.1017/S1816383121000151.

Marelli, Massimo (ed.)(2024), *Handbook on Data Protection in Humanitarian Action*, 3rd edition, Cambridge: Cambridge University Press.

Moynihan, Harriet (2019), *The Application of International Law to State Cyberattacks: Sovereignty and Non-Intervention*, London: The Royal Institute of International Affairs.

Obama, Barack (2020), *A Promised Land*, London: Penguin Books.

OCHA (2021), 'From digital promise to frontline practice: new and emerging technologies in humanitarian action'. [https://www.unocha.org/publications/report/world/digital-promise-frontline-practice-new-and-emerging-technologies-humanitarian-action].

Paracha, Anum, Junaid Arshad, Mohamed Ben Farah, and Khalid Ismail (2025), 'Deep Behavioral Analysis of Machine Learning Algorithms against Data Poisoning', *International Journal of Information Security*, vol. 24, article 29. doi:10.1007/s10207–10024–00940-x.

Rahman, Zara (2021), 'Rohingya Data Protection and the UN's Betrayal', *The New Humanitarian*, 21 June. [https://www.thenewhumanitarian.org/opinion/2021/6/21/rohingya-data-protection-and-UN-betrayal].

Reed, Michael (2003), 'The Agency/Structure Dilemma in Organization Theory: Open Doors and Brick Walls', in Haridimos Tsoukas and Christian Knudsen (eds), *The Oxford Handbook of Organization Theory*, New York: Oxford University Press, pp. 289–309.

Rid, Thomas (2013), *Cyber War Will Not Take Place*, New York: Oxford University Press.

Rodenhäuser, Tilman, and Kubo Mačák (2021), 'Even "Cyber Wars" Have Limits. But What If They Didn't?', *Humanitarian Law & Policy Blog*. [https://blogs.icrc.org/law-and-policy/2021/03/09/even-cyber-wars-have-limits/].

Schermers, Henry G., and Niels Blokker (2018), *International Institutional Law: Sixth Revised Edition*, Leiden/Boston: Brill Nijhoff. doi:10.1163/9789004381650.

Schmitt, Michael N. (ed.) (2017), *Tallinn Manual 2.0 on the International Law Applicable to Cyber Operations*, 2nd edition, Cambridge: Cambridge University Press. doi:10.1017/9781316822524.

Schmuck, Susanne, Andrej Zwitter, and Oskar J. Gstrein (2023), 'Big Data and the Humanitarian Sector: Emerging Trends and Persistent Challenges', in Andrej Zwitter and Oskar Gstrein (eds), *Handbook on the Politics and Governance of Big Data and Artificial Intelligence*, Cheltenham: Edward Elgar Publishing, pp. 41–63. doi:10.4337/9781800887374.00012.

Schneider, Jacquelyn (2016), 'Digitally-Enabled Warfare: The Capability-Vulnerability Paradox', CNAS. [https://www.cnas.org/publications/reports/digitally-enabled-warfare-the-capability-vulnerability-paradox].

Shanghai Cooperation Organization (2009), 'Agreement of SCO on Cooperation in the Field of Ensuring the International Information Security'. 16 June.

Sukumar, Arun (2017), 'The UN GGE Failed. Is International Law in Cyberspace Doomed As Well?', *Lawfare*. [https://www.lawfaremedia.org/article/un-gge-failed-international-law-cyberspace-doomed-well].

UN (1961), 'Vienna Convention on Diplomatic Relations'. [https://legal.un.org/ilc/texts/instruments/english/conventions/9_1_1961.pdf].

UN General Assembly (1946), 'Convention on the Privileges and Immunities of the United Nations'. doi:10.1163/9789004639096_050.

UN General Assembly (1948), 'Universal Declaration of Human Rights'. [https://www.un.org/en/about-us/universal-declaration-of-human-rights].

UN General Assembly (1966), 'International Covenant on Civil and Political Rights'. [https://www.ohchr.org/en/instruments-mechanisms/instruments/international-covenant-civil-and-political-rights].

UN General Assembly (1989), 'Convention on the Rights of the Child'. [https://www.ohchr.org/sites/default/files/crc.pdf].

UN General Assembly (2006), 'Convention on the Rights of Persons with Disabilities'. [https://www.ohchr.org/sites/default/files/Ch_IV_15.pdf].

UN General Assembly (2015), 'Group of Governmental Experts on Developments in the Field of Information and Telecommunications in the Context of International Security'. [https://docs.un.org/en/A/70/174].

UN General Assembly (2021a), 'Group of Governmental Experts on Advancing Responsible State Behaviour in Cyberspace in the Context of International Security'. [https://docs.un.org/en/A/76/135].

UN General Assembly (2021b), 'Official Compendium of Voluntary National Contributions on the Subject of How International Law Applies to the Use of Information and Communications Technologies by States'. [https://docs.un.org/en/A/76/136].

UN General Assembly (2021c), 'Open-Ended Working Group on Developments in the Field of Information and Telecommunications in the Context of International Security: Final Substantive Report'. [https://disarmament.unoda.org/open-ended-working-group/].

UN General Assembly, Report 76/135 (2021) and Resolutions 68/167 (2014), 69/166 (2015), 71/199 (2016), 73/27 (2018), 73/179 (2018), 73/266 (2018), 75/176 (2020), 75/240 (2020), and 76/19 (2021), 'United Nations Digital Library System'. [https://digitallibrary.un.org].

UNODA, 'Open-Ended Working Group'. [https://disarmament.unoda.org/open-ended-working-group/].

Väljataga, Ann, 'Back to Square One? The Fifth UN GGE Fails to Submit a Conclusive Report at the UN General Assembly', *CCDCOE*. [https://ccdcoe.org/incyder-articles/back-to-square-one-the-fifth-un-gge-fails-to-submit-a-conclusive-report-at-the-un-general-assembly/].

Zwitter, Andrej, and Oskar Josef Gstrein (eds), *Handbook on the Politics and Governance of Big Data and Artificial Intelligence*, Cheltenham; Northampton, MA: Edward Elgar Publishing Limited, 2023.

10 Without Borders, Within Boundaries

Learning How to Deliver Aid in Light of the Climate Emergency

*Bruno Jochum, Dikolela Kalubi, and Béatrice Godefroy**

The scientific community has been warning political authorities and public opinion about the severity of the climate and environmental crisis and the associated risks consistently for almost 40 years.[1] While the scale of global warming and local environmental damage has been described for decades, more recently, in 2009, researchers identified "planetary boundaries"[2] beyond which the Earth's systems that support human development may be irreversibly destabilised. They include rising temperatures, the collapse of biodiversity, disruptions to the water cycle, and other physical-chemical changes to the soil which, combined, quickly result in a genuine "planetary emergency". Over time, these processes can make parts of the planet uninhabitable and threaten the livelihoods of a large number of societies. All actors – including state structures, the private sector, and public service organisations – must, therefore, learn to operate within these planetary boundaries to stop contributing to the crisis through their own actions, anticipate their response to needs, and strengthen their resilience to foreseeable shocks and constraints.[3]

Like the rest of society – and given the political and social shortcomings in tackling the issue with the necessary determination – members of Médecins Sans Frontières (MSF) and the aid sector have only gradually become aware of the degree of severity of the climate emergency, its impact on the most vulnerable population groups, and their responsibility to act.[4] Increasing occurrences of droughts, floods, tropical storms, and heatwaves result in damage to infrastructure, a rise in displaced people, worsening food insecurity, and greater difficulties in accessing drinking water – conditions conducive to the spread of infectious diseases and tensions around ever-scarce natural resources.[5]

Although MSF has been providing a medical response to these needs for over 50 years, the organisation now faces new questions. What relevant interventions can it design in reaction to the growing scale and specific nature of these phenomena? How can it better incorporate climate and environmental issues into the development of health projects and the practices of healthcare and logistical support teams? Are these questions not an invitation to rethink a centralised "without borders" operating model, largely built around the rapid deployment of human and material resources and external quality standards, highly dependent on fossil fuels, and increasingly removed from the "medicine in remote

DOI: 10.4324/9781003542247-19

settings" of the early days? Finally, the political dimension cannot be ignored. Given the failings of the political sphere to act on the origins of the crisis, how should MSF react to governments' often deliberate investments in fossil fuels, condemning populations to predictable disaster? How should it respond to the inadequate allocation of resources for essential services – whose strengthening will prove critical for limiting harm – or address issues of social equity? Traditional humanitarian principles, particularly neutrality – which aims to facilitate the provision of assistance in times of war – are, by definition, of limited use as a basis for a humanitarian organisation to speak out when faced with such challenges.

Following a brief review of MSF's path to awareness of these issues, the first part of this chapter will question the implications of the climate emergency for humanitarian action and whether these challenge its traditional operating model. The second part will explore possible programmatic approaches and the necessary skills to tackle the changing health needs of vulnerable populations, as well as the requirement for high-quality care and environmental sustainability issues, emphasising both the dilemmas and the tensions associated with speaking out. Finally, the authors will set out the challenges that humanitarian organisations face in reducing their environmental footprint, the most common trade-offs this requires, the consequences for the viability of their operating model, and the frequently raised question of equity or justice in the distribution of effort.

The aim of this chapter is not to provide a neatly packaged set of thoughts on how to respond to climate change but to share reflections and possible adaptations for the humanitarian aid sector, through the specific example of MSF. First and foremost, it is an invitation to create space, provide means and consider ways of responding that are up to the challenge, face reality by exploring programmatic approaches, and take risks in terms of innovation and positioning.

I From Awareness to Accepting Responsibility

While humanitarian actors are no strangers to the issue of local environmental damage, the climate crisis is now attracting an unprecedented level of attention and debate, with the first reflections on the topic dating back to the early 2000s. The impacts of human activity are evident everywhere, and global heating levels are confirming the forecasts modelled by scientists. The Intergovernmental Panel on Climate Change (IPCC) noted in its 2023 Assessment Report that, based on the 2020 level of annual greenhouse gas emissions (GHG), the threshold of 1.5 °C average warming would be reached well before 2030, and the 2.0 °C threshold by the early 2040s.[6] The commitments made by states would, if they were applied effectively and immediately, result in warming close to 2.8 °C by 2100; however, the policies currently being implemented would take us to 3.2 °C – an unsustainable level far removed from the initial targets of the Paris Agreement.[7] Since 2020, the volume of emissions discharged into the atmosphere has continued to increase, and the speed of change observed may therefore exceed the forecasts.[8]

The 2002 creation, by the International Federation of Red Cross and Red Crescent Societies (IFRC), of the Climate Centre, which focuses on response, adaptation, and resilience as the logical corollary to its work on natural disasters, marked a groundbreaking step. As early as 2004, the International Committee of the Red Cross (ICRC) mentioned environmental damage and global warming as major factors that could aggravate future humanitarian crises. It also highlighted the uncertainty regarding the scale of the consequences and how to respond to them.[9]

Within MSF, an initial motion adopted by the General Assembly of the Swiss section in 2007 stated the necessity of taking steps to limit the environmental impact of its actions.[10] The Operational Centre calculated its carbon footprint and implemented technical projects, primarily in the field of renewable energy. In 2008, its research unit analysed the effects of the "resource curse" (mainly oil) on the structure of health systems in countries such as Nigeria, Chad, and Angola, and the resulting marginalisation of affected communities.[11] Since 2010, MSF Netherlands has been leading a number of initiatives, including one on environmental health aimed at the neglected medical needs of children who have suffered from lead pollution caused by artisanal mining activities in Nigeria.[12] An exploration of environmental health issues has thus made a tentative entry into the field of MSF's humanitarian action, on the periphery of its traditional interventions.

In response to scientists' warnings about the worsening of the climate crisis, numerous professional communities have organised themselves to mobilise their sectors, particularly health, including the Global Health and Climate Alliance (since 2011) and the US NGO Health Care Without Harm. Humanitarian organisations such as Oxfam, Care, and, later, the IFRC, joined forces with environmental organisations in 2009 for public campaigns calling for the conclusion of an ambitious, fair, and equitable agreement at the Conference of the Parties (COP) in Copenhagen.[13] These campaigns would intensify in the period leading up to COP21 and the Paris Agreement of 2015, revealing marked differences in the respective approaches and decisions taken by actors in the humanitarian aid sector, although they were often complementary to one another.

In 2014, Rony Brauman and Bruno Rebelle, former presidents of MSF France and Greenpeace, respectively, examined the commitment of medical humanitarian and environmentalist NGOs to ecological issues and the different timescales on which they operate: urgency and saving lives in the here and now for the former, and longer-term issues and impacts for the latter.[14] During this conversation, the legitimacy of MSF speaking out on critical topics of which – at the time – it had only very limited experience was called into question, insofar as they arose from political and economic decisions over which it had little leverage. The article ends on a humble note regarding issues seen as far exceeding the practice of humanitarian medicine, but emphasises that the organisation cannot be exonerated from its own responsibility as an actor that causes environmental damage.

Within MSF, collaboration between the Canadian and Swiss sections resulted in publications that contributed to the institution's awareness of the topic.[15] In 2020, the MSF movement adopted an Environmental Pact that identifies adapting operations, reducing its environmental footprint, and speaking out on the impacts of climate change as priorities.[16] Shortly afterwards, MSF committed to halving its GHG emissions by 2030. As a director of operations put it, "*We didn't know how to do it but we knew we had to.*"[17] The recent climate and environmental roadmaps, approved by the purchasing centres and boards of several MSF sections between 2022 and 2024, reflect this determination.[18] This coincides with a wide consultation launched by the International Red Cross and Red Crescent Movement, which would lead to the adoption, in 2021, of the "Climate and Environment Charter for Humanitarian Organizations", signed by numerous actors, including MSF.[19] Later, several governments would sign a "Humanitarian Aid Donors' Declaration on Climate and Environment", marking their intention of incorporating these issues more effectively into their funding frameworks.[20]

Now that the humanitarian sector has largely shown a willingness to act, new challenges are appearing around the practical implementation of these commitments, which are far from straightforward. Rethinking working methods and human resources and supply systems creates upheaval in well-established operating patterns. In practice, delivering humanitarian aid while respecting planetary boundaries means systematically identifying alternative ways of achieving the same end. This implies questioning what is an operational necessity, and what are critical quality standards, essential values, or simply professional culture. Implementation also raises the issue of the acceptable "price" of considering climate and environmental responsibility within an organisation's budget, in a society where actors such as businesses, institutions, and aid agencies can easily impose the consequences of their negative externalities (in terms of emissions or a large proportion of their waste) on the community (or "commons"), especially in contexts where processing and recycling services are inadequate or may not even exist.

Yet impacts and risks are worsening at an unprecedented pace, are already affecting the health of populations, and need mitigation and adaptation actions to be implemented faster.[21] Apart from the scale and frequency of extreme weather events, the World Health Organization (WHO) anticipates an increase in respiratory and cardiovascular diseases, the spread of vector-borne diseases such as malaria and dengue fever, and waterborne diseases such as cholera, and the emergence of new zoonoses.[22] The seasonality and geographical distribution of epidemics are increasingly variable, while the link between climate change, biodiversity loss, falling agricultural yields,[23] and worsening food security for populations is well established.[24] Finally, global warming not only amplifies needs; it also exacerbates existing vulnerabilities, exposure to violence, and social and political instability, forcibly displacing a growing number of people.[25] Faced with the combination of specific challenges and the possible emergence of a "permanent state of crisis", which adaptations and innovations should be prioritised for humanitarian organisations working primarily in the countries that are most vulnerable to climate change?

In light of this, it is hardly surprising that the debate around the role of humanitarianism and its limitations has been rekindled. Some authors advocate for reforms to the aid system and organisational mandates to better incorporate environmental issues, even to the point of a complete overhaul, by suggesting a symbolic merger between MSF and environmental organisations to link – in strategic terms – commitments that until now have been considered separately.[26] Conversely, a research director in an MSF section recently commented that the organisation should remain "human-centred" because of the inherent nature of its medical activities, though without denying the responsibilities arising from them. Beyond the necessity of adapting operations or reducing MSF's environmental footprint, it is ultimately the definition of the legitimate scope of humanitarian action and establishing priorities in resource allocation that are currently generating the most significant differences of opinion, as well as the need to recall the distinction between various agendas.[27]

II Adapting Operations for More Effective Action in the Climate Emergency: Opportunities and Dilemmas

Natural disasters, forced displacements, and epidemics existed well before the acceleration of the climate crisis and, indeed, triggered the implementation of humanitarian programmes. But global heating and its implications create new operational challenges and, in particular, a change of scale in the needs of the populations affected.

First, the recurrence of extreme weather events in some geographical regions, the probability of chaotic phenomena such as heat domes or torrential rains, and early signs of food insecurity or changes in epidemiology accentuate the foreseeable nature of crises and, therefore, the preparedness that needs to be activated to limit the damage. In the most fragile contexts, the specific consequences of heatwaves in urban areas, repeated flooding, or the salination of the land call for more relevant, innovative approaches that draw on successful local experiences. Finally, the expected scale of the climate crisis is such that the volume of assistance required could reach significant levels in the coming years. According to the 2024 *Global Humanitarian Overview*, climate-related disasters have multiplied 2.5 times during the last decade compared with the 1980s, with three times more floods and four times more heatwaves, and population displacements on the rise.[28] These trends are all the more disturbing when combined with other social and political factors, especially in societies where governance is fragile and infrastructure precarious, or in conflict situations.[29] Humanitarian actors must, therefore, develop new areas of expertise ("skilling up") as well as increase their operational capacity ("scaling up") in an unstable geopolitical context that has become unfavourable to international aid since the budget cuts introduced by the main donor countries.[30] This perspective invites a more modest approach to their capacity to mitigate suffering, seeing as they often lack experience supporting national partners for the reinforcement of local frameworks and have neither the resources nor all the necessary skills.[31] Above all, it emphasises the prime relevance, for the purpose of mitigating the severity of such crises, of making efforts to adapt and strengthen services in the general interest under the authority of governments and private sector actors. It also highlights the importance of climate justice to ensure a better distribution of the financial burden on an international scale.

The example of Bangladesh shows the extent to which the adaptability of national actors (the state, public services, and NGOs) can limit the consequences of extreme weather events for the most vulnerable populations. In 1970, tropical cyclone Bhola caused the deaths of at least 150,000 people (up to 500,000, according to some estimates),[32] while the 1974 famine due to flooding along the Brahmaputra River in the period after the civil war resulted in hundreds of thousands of victims. Following these traumatic events, the authorities implemented an extremely ambitious risk reduction, emergency preparedness, and food sovereignty plan. Consequently, the country became a pioneer in early warning systems and local cyclone preparedness programmes,[33] helping to reduce cyclone-related mortality by a hundredfold,[34] despite a threefold increase in their seasonal frequency as a result of global warming. Numerous national NGOs, such as Friendship or BRAC, have a good understanding of the issues, along with superior access and networks compared to those of their international counterparts, and are developing innovative community programmes that simultaneously incorporate climate adaptation, resilience, and mitigation. Along with anti-cyclone shelters, raising infrastructure, access to drinking water in areas being infiltrated by seawater, changes in agricultural practices, and the mobility needed to provide health services, the response also involves activating socio-economic safety nets (rapid cash transfers, either following a shock or even on a preventive basis, and insurance for the most vulnerable) and pooling costs within society. Today, these actors are rightly claiming to be given priority as recipients of international funds, in line with the "Grand Bargain" of 2015, but they continue to be allocated a minimal share.[35] Above all, they expect international aid organisations to provide technical support to promote the results achieved in the field, and access useful technologies and funding to facilitate the required scale-up. By the middle of the century, Bangladesh could have lost up to 15–20% of its territory, displacing tens of millions.[36] This perspective clearly illustrates the scale of the upheaval that will have to be adapted to; the criticality of predictability and preparedness; the influence of collective decisions and investments; and the potential role of international cooperation on the evolution of future scenarios regarding the number of victims associated with the climate emergency.

The issue of predictability concerns not only states but also international organisations, including emergency humanitarian organisations such as MSF, through a more systematic incorporation of risks in their programme design, as well as early warnings and preparedness in emergency response plans faced with repeated or prospective emergencies. This may include better use of the meteorological and climate data available, in anticipating extreme events or epidemiological surveillance, in order to deploy upstream and downstream actions that enable an improved response to impacts, in conjunction with local communities. Furthermore, practical methodologies have recently been developed for clearer identification of the main vulnerabilities in health projects, using an "all-hazard" approach and prioritising actions that ensure better, cross-cutting adaptations of care, medical services and their seasonality, infrastructure, staff skills, and preparedness for recurring or exceptional emergencies.[37] This involves making health services more useful to populations, more resilient to climate shocks, and more sustainable, with most practical solutions supporting all three objectives at the same time. The traditional opposition between the short and long term becomes less relevant when the actions chosen to strengthen health services also offer important and immediate benefits to patients and populations. Better heat management in hospitals, raising buildings to deal with flooding, access to care in remote areas, preventive strategies for malaria and malnutrition, improving blood banks, or using local/regional anaesthesia protocols where appropriate, and energy independence to address the risk of a shortage of petrol supplies are all measures that strengthen access and the quality of patient care. They also support the continuity of medical services, contribute to the achievement of programme targets, and favour greater sustainability.[38]

Conversely, strategic and technical innovation remains essential for tackling specific operational situations and new scenarios in which the international aid sector currently has only limited experience. How should organisations respond to the effects of long-term heatwaves, particularly when they occur in heavily polluted urban areas with high atmospheric humidity, and in countries where access to care is highly unequal? What strategies should be deployed to tackle more intense and recurrent flooding over wide areas, which destroys homes, prevents access to drinking water, disrupts agricultural production, and destabilises public services? What medical cares should be developed for populations affected by drinking chemically altered water in the event of local environmental pollution, as well as salinity aggravated by global warming, whose highly harmful impacts on reproductive health are often combined with greater social vulnerability of the women concerned? All these challenges should drive actors to identify the various operational scenarios; learn from the experience in the field of national actors, in particular; test new approaches; and develop the technical capacity to implement them successfully. The "non-linear" aspect of the risks associated with the acceleration in global warming, highlighted by scientists, also emphasises the need to prepare for the unknown, i.e. weather events on a very large scale, which are chaotic in nature and unprecedented in the places where they will occur. The expectation that tipping points in the Earth's physical systems will be crossed further accentuates this dimension.[39]

Anticipation, investing in adaptation, and the gradual acquisition of know-how can, therefore, contribute to limiting the impacts on people and the need for assistance. However, the response requires a significant increase in volume, mainly in well-known areas, such as providing care to displaced persons, and malnutrition. Adaptation cannot offset indefinitely the harmful effects of a sustained increase in the volume of GHGs in the atmosphere and temperatures, as long as those continue to be driven upwards by our political, economic, and social systems. And, in a context where several states are challenging the historical borders guaranteed by a weakened international order, and where conflictual power relationships are generating new needs in addition to climate threats, humanitarian actors will have to confront their limitations, with draconian choices regarding prioritisation. Given these complex dilemmas, the scarcity of available resources, and the "triage" of people in need it produces, some are calling for better protection against the impacts of climate change by reviewing the balance of means allocated to prevention and response. Is there not a case for an organisation such as MSF to develop more forcefully its preventive activities, following similar investments previously made in the areas of malnutrition, in the 2000s, or malaria? Taking into account capacity limits in emergencies, should the scope and timing of humanitarian interventions not include more efforts on adaptation and strengthening community resilience, giving these greater space in humanitarian aid?[40] In the health arena, this issue goes back to the traditional debate between public health approaches focused on a general responsibility to the whole population – and, as a consequence, an emphasis on efficiency to achieve the best health outcomes in a constrained environment – and humanitarian healthcare, centred on the limited responsibility to save lives through solidarity, through choice, or following an *"interim ethic"*,[41] in a situation of extreme negligence or particular victimisation. Despite its discourse often focusing on emergency interventions, MSF has frequently combined operational strategies and advocacy aimed at strengthening preventive measures and public health systems, such as access to medicines, political support for the launch of the Global Fund, or innovative initiatives to combat malnutrition, with variable outcomes depending on the choices made.[42] Humanitarian organisations will need to find a different balance based on their respective histories, social missions, and strategic decisions. Some will mainstream these issues into existing project frameworks and their usual operational policies, while others will develop new, dedicated programmes and corresponding public positions. In spite of these differences, the involvement of institutional actors is a decisive factor in scaling up and saving lives: mobilising local authorities and service organisations in the context of contingency plans, disaster risk reduction, and reinsurance mechanisms, both upstream and in response to shocks. Facilitating vulnerable countries' access to international development financial institutions and the Green Climate Fund, which is often challenging, is now critical in terms of accelerating funding at a time when other international solidarity budgets are drying up.

MSF's Environmental Pact is, therefore, part of a broader strategy recommending humanitarian action that is more anticipatory, more balanced between responding directly to the impacts of crises and strengthening resilience, and, finally, more collaborative and locally focused.[43] However, it is scarcely surprising that differences of opinion appear internally on a regular basis, given the still-limited extent of operational experience in these matters. These disagreements concern the relevance of various messages conveyed at COP-themed days dedicated to humanitarian or health issues;[44] the legitimacy of connecting, from the field, the occurrence of specific natural disasters with global warming; and the robustness of certain forecasts on future human impacts.[45] The organisation's ambition calls for more detailed guidance for teams in the field, but above all, increasing its experience so that it can confront chosen scenarios – such as heatwaves – to develop approaches that can then be scaled up and potentially amplified through public advocacy.[46] Finally, it requires greater consistency between the imperative of assisting victims of the crisis and the responsibility to act on its own contributions to environmental damage.

III Levers, Challenges, and Considerations on Reducing the Carbon Footprint of the Humanitarian Sector

While the recent consensus on reducing the environmental footprint of humanitarian action has led to a large number of institutional actors making commitments, implementing them presents several significant operational challenges. There are trade-offs to be made and specific benefits to be gained, along with a need for strategic continuity that clashes with a culture of urgency driven by the constant stream of genuine humanitarian crises, the considerable effort required to reach populations in need in the most challenging situations, and the sector's high levels of financial insecurity. Any environmental approach must, therefore, follow a "guiding thread", namely securing the quantity and quality of assistance for vulnerable populations and never acting to their detriment under any circumstances. It is a question of equipping organisations to achieve their humanitarian objectives as effectively as possible and anticipate the capacity risks associated with climate change, while fulfilling their responsibilities.

Annual emissions from international humanitarian assistance could reach 35 million tonnes of CO_2e (carbon dioxide equivalent), i.e. 1.5 times those of the British National Health Service.[47] Almost 60% are believed to come from the supply chain, with the remainder derived from travel and direct consumption of fossil fuels. In terms of activities, food aid would account for half; health and nutrition a quarter; and, including shelter and the distribution of basic relief items, these would collectively exceed 80% of the sector's emissions.

The MSF movement as a whole is thought to emit half a million tonnes of CO_2e every year,[48] which equates to the emissions of a European city of roughly 50,000 people and all their consumption of goods and services.[49] Around a fifth of these emissions are estimated to be linked to staff travel, mainly flights; almost a sixth to energy consumption, particularly the use of generators; and, unsurprisingly, well over half to the supply chain, notably for medical supplies. Humanitarian action can also impact on local ecosystems, with harmful consequences for health. As an example, the chemical components in medicines can pollute freshwater resources, especially in emerging countries, and contribute to antibiotic resistance.[50] The processing of some highly toxic waste resulting from medical treatments for cancer is unsatisfactory in countries that do not have the resources to deal with it appropriately. Above all, heavy reliance on single-use medical items generates considerable quantities of waste, the vast majority of which is incinerated, but not always at the required temperature. In MSF Switzerland, the consumption of medical examination gloves per patient admitted more than doubled in eight years to reach 4.5 gloves in 2019.[51] Reducing the environmental footprint associated with these items means establishing essential cross-cutting collaborations across roles and investing in the professional skills needed to do so.

In terms of more direct emissions produced by the aid sector, managing energy consumption, the thermal efficiency of infrastructure, and the use of lower-carbon energy sources rely on proven technical know-how. The issue is large-scale deployment through new operational standards and ensuring sufficient capacity to maintain them, either in-house or through outsourcing, or delegating responsibility to communities. The medium-term economic interest is unequivocal, as are several operational benefits, such as patient well-being, a stable energy supply, and price predictability, all of which are essential for the proper functioning of health services in vulnerable settings.[52] The situation is already working in favour of substantial growth in solar installations in low-income countries. Facing this challenge, the humanitarian sector has a huge comparative advantage: the limited lifespan of its projects and field offices means that most of its interventions can be reviewed every few years. This will make it easier to achieve a very significant proportion of the energy transition required by 2030, provided the new standards are systematically incorporated into the design and funding of new programmes, and logistics teams are trained.

Reducing travel requires trickier operational decisions and the ability to overcome the obstacles inherent in organisations' internal culture. Adhering to the principle of necessity demands stringent prioritisation of legitimate reasons to travel by plane, adapting recruitment policies in favour of a higher proportion of local staff and closer cooperation with national actors. Flying staff in is closely linked to the history of humanitarian action and the deployment of international volunteers, and was designed to offset the shortage of specialist local resources in crisis contexts, ensure accountability for the use of the organisation's financial means, and allow people to speak out to spur others into action. With the surge in the number of flights taken since the advent of low-cost air travel in the early 2000s, emissions related to flying now account for around 7% of emissions for the humanitarian sector as a whole and 20% of the MSF movement's carbon footprint.[53] Flying-related emissions can be limited by rationalisation efforts, such as reducing the number of international meetings, events, and in-person training courses, prioritising direct flights, or promoting rail transport in Europe – all measures that cause no real impact on the organisation's social mission. However, the majority of emissions from staff air travel remain linked to deployments or technical support from headquarters for interventions in the field. The predominance of international staff in management or specialist roles; centralised support from headquarters, with a rise in the number of "flying" technicians; and frequent rotations due to short contracts, resulting in several return trips a year, all contribute to a high level of travel. MSF, therefore, needs to question the human aspect of its operating methods and a support model that has led to an increased intensity of travel over time, in parallel with higher quality requirements and the level of operational technicality. While MSF managed to reduce staff air travel drastically during the period of restrictions caused by the COVID-19 pandemic, it did not result in a reappraisal of the main model or prevent a return to previous levels. Ultimately, policy choices will have to be made, and may be beneficial, with decisions taken closer to the ground, the development of locally recruited teams, greater stability, a limit on external technical recommendations that are sometimes difficult to absorb at project level, and, finally, improvement in the well-being of some staff who travel extensively.

In terms of procurement, projects aimed at limiting reliance on single-use products (particularly medical protection equipment) have shown that the quantities used are largely dependent on the choice of, and compliance with, certain protocols, medical staff responsibility, prevention and hygiene activities, and the composition of medical kits.[54] Working collaboratively with the professionals concerned to facilitate the transition towards more sustainable practices that provide the same level of quality for aid recipients is, therefore, necessary. As well as the volume of products consumed, prioritising procurement from suppliers that use more environmentally responsible manufacturing processes (low-carbon energy sources, limits on hazardous substances, etc.), or of alternative items with a lower impact, means strengthening "sustainability skills" in the procurement teams. It also implies a re-evaluation of their strategic role, shared responsibility mechanisms with other functions, and a consistent approach over the next 10 to 20 years. Such a transition is obviously not entirely straightforward. Establishing "green" procurement criteria for the energy sources, materials, or chemical procedures used by manufacturers may impact on other agendas, such as increasing regional procurement or affordability considerations. The decision to focus massively on certain production locations, such as India or China, for generic medicines sometimes results in the use of higher-carbon energy sources and less stringent environmental quality standards. While a small number of items is often responsible for the vast majority of emissions, organisations' capacity to express their requirements and select suppliers who are committed to reducing their environmental footprint will be crucial, as will businesses' ability to provide information about their products and certify their practices.

Cost is often cited as an obstacle to implementing these transitions, but it is important to take a nuanced view, since it is generally overestimated. According to a modelling exercise carried out with around 10 humanitarian organisations, the average net cost of deploying only decarbonisation solutions would be approximately 0.3% of their annual budget over seven years, including average savings of 1.5% and costs of 1.8%, within a wider range.[55] It is estimated that incorporating solutions to address local environmental damage, in particular related to waste processing, would result in a higher net average cost. Such orders of magnitude can be called on as part of normal organisational management, and financial feasibility hinges primarily on the political will of senior managers and their capacity for adhering to strategic decisions despite budgetary constraints. The savings generated by less flying and reduced use of air freight are significant and can fund investments in the transition. As an example, for MSF Switzerland, the inflation in the average cost of an airline ticket between 2019 and 2022 led to a 60% rise in the cost of a similar journey, i.e. an increase of CHF 3 million per year – the equivalent of the estimated annual investment needed to decarbonise the organisation. It is less an issue of the overall cost than a willingness to reallocate savings on certain items to support transformation efforts elsewhere, limiting the additional costs associated with better climate and environmental practices. The latter dimension should be highlighted in the context of the major funding crisis that has hit the humanitarian sector since the shutdown of USAID and the massive reallocation of cooperation funds from other essential donors, to defence, announced in early 2025. Forced to review their practices for financial reasons, particularly in terms of travel and procurement, MSF and other humanitarian actors can seize this opportunity to prioritise rationalisation measures which, as it happens, are also change levers for reducing their environmental footprint. The ability of so-called systemic actors[56] – institutional donors and United Nations organisations that handle the majority of humanitarian funding – to support these multiple efforts by adapting their frameworks is all the more important for organisations that are highly dependent on them.[57]

Lastly, the credibility of actions in terms of reducing the environmental footprint is established through compliance with certain principles[58] and international standards.[59] Every actor in society has the responsibility to take measures regarding what it controls and can influence. As large consumers of fossil fuels and goods, it is difficult for public service organisations to claim a level of exceptionalism that would exempt them from reviewing practices that are harmful to people and the environment. In the absence of a legitimate public authority allocating emissions rights equitably among different human activities based on their respective social roles, each actor must adopt a pragmatic approach to minimising its carbon and environmental footprint, in accordance with the IPCC's recommended trajectories and relevant standards. Guided by this voluntary, science-based approach, states, numerous businesses, and pioneering public services have adopted reduction targets relative to a past reference year, independently of future developments in their activity.[60] According to this approach, the stronger an organisation's growth, the more important it will be to gradually decouple its activities from carbon emissions to fulfil its target. Such efforts lie at the very heart of the stabilisation actions required to address this global emergency.

This ambition can sometimes be difficult to achieve for humanitarian organisations faced with a sharp increase in needs in their areas of intervention, and inflation limiting their financial flexibility. Other essential services, such as food production, health, transport, and even insurance, are also concerned. Their missions are obviously different from those of the major oil or mineral exploitation companies, but they continue to be highly dependent on fossil fuels and materials that are necessary for their day-to-day operations. In a context of increasingly scarce financial, energy, and material resources, accelerating the climate and environmental transformation and improving efficiency can protect the capacity of humanitarians to operate in the near future, as well as strengthen their room for manoeuvre for assisting populations. Ultimately, reducing CO_2 emissions by half by 2030 and beyond will rely on a combination of factors: internally, taking the necessary steps to bring about a change of organisational culture, providing technical support and implementing priority actions; and externally, the ability of businesses and states to speed up the decarbonisation of production chains for key items, so that humanitarian organisations can prioritise them as suppliers. Since the standard methodology for measuring emissions and following reduction targets is still based on estimates and contains uncertainties, complementary indicators should be considered to monitor progress, whether physical or in terms of action.[61] It is, therefore, a process of continuous learning which, without having to weaken the overarching objective, implies a dynamic adjustment of certain targets during the course of implementation, especially for procurement, depending on the actual timetable of actions, the progress achieved, and opportunities and changes in the organisation's level of activities. While the discussion on the impacts of MSF's growth on decarbonisation is legitimate, it should not obscure the considerable potential for emissions reductions.

IV Conclusion

Will the future of operating "without borders" and the emergency humanitarian response survive climate change, environmental challenges, and their multiple implications in a period marked by huge uncertainties and upheavals?[62] The discussion goes beyond the issue of MSF's operating model, which, in accordance with the ethics of responsibility, must change to help the organisation learn to function within planetary boundaries. It is also about humanitarian action – which has historically been "human-centred" and driven by the primary motivation of protecting human lives, regardless of the material consequences – (re) finding its legitimate place in a world undergoing a profound shift.

In operational terms, will the planetary emergency, combined with the destruction of the post-1945 global order, not fundamentally accelerate the reshuffling of the deck that is already under way to confront the growing needs to which the traditional international humanitarian sector is ill-equipped to respond? Within this redistribution between national and international actors, what role can be served by emergency humanitarian organisations, such as

MSF, which have limited experience of working in partnership with local actors and are not inclined to get involved in the disaster preparedness and response plans of national authorities or to consider their investments from a sustainability perspective? Yet becoming more relevant and efficient means making increasingly pressing choices as crises accelerate. The global arms race is directly soaking up the level of funding available for international aid, while the tensions around sovereignty and protectionism in certain countries are accentuating this dynamic. In most cases, the ethics of responsibility, incorporating environmental issues and the development of the capacity to provide emergency assistance on the ground, go hand in hand: by cooperating with local actors, exploiting the benefits of new operating practices, and reducing its dependence on fossil fuels, humanitarian action will protect itself from both specific capacity constraints and the effects of the increasing scarcity of materials and resources, namely volatility and the rise in numerous prices.

All over the world, from health systems to municipal authorities, public water and electricity distribution companies to civil protection and marine rescue organisations, many actors are engaged in these efforts, and are contributing to identifying possible solutions. Adaptation necessarily requires anticipation, strengthening and funding essential services in a world where the proportion of the population exposed to the risks and consequences of the climate crisis will vary considerably. It also calls for preventive or more agile money-transfer mechanisms, as well as insurance practices that protect the most vulnerable. From this point of view, humanitarian actors will mainly continue to be resources of last resort when the systems in place run out of capacity, offering a limited solution to inadequate public and private services. Nonetheless, they retain responsibility for incorporating risks in their emergency or rehabilitation programmes and their choice of services, infrastructure, cooperation with local actors, and community development, which in the longer term will support people's capacity for addressing the consequences of the planetary emergency while responding to their immediate needs.

To conclude, the scientific plea to respect the limits of a finite natural world as part of an equitable framework and the modern humanitarian imperative, which was born from a humanist revolt against mass crimes and the neglect of the vital needs of entire populations, can largely rejoin in protecting a *"safe and just space for humanity"*.[63] It is not biological life as such that is threatened, but human society in its current configuration, due to the increasing uninhabitability of the tropical zones associated with global warming, the collapse of biodiversity, and the loss of soil quality.[64] The political context is hardening considerably, with currents of thought from very diverse origins relegating the protection of people whose lives are under threat to the background and contesting the very concept of international solidarity.[65] Although their ideologies differ, the "techno-libertarians" proposing to dismantle the legacy of the Enlightenment to found a new, unequal society, the nationalist movements that support mass deportations of migrants, and extreme "anti-speciesists" who compare human dominance over the living world to the spread of a virus all display a wilful and growing anti-humanism. The political influence of the former is now having a genuine impact on both humanitarian and climate action, as evidenced by the abrupt shutdown of USAID and the ban imposed on various agencies on mentioning climate breakdown. It therefore falls to humanitarian actors to speak out and determinedly defend the legitimacy of their commitments, while avoiding an anthropocentric approach that might minimise the planetary emergency and the responsibilities associated with it. At a time when actual "heating policies" with a deliberate reinvestment in fossil fuels are being developed, and when international solidarity and climate action are under simultaneous attack,[66] with unprecedented attempts to dismantle them, humanitarian and environmental commitments are now linked in a common destiny, because of their most often shared humanist nature, the evolution in people's fundamental needs, and a principle of reality, which will, under the relentless pressure of physical events, impose itself.

Notes

* Translated from French by Karen Stokes.
1 The "environmental crisis" is not limited here to the climate emergency but also includes issues around biodiversity, water, and the harm associated with soil and air pollution.
2 See the research carried out at the Stockholm Resilience Centre, available at https://www.stockholmresilience.org/research/planetary-boundaries.html.
3 Resilience is the capacity of a system to return to its original state after it has been disrupted. More specifically, the UNISDR (United Nations International Strategy for Disaster Reduction) defines resilience as "*the ability of a system, community or society exposed to hazards to resist, absorb, accommodate, adapt to, transform and recover from the effects of a hazard [...], including through the preservation and restoration of its essential basic structures and functions*".
4 Buffet, 2009.
5 ICRC, 2021.
6 IPCC, 2023, p. 19, para. B.5.2.
7 Available at https://unfccc.int/process-and-meetings/the-paris-agreement.
8 Schmidt, 2024, p. 467.
9 ICRC, 2004.
10 Motion 5, MSF Switzerland General Assembly, 2007: "*The General Assembly requests a commitment from the Board to define and from the Executive to apply ecological practices in all our activities (missions and HQ) in order, as much as possible, to avoid contributing to the environment deterioration, which is a threat to populations.*"
11 Calain, 2008, p. 10.
12 MSF, 2022b.
13 Buffet, 2010.
14 Brauman et al., 2014, pp. 32–43.
15 Jochum et al., 2019; MSF, 2022a.
16 MSF, 2020. Available at https://www.msf.org/msfs-2020-environmental-pact.
17 MSF, 2021. Translated from French by Karen Stokes.
18 See, e.g. MSF Switzerland and Climate Action Accelerator, 2022: https://urgence-climatique.msf.ch/la-feuille-de-route/ and https://climatehub.msf.org/wp-content/uploads/2024/06/MSF_OCB_ROADMAP.pdf.

19 In December 2024, the Charter had 450 signatories. Humanitarian organisations agree unequivocally on a shared assessment and commitments: "*Today's climate and environmental crises threaten the survival of humanity [...] those who have contributed least to the problem are hit hardest [...] Our ability to protect the lives and the rights of present and future generations depends on whether we make the right choices now.*" Available at https://www.climate-charter.org/.
20 European Commission, 2022.
21 IPCC, 2014.
22 Van de Vuurst and Escobar, 2023; Carlson, et al., 2022, pp. 555–62.
23 Ritchie, 2024.
24 IPBES, 2020.
25 Damboeck et al., 2020.
26 Steinke, 2023; Slim, 2024.
27 See Weissman, 2020 and the interview with Pierre Krähenbühl, director of the International Committee of the Red Cross: Krähenbühl, 2024.
28 OCHA, 2023.
29 Al-Ansari, 2023.
30 Steinke, 2023.
31 Tholstrup and Vazquez, 2024.
32 Ouder, 2012.
33 Davison, 2022.
34 Haque et al., 2012, pp. 150–6.
35 See https://interagencystandingcommittee.org/grand-bargain; and Development Initiatives, 2023, p. 73.
36 Ministry of Environment, Government of the People's Republic of Bangladesh, 2022; and Germanwatch, 2004.
37 See WHO, 2020 and the Health Facility Climate Vulnerability and Capacity Assessment toolkit developed by the Climate Action Accelerator (2024d), available at https://climateactionaccelerator.org/climate-vca/.
38 More systematic incorporation of such methodologies and simplified checklists in the exploratory and design phases of new projects should be considered, to make a difference on a larger scale, regardless of the actors concerned.
39 Information on tipping points can be found here: https://www.pik-potsdam.de/en/output/infodesk/tipping-elements.
40 MSF Canada, 2024.
41 Rieff, 2003.
42 Bradol, 2011.
43 Tholstrup and Vazquez, 2024.
44 These days resulted in two new declarations: the "COP28 Declaration on Climate and Health" and the "COP28 Declaration on Climate, Relief, Recovery and Peace", the latter of which was written by the ICRC.
45 Weissman, 2020.
46 MSF Canada, 2024.
47 Climate Action Accelerator, 2024a.
48 Baseline emissions in 2019, available at https://climatehub.msf.org/mitigate/carbon-accounting/.
49 An average of 10.7 tonnes per inhabitant in the European Union: Eurostat, 2025.
50 Wilkinson et al., 2022.
51 Berthet, 2022.
52 See the Climate Action Accelerator pillar on assessing financial impacts, available at https://humanitarianplaybook.climateactionaccelerator.org/pillar-4/ and Global Platform for Action, 2022.
53 Climate Action Accelerator, 2024a, p. 18.
54 Berthet, 2022.

55 Considering only climate mitigation solutions (decarbonisation) and excluding other environmental solutions on a local scale (waste processing and recycling, water and sanitation): Climate Action Accelerator, 2024e, p. 66.
56 Actors who have the capacity to influence or act on the system as a whole.
57 See the recommendations to donors and United Nations organisations, Climate Action Accelerator, 2024b.
58 Climate Action Accelerator, 2024c, principle 1.
59 The Greenhouse Gas Protocol and the Science Based Targets initiative (SBTi) are well-recognised frameworks, both in terms of measuring carbon emissions and articulating reduction targets that are compatible with the IPCC's recommendations. Numerous actors, including United Nations organisations and donors, still need to align their practices with these international standards, by including their procurement in the scope of calculation of their carbon footprint and reduction trajectories. Based on these same frameworks, these institutions should also exclude carbon credits from the accounting of their reduction efforts and avoid claiming "carbon neutrality" without a legitimate basis, in the meantime spending amounts that could be better invested in their own transition.
60 See, e.g. NHS, 2020; the city of Copenhagen's 2025 climate plan, CPH, 2012; or the declaration of the International Maritime Rescue Federation, 2025.
61 Kaplan and Ramanna, 2022.
62 Pilling, 2025.
63 Rockström et al., 2023, pp. 102–11; Oliver et al., 2022, pp. e919–e927.
64 Xu et al., 2020, pp. 11350–5; Watts, 2020; Carrington, 2024.
65 As well as criticising a substantial proportion of initiatives associated with reproductive health, among others.
66 Duffau, 2025.

References

Al-Ansari, Nadhir (2023), 'Effondrement Des Barrages En Libye: Un Expert En Ingénierie s'interroge Sur La Gestion de l'ouvrage', *The Conversation*, 20 September. [http://theconversation.com/effondrement-des-barrages-en-libye-un-expert-en-ingenierie-sinterroge-sur-la-gestion-de-louvrage-213930].

Berthet, Corentine (2022), 'Masques et Gants à Usage Unique: Quelles Alternatives?', Unité de recherche sur les enjeux et pratiques humanitaires, MSF Switzerland Internal Report.

Bradol, Jean-Hervé (2011), 'Caring for Health', in Claire Magone, Michaël Neuman, and Fabrice Weissman (eds), *Humanitarian Negotiations Revealed: The MSF Experience,* London: Hurst & Co. [https://msf-crash.org/en/agir-tout-prix-negociations-humanitaires-lexperience-de-msf/ii-history].

Brauman, Rony, Bruno Rebelle, Boris Martin, and Christophe Buffet (2014), 'Le Politique, chaînon manquant entre humanitaires et environnementalistes?', *Humanitaire*, n° 38, pp. 32–43.

Buffet, Christophe (2009), 'Les humanitaires sont-ils prêts à relever le défi du changement climatique?', *Humanitaire*, n° 23. [https://0.journals.openedition.org/humanitaire/598].

Buffet, Christophe (2010), 'Humanitaires, verts et alters?', *Humanitaire*, n° 24. [https://journals.openedition.org/humanitaire/711].

Calain, Philippe (2008), 'Oil for Health in Sub-Saharan Africa: Health Systems in a "resource Curse" Environment', *Globalization and Health*, vol. 4, n° 1. doi:10.1186/1744-8603-4-10.

Carlson, Colin J., Gregory F. Albery, Cory Merow, Christopher H. Trisos, Casey M. Zipfel, Evan A. Eskew, Kevin J. Olival, Noam Ross, and Shweta Bansal (2022), 'Climate Change Increases Cross-Species Viral Transmission Risk', *Nature*, vol. 607, n° 7919, pp. 555–562. doi:10.1038/s41586–41022–04788-w.

Carrington, Damian (2024), '"Hopeless and Broken": Why the World's Top Climate Scientists Are in Despair', *The Guardian*, 8 May. [https://www.theguardian.com/environment/ng-interactive/2024/may/08/hopeless-and-broken-why-the-worlds-top-climate-scientists-are-in-despair].

Climate Action Accelerator (2024a), 'A Path to Climate-Smart Humanitarian Action'. [https://climateactionaccelerator.org/wp-content/uploads/2024/06/Sectoral-analysis-1.pdf].

Climate Action Accelerator (2024b), 'Enabling Change: How the UN & Donors Can Lead the Way'. https://climateactionaccelerator.org/wp-content/uploads/2024/06/Enabling-change-1.pdf.

Climate Action Accelerator (2024c), 'Guiding Principles for Effective Emissions Reduction'. [https://climateactionaccelerator.org/humanitarian-decarbonisation-roadmap/#guiding-principles-for-effective-emissions-reduction].

Climate Action Accelerator (2024d), 'Health Facility Climate Vulnerability and Capacity Assessment (VCA)'. [https://climateactionaccelerator.org/climate-vca/].

Climate Action Accelerator (2024e), 'Operational Playbook'. [https://climateactionaccelerator.org/wp-content/uploads/2024/06/Operational-playbook-1.pdf].

Climate Action Accelerator. 'Operational Playbook – Pillar 4'. [https://humanitarianplaybook.climateactionaccelerator.org/pillar-4/].

Climate Charter, 'The Climate and Environment Charter for Humanitarian Organizations'. [https://www.climate-charter.org/].

'COP28 Declaration on Climate, Relief, Recovery and Peace' (2023). [http://mptf.undp.org/news/cop28-declaration-climate-relief-recovery-and-peace].

'COP28 UAE Declaration on Climate and Health' (2023). https://www.who.int/publications/m/item/cop28-uae-declaration-on-climate-and-health.

Damboeck, Johanna, Kaori Oshima, Corey Pattison, and Nicolas Perrin (2020), 'Building Resilient Communities in West Africa in the Face of Climate-Security Risks', *World Bank Blogs*. [https://blogs.worldbank.org/en/dev4peace/building-resilient-communities-west-africa-face-climate-security-risks].

Davison, Catherine (2022), 'Cyclones – Bangladesh: le pays précurseur dans la lutte contre les catastrophes naturelles', *BBC News Afrique*. 23 July. [https://www.bbc.com/afrique/monde-62251425].

Development Initiatives (2023), 'Global Humanitarian Assistance Report 2023'. [https://devinit.org/resources/global-humanitarian-assistance-report-2023].

Duffau, Eléonore (2025), 'Les attaques de l'administration Trump II contre le climat, l'environnement et la biodiversité', *IRIS*. [https://www.iris-france.org/les-attaques-de-ladministration-trump-ii-contre-le-climat-lenvironnement-et-la-biodiversite/].

Eurostat (2025), 'EU Greenhouse Gas Footprint: 10.7 Tonnes per Capita'. [https://ec.europa.eu/eurostat/web/products-eurostat-news/w/ddn-20250219-1].

European Commission (2022), 'Humanitarian aid donors' declaration on climate and environment'. [https://civil-protection-humanitarian-aid.ec.europa.eu/what/humanitarian-aid/climate-change-and-environment/humanitarian-aid-donors-declaration-climate-and-environment_en].

Germanwatch (2004), 'Sea-Level Rise in Bangladesh and the Netherlands'.

Global Platform for Action (2022), *The State of the Humanitarian Energy Sector: Challenges, Progress and Issues in 2022*, Geneva: UNITAR.

Haque, Ubydul, Masahiro Hashizume, Korine N Kolivras, Hans J Overgaard, Bivash Das, and Taro Yamamoto (2012), 'Reduced Death Rates from Cyclones in Bangladesh: What More Needs to Be Done?', *Bulletin of the World Health Organization*, vol. 90, n° 2, pp. 150–156. doi:10.2471/BLT.11.088302.

ICRC (2004), 'ICRC Assistance Policy'. [https://www.icrc.org/sites/default/files/external/doc/en/assets/files/other/irrc_855_policy_ang.pdf].

ICRC (2021), 'World Humanitarian Day: Climate Change, Conflict and a Changing Humanitarian Response'. [https://www.icrc.org/en/climate-change-conflict-humanitarian-response].

Intergovernmental Panel on Climate Change (2014), 'Climate Change 2014: Synthesis Report. Contribution of Working Groups I, II and III to the Fifth Assessment Report of the Intergovernmental Panel on Climate Change', Geneva. [https://www.ipcc.ch/report/ar5/syr/].

Intergovernmental Panel on Climate Change (2023), 'Climate Change 2023: Synthesis Report. Contribution of Working Groups I, II and III to the Sixth Assessment Report of the Intergovernmental Panel on Climate Change', Geneva. doi:10.59327/IPCC/AR6–9789291691647.

International Maritime Rescue Federation (2025), 'Maritime SAR Organisations Join Forces to Advance Sustainability Efforts'. [https://www.international-maritime-rescue.org/news/maritime-sar-organisations-join-forces-to-advance-sustainability-efforts].

IPBES (2020), 'Key Messages from the IPBES Global Assessment of Particular Relevance to Indigenous Peoples and Local Communities'.

Jochum, Bruno, Carol Devine, François Delfosse, Léo Lysandre Tremblay, and Maria Guevara (2019), 'Choices at the time of the climate emergency', *Humanitarian Alternatives*, n° 11. [https://www.alternatives-humanitaires.org/en/2019/07/18/choices-at-the-time-of-the-climate-emergency/].

Kaplan, Robert S., and Karthik Ramanna (2022), 'We Need Better Carbon Accounting. Here's How to Get There', *Harvard Business Review*. [https://hbr.org/2022/04/we-need-better-carbon-accounting-heres-how-to-get-there].

Krähenbühl, Pierre (2024), interview, RTS, 28 May. [https://www.rts.ch/play/tv/la-matinale/video/linvite-de-la-matinale-video-pierre-kraehenbuehl-directeur-du-comite-international-de-la-croix-rouge-cicr?urn=urn%3Arts%3Avideo%3A14933928].

Ministry of Environment, Forest and Climate Change, Government of the People's Republic of Bangladesh (2022), 'National Adaptation Plan of Bangladesh (2023–2050)'. [https://moef.portal.gov.bd/sites/default/files/files/moef.portal.gov.bd/npfblock/903c6d55_3fa3_4d24_a4e1_0611eaa3cb69/National%20Adaptation%20Plan%20of%20Bangladesh%20%282023-2050%29%20%281%29.pdf].

MSF (2020), 'The Environmental Pact'. [https://www.msf.org/msfs-2020-environmental-pact].

MSF (2021), 'Urgence climatique: nous n'avons pas d'autre choix que d'agir'. [https://www.msf.ch/nos-actualites/communiques-presse/urgence-climatique-nous-navons-pas-dautre-choix-que-dagir].

MSF (2022a), 'MSF's Policy Brief for the Lancet Countdown on Health and Climate Change'. [https://www.msf.org/msf-policy-brief-lancet-countdown-health-and-climate-change].

MSF (2022b), 'Nigeria: Prevention is key to stop children from dying of lead poisoning'. [https://www.msf.org/nigeria-prevention-key-stop-children-dying-lead-poisoning].

MSF Canada (2024), 'Climats Hostiles: Relever Les Défis de l'acheminement de l'aide Dans Le Contexte Du Changement Climatique'. [https://www.msf.ch/media/6077].

MSF Climate Hub, 'Carbon Accounting'. [https://climatehub.msf.org/mitigate/carbon-accounting/].

MSF Switzerland and Climate Action Accelerator (2022), 'La feuille de route – Urgence climatique'. [https://urgence-climatique.msf.ch/la-feuille-de-route/].

NHS (2020), 'Delivering a "Net Zero" National Health Service'. [https://www.england.nhs.uk/greenernhs/wp-content/uploads/sites/51/2020/10/delivering-a-net-zero-national-health-service.pdf].

OCHA (2023), 'Global Humanitarian Overview 2024'. [https://www.unocha.org/publications/report/world/global-humanitarian-overview-2024-enarfres].

Oliver, Tom H., Bob Doherty, Andre Dornelles, Nigel Gilbert, Matthew P. Greenwell, Laura J. Harrison, Ian M. Jones, et al. (2022), 'A Safe and Just Operating Space for Human Identity: A Systems Perspective', *The Lancet Planetary Health*, vol. 6, n° 11, pp. e919–927. doi:10.1016/S2542–5196(22)00217–0.

Ouder, Paula (2012), 'NOAA Researcher's Warning Helps Save Lives in Bangladesh'. [https://web.archive.org/web/20120202150332/http://www.research.noaa.gov/spotlite/2007/spot_cyclone.html].

Pilling, David (2025), 'Can international aid survive in a crumbling world order?', *Financial Times*, 27 March. [https://www.ft.com/content/b3667445-a242-46fb-bcb3-0a21386ce355].

Potsdam Institute for Climate Impact Research, 'Tipping Elements – big risks in the Earth System'. [https://www.pik-potsdam.de/en/output/infodesk/tipping-elements].

Rieff, David (2003), *A Bed for the Night: Humanitarianism in Crisis*, New York: Simon & Schuster.

Ritchie, Hannah (2024), 'How Will Climate Change Affect Crop Yields in the Future?', *Our World in Data*. [https://ourworldindata.org/will-climate-change-affect-crop-yields-future].

Rockström, Johan, Joyeeta Gupta, Dahe Qin, Steven J. Lade, Jesse F. Abrams, Lauren S. Andersen, David I. Armstrong McKay, et al. (2023), 'Safe and Just Earth System Boundaries', *Nature*, vol. 619, n° 7968, pp. 102–111. doi:10.1038/s41586–41023–06083–06088.

Schmidt, Gavin (2024), 'Climate Models Can't Explain 2023's Huge Heat Anomaly — We Could Be in Uncharted Territory', *Nature*, vol. 627, n° 8004. doi:10.1038/d41586–41024–00816-z.

Slim, Hugo (2024), 'Saving Humans Is Not Enough. Humanitarian Purpose Needs to Change', *The New Humanitarian*, 9 September. [https://www.thenewhumanitarian.org/opinion/2024/09/09/saving-humans-not-enough-humanitarian-purpose-needs-change].

Steinke, Andrea (2023), 'Climate Change and Humanitarian Change', *Centre for Humanitarian Action*. [https://www.chaberlin.org/en/publications/climate-change-and-humanitarian-change/].

Stockholm Resilience Centre, 'Planetary Boundaries'. [https://www.stockholmresilience.org/research/planetary-boundaries.html].

Tholstrup, Sophie, and Mauricio Vazquez (2024), 'Humanitarian action on climate and conflict: Narratives, challenges and opportunities', ODI Report, London: ODI: [https://media.odi.org/documents/Report_Humanitarian_action_on_climate_and_conflict.pdf].

UNFCC, 'The Paris Agreement'. [https://unfccc.int/process-and-meetings/the-paris-agreement].

Urban Development (2012), 'The CPH 2025 Climate Plan'. [https://urbandevelopmentcph.kk.dk/climate].

Van de Vuurst, Paige, and Luis E. Escobar (2023), 'Climate Change and Infectious Disease: A Review of Evidence and Research Trends', *Infectious Diseases of Poverty*, vol. 12. doi:10.1186/s40249–40023–01102–01102.

Watts, Jonathan (2020), 'One Billion People Will Live in Insufferable Heat within 50 Years – Study', *The Guardian*, 5 May. [https://www.theguardian.com/environment/2020/may/05/one-billion-people-will-live-in-insufferable-heat-within-50-years-study].

Weissman, Fabrice (2020), 'Should Médecins Sans Frontières join the fight against global warming?', *Humanitarian Alternatives*, n° 13. [https://www.alternatives-humanitaires.org/en/2020/03/18/should-medecins-sans-frontieres-join-the-fight-against-global-warming/].

WHO (2020), *WHO Guidance for Climate-Resilient and Environmentally Sustainable Health Care Facilities*, 1st ed., Geneva: WHO.

Wilkinson, John L., Alistair B. A. Boxall, Dana W. Kolpin, Kenneth M. Y. Leung, Racliffe W. S. Lai, Cristóbal Galbán-Malagón, Aiko D. Adell, et al. (2022), 'Pharmaceutical Pollution of the World's Rivers', *Proceedings of the National Academy of Sciences*, vol. 119, n° 8. doi:10.1073/pnas.2113947119.

Xu, Chi, Timothy A. Kohler, Timothy M. Lenton, Jens-Christian Svenning, and Marten Scheffer (2020), 'Future of the Human Climate Niche', *Proceedings of the National Academy of Sciences*, vol. 117, n° 21, pp. 11350–11355. doi:10.1073/pnas.1910114117.

Epilogue

Negotiating Spaces, Defending Convictions

*Françoise Duroch**

"You cannot help the poor by destroying the rich", wrote William J. H. Boetcker in a leaflet published in 1916:[1] a maxim that clearly evokes the beliefs that appear to underpin the events currently affecting the international aid system. Indeed, over 150 years later, the financial affluence enjoyed by most of the humanitarian sector at the end of the twentieth century is now a distant memory. This period of abundance had allowed some organisations to embark on large-scale aid interventions in countries such as Rwanda or Somalia, in the heart of areas prey to conflicts and violence, alongside peacekeeping operations. It was, therefore, not uncommon to hear criticism of what some called the "humanitarian circus", meaning a multiplicity of poorly coordinated actors working in the same area of operations. This model is now in crisis, as evidenced not only by the reduction in aid budgets in the US, but also the emergence of political classes who are challenging the notions that have long been the bedrock of humanitarian action. These include international solidarity, which – in the eyes of Médecins Sans Frontières (MSF) since its creation in 1971 – should be embodied in the provision of meaningful medical assistance beyond the administrative borders of the countries of origin of emergency aid workers.

Prior to the US decisions, Germany, the world's second-largest donor, reduced its funding by half, calling for aid to be more "effective". France and the United Kingdom have adopted a similar approach, with the latter reallocating budgets to defence. Today, in Chad, Sudan, and the eastern Democratic Republic of the Congo, international organisations are scarce, funding inadequate, and the needs immense. The imperative to do more with less, already under way in some United Nations agencies, is only a matter of time.[2] For the millions of people who rely on vital international aid, the consequences are becoming critical. Numerous national and local organisations that played a central role in deploying aid on a day-to-day basis will not be able to survive if deprived of the funds needed to pursue their activities.

Futurology is an inherently uncertain discipline, and it is currently complex, if not impossible, to predict the future of the humanitarian landscape in the short term, given the disappearance of a number of organisations with which MSF used to collaborate. In this respect, the concept of "humanitarian space" still refers to the space that the organisation will be able to negotiate, not only

DOI: 10.4324/9781003542247-20

with external actors, but also based on its human and financial resources, without straying outside its legitimate sphere of action. Similarly, it is difficult to express a view on the emergence of some sort of "multilateralism 2.0" that might rise from the ashes of the unipolar order that was established at the end of the Cold War, in which new donors would be quick to fill the gap left by the US withdrawal. More critical still will be the repercussions of the cessation of US funding on the populations of countries in crisis, the breakdown in the supply of medicines used to treat certain chronic diseases, and the return of the "global gag rule"[3] and its consequences for sexual and reproductive health, support for migrants, or aid allocated to LGBTQI+ people. Separately from financial considerations, the whole moral economy of the aid sector is currently being undermined. The portrayal of refugees has been distorted, women's rights to control their own bodies disregarded, and organisations that support sex workers forced to close down. Far from being isolated incidents, negative attitudes towards certain groups can be found in much of Europe and should drive humanitarian organisations to speak out strongly and reaffirm their commitment to independent international aid, regardless of the gender or sociopolitical status of the recipients.

During the 1990s and 2000s, MSF challenged the propensity of Western democracies to enter into *"just wars"*[4] in the name of an allegedly universal set of rights. At the time, it was a question of protecting independent humanitarian aid, being *"where others are not"* and working with *"populations in danger"*[5] abandoned at the edge of conflicts. Humanitarian action was supposed to stay well away from political considerations and avoid any temptation to establish democratic values forcefully on the other side of the world. A new reality is currently emerging, marked by the return of war in Europe, where the Ukrainian conflict has taken the place of those in Bosnia and Chechnya.

USAID – once, along with Hollywood, a symbol of US soft power – has now been dismantled, and with it a large part of a system that relied on the financial generosity of a single organisation and country. Created in 1961, in response to the sense of insecurity imposed by the Cold War, and which appeared to threaten the American people, the Truman Doctrine saw it as a means of combating communism. The creation of USAID thus enabled other bilateral agencies to open in the West. The cuts to the US aid budget currently taking place amount to USD 60 billion, representing a 40% reduction in global humanitarian assistance. One of the most significant cuts is affecting Ukraine, which has lost almost USD 1.5 billion. The signal is not only unambiguous; it also serves as a reminder of the disproportionate importance of the US contribution to the global humanitarian aid budget, and the fragility of a sector that is so heavily dependent on the political whims of a head of state. For some countries, this could mean the collapse of already precarious health systems, prompting fears of disastrous human consequences.

Sovereigntist tensions, cultural isolationism, protectionism, and the rise in nationalism are now widespread in both Europe and the rest of the world. Western generosity appears to have reached its limits.

This book comes to an end as these events unfold. While all the contributors attempt to be critical, they nonetheless remain attached to an organisation which, as well as providing emergency aid, will always oppose moves towards nationalism and identity politics, exclusionary practices, and double standards in how refugees are treated.

The examination of MSF's practices proposed by the various authors of this book highlights the multiple tensions and paradoxes inherent in contemporary humanitarian action. Long seen as an emblematic figure in the humanitarian aid sector, MSF still constantly redefines itself in its attempts to reconcile operational efficiency with ethical and humanist principles. Although it remains independent, it nevertheless forms part of a vast aid system that it cannot ignore and maintains often close relationships with the various political actors in the countries where it operates. Its capacity for adapting to social and environmental change is both its trademark and an essential condition of its survival, despite its soaring growth and its governance, which sometimes negatively affect its agility. The illusion of believing that the organisation could expand sufficiently to respond to the world's infinite humanitarian needs – "the sky's the limit" – contrasts with a lucid, pragmatic vision designed to confine it to a marginal role: that of a straightforward emergency aid organisation, an actor of last resort when societies collapse, services and structures fail, and civilian populations are abandoned. Within MSF, currents of thought sometimes coincide, but at other times clash, in areas such as environmental issues or the interpretation of international humanitarian law. These themes are regularly addressed in debates on whether a medical organisation has the legitimacy to speak out on such vast and complex topics. Part of MSF's identity, therefore, still remains anchored in its capacity to question its own practices, a salutary exercise made necessary by the difficulty of the task of helping people in need, since *"it is not enough to do good, it must also be done well".*[6]

The different contributions in each of the chapters of this book have emphasised the complexity of unavoidable trade-offs, either in terms of the types of activities implemented, partnerships formed, or compromises made. Such dilemmas are inherent in humanitarian action, and organisations bear a heavy responsibility when it comes to making decisions.

The protest movements that have arisen in numerous countries, from Sudan to Iran and Myanmar, are representative of dilemmas over the type of support to offer to victims of political repression. MSF's reticence to take a stand on such events, which often fall outside its traditional sphere of activity, is echoed in the questions raised by locally recruited teams, who sometimes resent its apathy towards the violence that impacts them directly.

Moreover, the organisation faces internal criticism on the standardisation of its actions, a level of technicity that can at times be far removed from the local reality, and its role in broader power dynamics, including the geopolitics of conflicts or systemic inequalities in health and the treatment of refugees. On this last point, MSF should remain vigilant to ensure its actions are not appropriated – a constant concern in the course of aid operations – for political or security purposes by states that have demonstrated, especially during the Ukrainian crisis, their ability to show a particularly selective form of solidarity.

The authors also insist on the necessity of MSF distancing itself from an overarching view of aid and focusing on implementing projects jointly with affected populations, taking the specific cultural, social, and political characteristics of each country into account. This change further implies continuing to combat the racial or gender discrimination that exists within the organisation and sometimes unconsciously influences medical and operational decisions, as well as its way of speaking out and the images it communicates. The various scandals and social movements that have marked the last decade, such as #metoo and Black Lives Matter, have prompted profound questions about the organisation, in areas including its human resources policies and how it has managed abuse internally. This is a complex and sometimes painful exercise, but MSF continues to make progress on these sensitive subjects while attempting to maintain unity and avoid ideological pitfalls. New sections are emerging in the Global South, and the organisation is gradually getting the measure of the sociocultural diversity of its staff and the major role they play in aid deployment and security management.

The COVID-19 pandemic also reshuffled the deck and highlighted the limitations of a centralised humanitarian system. Health security remains a concept in constant flux that emphasises the massive inequalities in terms of access to care suffered by the most vulnerable populations. On the other hand, in line with international directives on environmental protection, the organisation has implemented procedures to limit its carbon footprint. These sometimes collide with an internal culture that is somewhat unaccustomed to restricted mobility, and with a modus operandi that is highly dependent on fossil fuels, often working to timescales driven by medical emergencies.

MSF, like other actors, must come to terms with major emerging issues, such as the climate crisis, protecting its digital data, or managing risks that affect its staff, which will force it to change its ways of working. Moreover, the development of social media has created a vast echo chamber that requires multiple actors to engage in constant critical reflection, obliging the organisation to increase its level of vigilance and be permanently accountable for its actions. In this respect, the risks of disinformation represent a new threat for MSF, in terms of both security and reputational damage.

This book, therefore, comes at a time of profound upheaval in the humanitarian landscape that unquestionably invites MSF to seize the opportunity to transform itself, as it is already doing. This is not about embarking on a fresh reform of the aid sector – previous attempts having achieved mixed results – but continuing to think, adapt, and engage, and thus defend a set of convictions against the rise in identity politics. Far from being complacent, it is in its capacity to evolve pragmatically and learn from its mistakes that the strength of the organisation lies. Sometimes viewed as arrogant within non-governmental organisations, it can antagonise others by its claim to be different and its reluctance to join the main platforms in the humanitarian sector. That said – and as some aid workers are amused to point out – the harshest criticisms of MSF come from MSF itself.

Notes

* Translated from French by Karen Stokes.

1 William J. H. Boetcker was an American religious leader and an influential public speaker. He was the author of a leaflet called *The Ten Cannots*, published in 1916. The quote is often misattributed to Abraham Lincoln.

2 United Nations Development Programme, 2025.

3 The "global gag rule" prevents foreign non-governmental organisations in receipt of US funds from providing services or information concerning, or advocating in favour of, legal abortion.

4 Weissman, 2004.

5 Jean, 1992.

6 Denis Diderot, French writer and philosopher, in a letter of 1762. Translated from French by Karen Stokes.

References

Jean, François (1992), 'Populations in Danger'. [https://msf-crash.org/en/war-and-humanitarianism/populations-danger].

United Nations Development Programme (2025), 'Making funds go further as Sudan's war continues'. [https://stories.undp.org/making-funds-go-further-as-sudans-war-continues].

Weissman, Fabrice (ed.) (2004), *In the Shadow of 'Just Wars': Violence, Politics and Humanitarian Action*. London: Hurst & Co.

Appendix

The Charter of Médecins Sans Frontières

Médecins Sans Frontières (MSF) is a private international association. The association is made up mainly of doctors and health sector workers and is also open to all other professions which might help in achieving its aims. All of its members agree to honour the following principles:

- Médecins Sans Frontières provides assistance to populations in distress, to victims of natural or man-made disasters and to victims of armed conflict. They do so irrespective of race, religion, creed or political convictions.
- Médecins Sans Frontières observes neutrality and impartiality in the name of universal medical ethics and the right to humanitarian assistance and claims full and unhindered freedom in the exercise of its functions.
- Members undertake to respect their professional code of ethics and maintain complete independence from all political, economic or religious powers.
- As volunteers, members understand the risks and dangers of the missions they carry out and make no claim for themselves or their assigns for any form of compensation other than that which the association might be able to afford them.

Index

abortion: access 13; care 82; programme 139
acceptance 44, 60–1, 69; community 106
access 42, 54–60, 69, 71, 79, 82, 114, 119, 123, 147, 186–7, 192, 194; to asylum 24; Campaign 89; to communities 146; to populations 52, 58, 68–9, 139–40, 147, 183; to treatment 39–40, 44, 85; unauthorised 189–90; *see also* access to care
access to care 19, 25–6, 91, 99, 103, 117–18, 168, 180, 209, 227
accountability 18, 31–47, 56–8, 105–7, 161–2, 212, 227; to affected populations 33–4, 47; lack of 102, 182; legal 57; moral 169; sectoral 35; systems 115
advocacy 27, 37, 100, 132, 136–46
Afghanistan 40, 56–61, 103, 138
aid sector 1–4, 31, 54, 59, 148, 166, 203, 209, 212, 225–7; humanitarian 157, 160, 204–5, 226
aid system 168, 207; international 224, 226
AIDS 16, 31, 38–44, 98–101, 167; *see also* HIV
anti-racism 161–5; training 162; *see also* racism
artificial intelligence 130, 184–6

Bahrain 117
Bangladesh 28, 146, 185, 208
bear witness 10, 42, 121, 135–48; *see also* speak out
Biafra 2, 37, 52–3, 135
Brazzaville 10–16

Central African Republic 104, 132
Chad 138, 205, 224
Charter 2, 32–3; Climate and Environment 206; Humanitarian 32; MSF 36, 106
Chechnya 18, 69, 135
cholera 33, 89, 206
chronic disease 80–2, 100
civil society 116, 124–5, 168; actor 120, 131; alliances 105; expectations 120; movements 121; organisations 44, 118, 184
climate crisis 10, 204–16, 227; *see also* climate emergency; planetary emergency
climate emergency 204–8; *see also* climate crisis; planetary emergency
climate: change 204–15; crisis 10, 204–16
colonialism 2, 89, 162–3, 167, 169; Western 168; *see also* neocolonial
communication 84, 132, 139, 186–90; public 135; strategy 131
community-inclusive 114–15
consent 137–8, 143; informed 137, 140, 192
counterterrorism 24, 56–7, 191
COVAX 89–91, 103
COVID-19 1, 25, 85–91, 97–106, 114, 129, 167, 172, 213
Cox's Bazar 28, 146
criminalisation 25–6, 147
cybersecurity 184, 192

Darfur 68, 70, 121
data management 185, 192
decolonisation 166–72
Democratic Republic of the Congo 102–4, 115, 129, 161, 224
development 1, 31, 34–44, 77–8, 92, 210; international 158
discrimination 16, 138, 143, 161, 164, 169, 177–81; racial and gender-based 19, 177, 227
disinformation 129–33, 147

displaced people 117, 203; *see also* displacement
displacement 26, 81, 207; *see also* displaced people
diversity 158, 168, 170, 177–81, 227; sociocultural 19; training 162
duty of care 59, 191

Ebola 97–102, 114, 129, 161
Egypt 28
environmental damage 203–14; *see also* environmental impact
environmental impact 205; *see also* environmental damage
epidemic 15, 89, 109, 206; Ebola 99, 114; HIV 40, 98, 101
equity 177–81, 204; global 100; health 96, 101, 103; social 204; *see also* inequity
ethical dilemma 85, 93, 96–8, 103, 107
Ethiopia 53, 130–1, 139, 142, 145
exclusion 25–8

field hospitals 79–82
footprint: carbon 205, 212, 227; environmental 204–14
funding 18, 27, 35, 38, 102, 210, 214, 216, 224–5; EU 26; institutional 40; private 14, 33; reductions 103
fundraising 11, 14–15, 142

Gaza 1, 51–2, 56–7, 82–91, 130, 186
Geneva Conventions 54, 60
global health 98, 157–71; actors 90; and Climate Alliance 205; funds 96; governance 105; inequities 97, 99, 103; reform of 161; security 24, 96–107; Security Agenda 99; Security Initiative 108
global heating 204, 207; *see also* global warming
Global South 24, 71, 89, 91, 138, 141, 142, 227
Global War on Terror 31–40, 59
global warming 203–16; *see also* global heating
Grand Bargain agreement 34, 208

Haiti 68
health system 25, 78–92, 98, 102, 104, 117, 185, 205, 216; local 92, 102; public 96, 123; strengthening 100, 115, 210
HIV 10, 16, 31, 38–45, 103, 167; epidemic 40; prevention 13, 41; treatment 38–41, 99, 44; *see also* AIDS

Hong Kong 118–19, 131
hostility 51–61, 70, 129
human rights law 187, 190–7
humanitarian imperative 96–107, 216
humanitarian information 183–94
humanitarian medicine 77–8, 91, 99, 205
humanitarian space 27, 60, 69, 72, 224
Humanitarian-Development-Peace Nexus 35–43
humanitarianism 1, 27, 31–45, 52–3, 77, 92, 119, 137, 158–67, 186, 207

identity 4, 33–45, 121, 124, 131, 135–6, 141, 160–71, 184, 226; group 157–8, 167; politics 166, 226–7; racial 179
IFRC 34, 102, 114, 205
impartiality 2, 4, 32–42, 71–2, 165, 172
inclusion 27, 158, 177–81; training 170; *see also* community-inclusive; inclusive care models; inclusivity
inclusive care models 44
inclusivity 148
independence 18, 27, 31–45, 72, 183–95; financial 2, 33, 39, 40, 45; image of 18; interpretation of 40; loss of 193; perception of 186, 193; reputation of 131; threat to 192; understanding of 38
individuals recruited locally 138; *see also* locally hired staff
inequality 24, 78, 80, 89, 137, 157–70; economic 158, 166; gender 97, 180; racial 168, 178; social 157; structural 158; systemic 158, 161, 226–7
inequity 78, 159, 171; health 96–107; *see also* equity
insecurity: food 203, 207; normalisation of 56; perception of increased 53; *see also* security
International Committee of the Red Cross 33, 51, 57, 59, 135, 184–95, 205
international humanitarian law 1, 51–61, 187–94, 226; dismissal of 62; protection 189; violation of 61
international law 36, 52–3, 58, 187–90
intubation 87
Israel 52, 56–8, 82–3, 130, 186

Kosovo 11–18, 53
Kunduz 56–7, 138

La Mancha Agreement 33–42, 177
Lebanon 131
legitimacy 17, 39, 54–9, 121, 124–5, 138, 145–6, 205–7, 211, 217, 226

locally hired staff 68–72, 118, 122–5, 131, 139–40, 177, 180, 182, 213, 226; *see also* individuals recruited locally

malaria 89, 102–3, 107, 206, 209–10
malnutrition 10, 89, 209–10
measles 89–90
mental health 14, 18, 26
migrants 9, 24–8, 119, 129; racialised 24; securitisation 27; *see also* migration
migration 18, 24–8, 38; forced 103; *see also* migrants
Ministry of Health 40–1, 44, 54, 83–6, 104, 117, 123–4, 131
minorities 97–107, 169; racial 164; *see also* minority communities and minority groups
minority communities 101
minority groups 106, 162
misinformation 119, 129
Myanmar 117–24, 130–1, 147, 185

natural disasters 11–16, 205, 207, 211
negotiation 17, 27, 54, 58, 68–70, 81
neocolonial 61, 169; heritage 137; *see also* colonialism
neutrality 2, 4, 32–43, 53, 70–2, 141, 165, 172, 204; carbon 219; hospital 57; reputation of 131
Niger 88–91
Nigeria 17, 52–3, 137–40, 146, 205
non-state armed actors 69, 70; *see also* non-state armed groups
non-state armed groups 51, 54; *see also* non-state armed actors
North Atlantic Treaty Organization (NATO) 11–13, 18

patient-centred care 36, 42
perception 1–2, 40, 53, 180; data 114; negative 58
philanthropy 158, 162, 171
planetary boundaries 203, 206, 215
planetary emergency 203, 215–17; *see also* climate crisis; climate emergency
principles 28, 31–45, 58, 60, 70–1, 104, 119, 136–40, 159–73, 187–91, 204; Chantilly 33, 36–7, 43, 46; ethical 100, 226; humanitarian 32, 34, 45, 47, 171, 190, 204; universal 157, 168
profiling 69
protection 26–7, 37–8, 54–60, 71, 82, 121, 131, 187–93; data 191–3; of healthcare 52; international 24, 37

racism 97, 161–70, 177–9; institutional 164, 169, 178; structural 177–8; systemic 164, 168; *see also* anti-racism
refugees 11–12, 18, 24–8, 33, 101, 103
Republic of the Congo 12
reputation 4–5, 70, 103, 121, 131–2, 146
rights: -based Agenda 41–4; -based approach 31–43; civil 157, 165, 172; equal 169; human 25, 36–8, 43, 98, 101, 147–8, 157–68, 191, 197; individual 165, 168, 173; universal 157, 159; women's 165, 168, 225
risk 14, 19, 56–61, 69–71, 81, 98, 129, 138–40, 183–5, 206, 216; aversion 46, 59; exposure 59; of instrumentalisation 186–7, 192; management 59, 192; perception of 59, 68; reduction 208, 210; reputational 39, 118, 147; residual 60; transfer of 61, 71–2
Rwanda 25, 33, 37, 44, 136

Sahel 69, 131
security 24, 56, 60, 69–72, 96, 98, 101, 132; agendas 24; border 28; cyber 184, 192; false sense of 60; incidents 55, 60; internal 53; international 187; management 59, 61, 68, 71; national 1, 24, 98, 191; paradox 60
social justice 105, 157–71
social media 119–22, 129–32, 136, 147, 227
social mission 4, 38, 165, 210, 213
solidarity 14, 18, 28, 85, 117–22, 146, 158, 167, 210; activists 119; budgets 210; criminalisation of 26; financial 14; global 1; international 102–3, 141, 216–17, 224; mockery of 162; selective 26
Somalia 69
South Africa 38–9, 44, 118, 167
speak out 32–3, 55, 103, 118, 125, 135–47, 205–6, 217, 225–7; *see also* bear witness
Sphere Project 32–44
standards 31–44, 92, 142, 193, 212; international 61, 214; medical 78; quality 84, 204, 206, 213
stereotypes 19, 137, 142; gender or racial 139
Sudan 28, 51–8, 68, 70, 117–24, 130, 138, 146–7
surgery 80, 83; reconstructive 83–4, 91; trauma 79, 81–2; wartime 16
surveillance 3, 103, 188–91, 209
sustainability 204–16; financial 39
Syria 54, 61, 79–82, 145–6

témoignage 33, 42–3, 135–48; visual 141, 145
Tigray 131, 139, 145
tsunami 11–18
tuberculosis 16, 37, 102–3, 185
Turkey 18, 25–6, 79–82

Ukraine 13–16, 26, 51, 130, 225
United Nations 11, 123, 166, 188, 213, 224; General Assembly 32; High Commissioner for Refugees 16, 185; Security Council 52, 54, 99, 101, 105

vaccination: campaigns 58, 105; measles 90; programme 89–90; routine 102; teams 90
vaccine 89–90; access 89; COVID-19 89, 103, 107; distribution 91, 103; hesitancy 129; hoarding of 1; race-based 172; technologies 89
ventilation 87
violence 26–7, 51–62, 70, 79–85, 116–23; against healthcare structures 51; against humanitarian staff 70; against migrants 25; border 28; community 114; domestic 99; gender-based 99; incitement of 129; political 97; sexual 13, 16–17, 20, 138, 146; state-perpetrated 26; structural 26, 99, 104

World Food Programme 131
World Health Organization 11, 15, 37, 41, 84, 89–90, 93, 96–105, 206
World Humanitarian Summit 34–6

Yemen 85–91

For Product Safety Concerns and Information please contact our EU representative GPSR@taylorandfrancis.com Taylor & Francis Verlag GmbH, Kaufingerstraße 24, 80331 München, Germany